# Pharmacotherapy for Complex Substance Use Disorders

## A Practical Guide

# Pharmacotherapy for Complex Substance Use Disorders

## A Practical Guide

Edited by

Thanh Thuy Truong, M.D.

Benjamin T. Li, M.D.

Daryl Shorter, M.D.

Nidal Moukaddam, M.D., Ph.D.

Thomas R. Kosten, M.D.

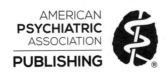

AMERICAN
PSYCHIATRIC
ASSOCIATION
PUBLISHING

If you wish to buy 50 or more copies of the same title, please go to www.appi.org/specialdiscounts for more information.

Copyright © 2024 American Psychiatric Association Publishing

ALL RIGHTS RESERVED

First Edition

Manufactured in the United States of America on acid-free paper
27   26   25   24   23      5   4   3   2   1

American Psychiatric Association Publishing
800 Maine Avenue SW, Suite 900
Washington, DC 20024-2812
www.appi.org

**Library of Congress Cataloging-in-Publication Data**
Names: Truong, Thanh Thuy, editor. | Li, Benjamin T., editor. | Shorter, Daryl, editor. | Moukaddam, Nidal, editor. | Kosten, Thomas R., editor. | American Psychiatric Association, issuing body.
Title: Pharmacotherapy for complex substance use disorders : a practical guide / Thanh Thuy Truong, Benjamin T. Li, Daryl Shorter, Nidal Moukaddam, Thomas R. Kosten.
Description: Washington, D.C. : American Psychiatric Association Publishing, 2023. | Includes bibliographical references and index.
Identifiers: LCCN 2023018637 (print) | LCCN 2023018638 (ebook) | ISBN 9781615374953 (paperback) | ISBN 9781615374960 (ebook)
Subjects: MESH: Substance-Related Disorders—drug therapy
Classification: LCC RC564 (print) | LCC RC564 (ebook) | NLM WM 270 | DDC 616.86—dc23/eng/20230630
LC record available at https://lccn.loc.gov/2023018637
LC ebook record available at https://lccn.loc.gov/2023018638

**British Library Cataloguing in Publication Data**
A CIP record is available from the British Library.

# Contents

# Contributors

**Tabark Altai, M.D.**
Resident, University of San Francisco, Fresno, California

**M. Asif Khan, M.D., M.R.O.**
Assistant Professor, Menninger Department of Psychiatry and Behavioral Sciences, Baylor College of Medicine, Houston, Texas

**Britney Lambert, M.D.**
Assistant Professor, Menninger Department of Psychiatry and Behavioral Sciences, Baylor College of Medicine, Houston, Texas

**Benjamin Li, M.D.**
Associate Professor, Menninger Department of Psychiatry and Behavioral Sciences, Baylor College of Medicine, Houston, Texas

**Claire K. Morice, M.D.**
Assistant Professor, Menninger Department of Psychiatry and Behavioral Sciences, Baylor College of Medicine, Houston, Texas

**Nidal Moukaddam, M.D., Ph.D.**
Associate Professor, Menninger Department of Psychiatry and Behavioral Sciences, Baylor College of Medicine; and Director of Adult Psychiatry Outpatient Services, Harris Health System, Houston, Texas

**Crystal Obiozor, M.D.**
Child and Adolescent Psychiatry Fellow, Menninger Department of Psychiatry and Behavioral Sciences, Baylor College of Medicine, Houston, Texas

**Andres Ojeda, M.D.**
Assistant Professor, Menninger Department of Psychiatry and Behavioral Sciences, Baylor College of Medicine, Houston, Texas

**Edore Onigu-Otite, M.D.**
Associate Professor, Menninger Department of Psychiatry and Behavioral Sciences; Medical Director, Pediatric Addiction Clinic; and Associate Course Director, Ben Taub Mental Health Services, Baylor College of Medicine, Houston, Texas

**Hazem Shahin, M.D.**
Assistant Professor, Menninger Department of Psychiatry and Behavioral Sciences, Baylor College of Medicine, Houston, Texas

**Nancy C. Shenoi, M.D.**
Addiction Psychiatry Fellow, Menninger Department of Psychiatry and Behavioral Sciences, Baylor College of Medicine, Houston, Texas

**Daryl Shorter, M.D.**
Medical Director, Addiction Services, The Menninger Clinic, and Associate Professor, Menninger Department of Psychiatry and Behavioral Sciences, Baylor College of Medicine, Houston, Texas

**Thanh Thuy Truong, M.D.**
Assistant Professor, Menninger Department of Psychiatry and Behavioral Sciences, Baylor College of Medicine, Houston, Texas

**Richa Vijayvargiya, M.D.**
Assistant Professor, Department of Psychiatry, University of Florida, Gainesville, Florida

**Mark Yurewicz, M.D.**
Assistant Professor, Menninger Department of Psychiatry and Behavioral Sciences, Baylor College of Medicine, Houston, Texas

# Disclosures

*The contributors to this volume have indicated they have no financial interest in or other affiliation with a commercial supporter, manufacturer of a commercial product, and/or provider of a commercial service.*

# Preface

*Welcome to* Pharmacotherapy for Complex Substance Use Disorders: A Practical Guide. Our goal for this text is to provide practical clinical pearls and evidence-based recommendations to help clinicians feel more confident in their management of patients with complex substance use disorders (SUDs). Our team of addiction psychiatrists identified relatively limited literature on the pharmacotherapy of multi-substance use disorders and special populations such as adolescents, pregnant patients, and members of the LGBTQ+ community. With few FDA-approved treatments for SUDs and no explicit treatment guidelines, we hope to bring our clinical experience to mental health and primary care clinicians. Most of all, we hope to allay fears and instill hope in clinicians and patients during their recovery journeys.

## How to Use This Book

In this text, we primarily review maintenance pharmacological treatment for SUDs. We do not detail the management of intoxication and withdrawal syndromes and defer that information to other texts, such as *The ASAM Principles of Addiction Medicine* (Miller 2018). The authors of Chapter 5, "Alcohol and Co-occurring Substance Use"; Chapter 6, "Stimulants and Co-occurring Substance Use"; and Chapter 7, "Opioids and Co-Occurring Substance Use" review pharmacotherapeutic interventions for the substances mentioned in their respective chapter titles as the primary substance, while considering the co-occurring substances as secondary. We determine the primary substance based on factors such as the most significant functional impairment, the strongest craving, or as perceived by the patient. The authors of Chapter 12, "Substance Use Disorders in Pregnancy"; Chapter 13, "Addictive Disorders in Adolescents"; and Chapter 14, "Substance Use Disorders in the LGBTQ+

Population" examine common SUDs and unique considerations in selecting pharmacological or behavioral interventions for these patient populations.

Because the nomenclature and criteria for SUDs changed from DSM-IV (American Psychiatric Association 1994) to DSM-5 (American Psychiatric Association 2013), we use words such as *abuse, dependence,* and *relapse* when citing older studies that followed DSM-IV criteria or used older terminology. Otherwise, we prefer *substance use disorder, recurrence,* and *return to use.*

# References

American Psychiatric Association: Diagnostic and Statistical Manual of Mental Disorders, 4th Edition. Washington, DC, American Psychiatric Association, 1994

American Psychiatric Association: Diagnostic and Statistical Manual of Mental Disorders, 5th Edition. Arlington, VA, American Psychiatric Association, 2013

Miller S: The ASAM Principles of Addiction Medicine, 6th Edition. Philadelphia, PA, Lippincott Williams and Wilkins, 2018

# 1

# Overview of Substance Use Disorders

Thanh Thuy Truong, M.D.

## Defining Addiction

Many definitions and models of addiction have been formulated over the years, including moral failing, brain disease, physiological dependence, self-medication, compulsive behaviors, and social contagion (West 2013). While any combination of these models may resonate for any one individual, no single perspective captures the complexity of addictive disorders. Taking these models together, we define *addiction* in this book as a powerful motivation to engage in a behavior or use a substance despite persistent harmful consequences.

## Epidemiology

Substance use disorders (SUDs) and related disorders are significant public health challenges worldwide that have devastating impacts on the economy, health care, and individual lives. In 2021, the National Survey on Drug Use and Health estimated that 46.3 million Americans ages 12 and older (16.5%) met the criteria for an SUD during the prior year; 24 million had a drug use disorder, and 7.3 million had both alcohol use disorder (AUD) and a drug use disorder (Substance Abuse and Mental Health Services Administration 2021).

### Alcohol

In 2021, 133.1 million Americans ages 12 and older reported using alcohol in the past month (representing current alcohol users). Among these, 60 million

(45.1%) were classified as binge drinkers, and 16.3 million (12.2%) were classified as heavy drinkers (Substance Abuse and Mental Health Services Administration 2021). Approximately 29.2% of adults ages 18–25, 22.4% of adults ages 26 and older, and 3.8% of adolescents ages 12–17 reported binge alcohol use. Approximately 29.5 million people ages 12 or older (10.6%) met DSM-5 criteria for AUD in the past year (American Psychiatric Association 2013).

## Tobacco

In 2021, 61.6 million people ages 12 and older (22% of the population) reported using nicotine products such as tobacco products or had vaped nicotine in the past month. Among current users, approximately 86.2% of those age 26 or older reported using only tobacco products, whereas nearly 60.5% of adolescents ages 12–17 only vaped nicotine. Approximately 28.2 million people age 12 or older (10.1%) reported nicotine dependence in the past month. Among past-month cigarette users, approximately 64.7% had nicotine dependence; approximately 89% of users ages 26 and older had used only tobacco products, whereas nearly two-thirds of adolescents ages 12–17 had vaped nicotine (Substance Abuse and Mental Health Services Administration 2021). In 2019, legislation raised the federal minimum age for the sale of tobacco products, including e-cigarettes, from 18 to 21 to reduce underage nicotine use.

## Cannabis

In 2021, approximately 52.5 million individuals ages 12 and older (18.7% of the population) reported marijuana use within the past year. Additionally, around 16.3 million people met the criteria for cannabis use disorder (CaUD), with the highest percentage observed among young adults ages 18–25 (Substance Abuse and Mental Health Services Administration 2021).

## Stimulants

In 2021, approximately 4.8 million individuals (1.7% of the population) ages 12 and older reported using cocaine or crack cocaine within the past year. Among them, 1.4 million people (0.5%) met the criteria for cocaine use disorder (CUD). Furthermore, 2.5 million (0.9%) reported methamphetamine use, with 1.6 million (0.6%) experiencing methamphetamine use disorder.

The survey also revealed that a total of 3.7 million people (1.3%) reported misusing prescription stimulants, and 1.5 million (0.5%) had a prescription stimulant use disorder (Substance Abuse and Mental Health Services Administration 2021).

## Opioids

In 2021, approximately 1.1 million individuals (0.4% of the population) age 12 or older reported using heroin within the past year, while 1 million (0.4%) met the criteria for heroin use disorder. Regarding prescription opioids, 8.7 million people (3.1%) reported misuse, and 5.6 million (2%) had an opioid use disorder (OUD), including both heroin and prescription opioids (Substance Abuse and Mental Health Services Administration 2021).

## Novel Psychoactive Substances

In 2021, approximately 1.7 million individuals (0.6% of the population) age 12 or older reported using kratom within the past year. Additionally, 483,000 (0.2%) reported using synthetic marijuana, also known as spice or K2. The use of synthetic stimulants chemically related to cathinones, commonly referred to as bath salts, was reported by less than 0.1% of the population (Substance Abuse and Mental Health Services Administration 2021).

## Multi-substance Use Disorders

In a 2018 analysis of 2,000 adult primary care patients, 13.8% reported multi-substance use disorder (MSUD). Among those with AUD, OUD, CUD, or CaUD, a much larger percentage reported MSUD than did those with a tobacco use disorder (TUD) (i.e., 93.8% of patients with heroin use had another SUD). However, patients with a higher severity of TUD or AUD had greater odds of having another SUD. TUD was the most common comorbid SUD (John et al. 2018). A national survey of U.S. adults identified a prevalence of 7.8% for lifetime MSUD. It indicated that most adults reporting past-year non-alcohol SUDs had at least one co-occurring SUD, although the survey did not include comorbid TUD (McCabe et al. 2017). Considered the fourth wave of the opioid epidemic, the combined use of methamphetamine and opioids (mostly synthetic opioids such as fentanyl) resulted in markedly increased overdose death rates between 2012 and 2019 (National Institute on Drug Abuse 2021).

## Co-occurring Substance Use Disorders and Psychiatric Disorders

Multiple studies have found high rates of co-occurring SUDs and psychiatric disorders such as depression and bipolar disorder, ADHD, and psychotic disorders. It is estimated that half of adults experiencing a mental illness also have an SUD, and vice versa. Comorbidities are also common among youth with SUDs. In a survey of community-based SUD treatment programs, more than 60% of adolescents also met criteria for another mental illness (Hser et al. 2001; Substance Abuse and Mental Health Services Administration 2021).

## Suicide

Suicide continues to be a leading cause of death in the United States, increasing by 33% between 1999 and 2019. It is the second leading cause of death for individuals ages 10–34. In 2020, approximately 46,000 people in the United States died from suicide. Among youth ages 12–17, 12% reported having serious thoughts of suicide, 5.3% reported making a suicide plan, and 2.5% reported attempting suicide. Among adults ages 18 and older, 4.9% reported having serious thoughts of suicide, 1.3% reported making a suicide plan, and 0.5% reported attempting suicide (Substance Abuse and Mental Health Services Administration 2021). SUDs significantly increase the risk of suicide, particularly among those with psychiatric conditions. A case-control study by Lynch et al. (2020) found that the odds of suicide were 2 times higher for participants with TUD; 5.8 times higher for those with AUD; 5.3 times higher for those with drug use disorders; and 11.2 times higher for those with combined AUD, TUD, and drug use disorders. The authors calculated these odds after adjusting for age, sex, education, poverty level, psychiatric conditions, and, notably, the Charlson Comorbidity Index, an instrument developed to predict the 10-year survival of patients with multiple nonpsychiatric medical comorbidities. Lynch and colleagues also identified sex differences, with males having adjusted odds of suicide ranging from 1.8 times higher for those with TUD to 7.9 times higher for those with combined AUD, TUD, and drug use disorder. The odds of suicide for females ranged from 2.5 times higher for those with TUD to 16.7 times higher for those with combined AUD, TUD, and drug use disorder. TUD alone increases the risk of suicide. Other studies have found an association between tobacco use and suicidality, even after controlling for mental disorders and sociodemographic covariates (Han et al. 2017). Moreover, MSUD is more prevalent among adults with other psychiatric disorders, including mood disorders, personality disorders, and PTSD.

The odds of MSUD are more than 9 times higher in individuals with multiple lifetime psychiatric disorders than in those with no lifetime psychiatric disorders (McCabe et al. 2017).

# Screening for Multi-substance Use and Co-occurring Disorders

Screening for SUDs is essential in any medical setting. The National Institute on Drug Abuse (NIDA) Quick Screen accurately identifies high-risk patients by using a single question. For illicit drug use, the question is: "How many times in the past year have you used drugs or used a prescription medication for nonmedical reasons?" For alcohol use, the screener asks, "How many times in the past year have you had five or more [for men] or four or more [for women] drinks in a day?" For tobacco use, the question is, "How many times in the past year have you used any tobacco products?" A response of *never* requires no further evaluation, and the clinician should affirm the patient for making healthy choices. If the patient answers with a positive number, a detailed evaluation is needed to assess the risk and presence of an SUD (National Institute on Drug Abuse 2014). Alternatively, patients may fill out a screening questionnaire for substance use before the appointment. Evidence-based assessment tools from the NIDA are also available online for patients and clinicians (www.drugabuse.gov), including the Tobacco, Alcohol, Prescription medication, and other Substance use (TAPS) screener for adults and the Brief Screener for Tobacco, Alcohol, and other Drugs (BSTAD) for adolescents. Patients are more comfortable sharing when they are informed that inquiry includes all substances, including commonly used substances such as caffeine. They are also more likely to provide detailed information when asked open-ended questions (i.e., "How has this substance impacted your life? In what way?"). In the extended evaluation, clinicians should assess for current and past use, average and peak use, route(s) of administration, age at onset of use, and age at onset for an SUD.

## Medical Consequences

Inquiry and testing for medical consequences of substance use are necessary to engage patients in less harmful behaviors. A physical examination should include assessing pulmonary and cardiac function and dermatological signs of use (i.e., track marks and pock marks) with possible infection (i.e., abscesses). Laboratory testing should include a complete blood count, serum chemistry panel, hemoglobin A1C, lipid profile, liver function test, urine toxicology screen, pregnancy screen (if indicated), and sexually transmitted infection screen that includes HIV and hepatitis B and C. Specific laboratory markers related to substance use are discussed in Chapter 4, "Laboratory Testing."

### Psychiatric Disorders

Given the high comorbidity of psychiatric conditions such as mood, anxiety, and personality disorders, screening for these conditions in the primary care setting is essential for determining the need for a referral to specialty psychiatric and addiction treatment. Although numerous screening tools are available, primary care physicians should choose screening instruments based on the most prevalent conditions in their respective population and the measure's sensitivity and specificity. To screen and assess the severity of depression and anxiety, respectively, the Patient Health Questionnaire–9 (PHQ-9) and General Anxiety Disorder–7 (GAD-7) are simple to administer during or before the appointment. Scores may be trended over time to assess response to treatment. For time-constrained clinicians, ultrabrief versions such as the GAD-2 or PHQ-2 are available (Kroenke et al. 2001; Mulvaney-Day et al. 2018; Spitzer et al. 2006).

# Harm Reduction as a Treatment Philosophy

*Harm reduction* is a person-centered approach that aims to reduce harm from substance use to individuals and communities and increase engagement with health care resources. Examples of strategies include encouraging use of clean needles, providing opioid agonist treatment, and offering supervised facilities for active users (Table 1–1). Although some of these methods are controversial, many adverse health consequences are due not to substance use but to other factors. Therefore, practical strategies can significantly improve short- and long-term economic, health, and social outcomes. The patient-centered approach also reduces stigma and improves the therapeutic alliance, particularly when treating patients with MSUD (Stancliff et al. 2015). In our clinical experience, these patients face more significant barriers to consistent engagement in treatment because of financial strain, intoxication, or cognitive impairments from their substance use. Therefore, we approach recovery as a continuum, with the initial goals for all patients being attendance at appointments and working collaboratively. Although abstinence is one approach to

**Table 1–1.    Examples of harm reduction strategies**

Designated drivers

Safe housing

Pre-exposure HIV prophylaxis

Post-exposure HIV prophylaxis

Syringe needle access programs

Supervised drug consumption venues

Transition from intravenous use to another method (e.g., snorting)

Naloxone kits for overdose prevention

Opioid agonist or antagonist treatment

Medication for various substance use disorders

reducing harm, complete abstinence from all substances at once may not be possible or preferred by the patient. We focus on improved health and functioning as individuals work toward their goals. Some patients choose to first address current substances and behaviors that are most impairing and to address others at a later point in treatment. The philosophy of harm reduction creates flexibility, encourages collaboration, and empowers the patient.

# Stigma and Recommended Terminology

*Stigma* is discrimination against an identifiable group of people. Stigma about people with SUD might include believing that they are dangerous, have character defects, or engage in immoral behavior. Stigma in society and the medical community poses a substantial barrier to seeking care for people with SUDs. In medical charts, stigmatizing terminology such as *abuse, addict,* and *junkie* can induce negative bias in the clinician that can affect the quality of care. Research has shown that clinicians are more likely to recommend punitive rather than therapeutic solutions when a clinical vignette uses *substance abuser* versus *person with substance use disorder* (Ashford et al. 2018; Kelly and Westerhoff 2010). Using person-first language reminds patients, families, and clinicians that the person is not simply defined by their SUD (Table 1–2).

# Ongoing Challenges

There have been increasing challenges to addressing common substances that now have greater potency and lethality (i.e., methamphetamine) and the

Table 1–2.    Recommended terminology

| Terms to avoid | Recommended alternative terms |
| --- | --- |
| Addict, junkie, abuser | Person with substance use disorder (e.g., alcohol use disorder), user |
| Abuse, habit | Use, unhealthy use, at-risk or high-risk use, harmful use, substance use disorder |
| Alcoholic | Person with alcohol use disorder |
| Clean or dirty urine | Negative or positive results |
| Clean or dirty, referring to current use | Abstinent, not actively using, person in recovery |
| Medication-assisted treatment | Opioid agonist treatment, medication for substance use disorder |
| Relapse | Recurrence, return to use |
| Binge | Heavy-drinking episode |
| Detoxification, detox | Withdrawal management |

emergence of novel psychoactive substances that often evade detection by standard toxicology screens. In recent years, the combination of stimulants and other substances with illicitly manufactured fentanyl has been a major cause of overdoses (National Institute on Drug Abuse 2021). This trend continued during the coronavirus SARS-CoV-2 disease (COVID-19) pandemic, with studies showing a marked increase in urine drug screens being positive for fentanyl (35%) and amphetamine (89%) (Niles et al. 2021). Entry and retention of patients in treatment for addictive disorders continue to be low. In 2020, only 6.5% of individuals ages 12 and older with an SUD received any substance use treatment (Substance Abuse and Mental Health Services Administration 2021). Altogether, assessment and treatment for MSUD are essential for all patients who use substances, including tobacco and alcohol, because they are at risk of worse outcomes from overdose, suicide, high-risk behaviors, and medical comorbidities that constitute barriers to treatment (Connor et al. 2014).

# References

American Psychiatric Association: Diagnostic and Statistical Manual of Mental Disorders, 5th Edition. Arlington, VA, American Psychiatric Association, 2013

Ashford RD, Brown AM, Curtis B: Substance use, recovery, and linguistics: the impact of word choice on explicit and implicit bias. Drug Alcohol Depend 189(Aug):131–138, 2018 29913324

Connor JP, Gullo MJ, White A, et al: Polysubstance use: diagnostic challenges, patterns of use and health. Curr Opin Psychiatry 27(4):269–275, 2014 24852056

Han B, Compton WM, Blanco C: Tobacco use and 12-month suicidality among adults in the United States. Nicotine Tob Res 19(1):39–48, 2017 27190402

Hser Y-I, Grella CE, Hubbard RL, et al: An evaluation of drug treatments for adolescents in 4 US cities. Arch Gen Psychiatry 58(7):689–695, 2001 11448377

John WS, Zhu H, Mannelli P, et al: Prevalence, patterns, and correlates of multiple substance use disorders among adult primary care patients. Drug Alcohol Depend 187(June):79–87, 2018 29635217

Kelly JF, Westerhoff CM: Does it matter how we refer to individuals with substance-related conditions? A randomized study of two commonly used terms. Int J Drug Policy 21(3):202–207, 2010 20005692

Kroenke K, Spitzer RL, Williams JB: The PHQ-9: validity of a brief depression severity measure. J Gen Intern Med 16(9):606–613, 2001 11556941

Lynch FL, Peterson EL, Lu CY, et al: Substance use disorders and risk of suicide in a general US population: a case control study. Addict Sci Clin Pract 15(1):14, 2020 32085800

McCabe SE, West BT, Jutkiewicz EM, et al: Multiple DSM-5 substance use disorders: a national study of US adults. Hum Psychopharmacol 32(5), 2017 28750478

Mulvaney-Day N, Marshall T, Downey Piscopo K, et al: Screening for behavioral health conditions in primary care settings: a systematic review of the literature. J Gen Intern Med 33(3):335–346, 2018 28948432

National Institute on Drug Abuse: NIDA Quick Screen V1.0. Bethesda, MD, National Institute on Drug Abuse, 2014. Available at: https://nida.nih.gov/sites/default/files/pdf/nmassist.pdf. Accessed February 13, 2023.

National Institute on Drug Abuse: Drug Overdose Death Rates. Bethesda, MD, National Institute on Drug Abuse, 2021. Available at: https://www.drugabuse.gov/drug-topics/trends-statistics/overdose-death-rates. Accessed January 29, 2021.

Niles JK, Gudin J, Radcliff J, et al: The opioid epidemic within the COVID-19 pandemic: drug testing in 2020. Popul Health Manag 24(S1):S43–S51, 2021 33031013

Spitzer RL, Kroenke K, Williams JBW, et al: A brief measure for assessing generalized anxiety disorder: the GAD-7. Arch Intern Med 166(10):1092–1097, 2006 16717171

Stancliff S, Phillips BW, Maghsoudi N, et al: Harm reduction: front line public health. J Addict Dis 34(2–3):206–219, 2015 26080038

Substance Abuse and Mental Health Services Administration: Key Substance Use and Mental Health Indicators in the United States: Results From the 2020 National Survey on Drug Use and Health. Rockville, MD, Substance Abuse and Mental Health Services Administration, 2021, p 156. Available at: https://www.samhsa.gov/data/sites/default/files/reports/rpt35325/NSDUHFFRPDFWHTMLFiles2020/2020NSDUHFFR1PDFW102121.pdf. Accessed February 15, 2023.

West R: Models of Addiction (EMCDDA Insights). Lisbon, European Monitoring Centre for Drugs and Drug Addiction, 2013

# 2

# General Approach to Patients With Multi-substance Use Disorders

Hazem Shahin, M.D.

*Substance use* affects multiple aspects of a person's life and health. Thus, the optimal approach to substance use patients is multidisciplinary and multimodal. It should include screening for substance use, conducting a complete medical and psychiatric assessment, treating intoxication and withdrawal syndromes when necessary, and managing co-occurring psychiatric and general medical conditions. Clinicians can use this information to develop a realistic, individualized, and practical treatment plan that also addresses social needs that might be contributing to the existing pathology. Treatment goals should be the reduction of physiological, psychological, and social risks associated with the substance use, which might be achieved through abstinence, reduction of use frequency and severity, reduction in the possibility of overdoses, prevention of return to use, and/or improvement in psychological and social functioning.

Compared with single-substance use disorder, which is already known to be complex and to require a multifaceted approach, multi-substance use disorder (MSUD) further complicates recovery because patients could present with atypical symptomatology, experience a more complicated course of illness, and require a more intensive treatment plan that addresses the variety of substances used and the intricate relationships between them. Available research demonstrates that, when compared with single-substance use, multisubstance use is associated with higher rates of the following:

- Risk of trauma exposure and consequences (Johnson et al. 2006)
- Lifetime suicide attempts and financial/legal problems (Bhalla et al. 2017)
- Likelihood of overdose (Coffin et al. 2003)
- More severe medical and psychiatric comorbidities (Shaffer et al. 2004)

A comprehensive psychiatric evaluation is essential to guide the treatment of patients with substance use disorder (SUD). The assessment should include the following:

- Detailed history of past and present substance use and the effects of substance use on cognitive, psychological, behavioral, and physiological functioning
- General medical and psychiatric history and examination
- History of psychiatric treatments (i.e., residential treatment) and outcomes
- Family and social history
- Toxicology screening of blood, breath, or urine for substances
- Other laboratory tests to help confirm the presence or absence of conditions that commonly co-occur with SUDs
- Additional information from family or close relations (obtain the patient's permission to contact)

# Setting the Stage

Prior to the interview, a few steps may be taken to help make the evaluation smoother, more comprehensive, and more productive. These steps focus on understanding the acuteness or chronicity of the patient's condition and on directing the approach based on the setting. The clinician's approach in each setting is different and requires different sets of tools and skills. For example, in the acute setting, patients might present with intoxication or withdrawal, whereas in the chronic setting, they may present for routine medical or psychiatric care. With acute presentations, patients might readily report their use and ask for help but also might be in a poor mental state that prevents them from engaging in meaningful conversation or tolerating a lengthy interview. In chronic presentations, patients might not be ready to report substance use or might minimize their use because they fear stigma and judgment. Without systematic screening, patients' struggles may be missed. Some of the important steps that can be taken before the interview include, but are not limited to, the following:

- *Conduct a comprehensive review of electronic medical records.* This should include the patient's prior diagnoses, presentations, drug screening results, and prescription drug monitoring program reports. For example, a patient with a history of multiple emergency department visits for psychosis or bizarre behavior and drug test results that were positive for multiple substances would indicate a higher severity of substance use and treatment resistance. In patients with comorbid chronic psychiatric diagnoses, multisubstance use might suggest self-medication for symptoms that require a higher level of care. Patients with opioid and sedative use disorders may frequently express pain or anxiety in order to acquire opioid or benzodiazepine medications for withdrawal management. Some patients with MSUD are unaware that they are taking multiple substances because the medications have been prescribed; for example, patients with alcohol use disorder who have also been prescribed opiates or benzodiazepines may not report the medications and instead report only the alcohol use. Therefore, the clinician should review the prescription drug monitoring program report before the appointment.
- *Prepare the appropriate screening or assessment tools.* Having reviewed the patient's records and understood the acuity versus the chronicity of their presentation, the clinician can decide on the appropriate tools to utilize. In the acute setting, brief clinician-administered tools may be preferred compared with comprehensive but lengthy tools that are more suitable for use in chronic or outpatient settings. Self-administered tools are more useful in addiction clinics than in other settings because patients are more realistic and forthcoming.
- *Prepare the location of the interview.* Evidence has shown that maintaining a high level of security and confidentiality in the interview room is essential to completing an accurate substance use assessment (Vendetti et al. 2017). Patients who feel uneasy or do not trust that their medical records will be secure will likely be reluctant to provide frank and full disclosure of their substance use and its negative consequences. Interviewing the patient in an open space, such as the emergency department or a hospital room, or in front of a large treatment team may not be perceived as safe and private, leading them to minimize or deny substance use (Schaper et al. 2016).

# Approach to History Taking

Substance use patients who are reaching for help and experiencing guilt may feel ambivalence, resistance to change, and sometimes denial. The clinician's approach can significantly affect whether the patient will leave the assessment in a position to take the next step forward. The conversation should be direct, empathetic, and nonjudgmental. Clinicians can expect verbal cues from patients, such as giving contradicting accounts, placing and displacing the blame on circumstances and others, and minimizing their use or the consequences. Nonverbal cues may include appearing irritable, frequently attempting to change the subject, or refusing to talk. Interviewers must not use language that implies presumption or prejudice, not appear rushed or emotionally detached, and be aware of their tone and body language. They should start with open-ended questions and avoid negative terms such as *alcoholic, addict,* and *abuser*. Using empathetic, reflective phrases can invite patients to continue the conversation without feeling interrogated. One example of a simple, reflective statement is as follows:

> **Patient:** I tried to stop on my own, but I couldn't.
> **Interviewer:** I understand how that can be difficult.

Making a point to ask about some positive experiences early in the interview builds rapport and allows the clinician to get a comprehensive assessment of the patient. Such experiences might include past periods of successful sobriety, coping skills, support systems, and spirituality (Morgen 2017). This approach might help decrease patient dropout after the initial assessment; the average dropout rate within 30 days of initial assessment across SUDs is approximately 50%, with estimates ranging from 26% to 80% (Basu et al. 2017). Although using multiple substances is common, patients usually seek help and talk freely about only those they believe to be problematic and omit mention of other substances. For example, an intravenous heroin user might be willing to speak in detail about all aspects of their heroin use but resist discussing their daily cannabis use. Clinicians should assess readiness for change in each area and ask about the patient's goals. This approach helps keep patients engaged. Patients already feel a loss of control over their substance use, so letting them guide treatment gradually restores their sense of empowerment.

Recruiting family and friends as a source of collateral information or motivation and support is essential. However, clinicians must maintain their patient's trust and autonomy by obtaining written consent for these contacts and explaining the scope of the informant's interview. Understanding the relationship dynamic between patients and their support network is important because patients' goals might not be the same in different treatment stages as those of their family and other supporters. It is important for patients to not feel alienated and to believe the treatment is in line with their goals.

Finally, given the natural course of SUDs and their tendency toward chronicity, the assessment becomes an ever-evolving process and should not be limited to one interview. The clinician must keep a log of changes and further findings because patients' presentation and their willingness to discuss multiple facets of their lives could vary as the collaboration progresses. Repeated evaluations are necessary to clarify co-occurring conditions and past traumatic experiences. Keeping an open mind about new information also helps the clinician stay abreast of the phases of the disorder.

# Approach to the General Medical Evaluation

Substance use can lead to impaired function in any biological system of the body. Patients might present with multiple medical problems resulting from toxicity (including overdose), withdrawal, the consequences of the route of administration, or engagement in high-risk behaviors associated with their use (i.e., needle sharing, unprotected sexual encounters, poor hygiene). The medical sequelae of using multiple substances depend on the combination of substances involved. For example, mixing stimulants increases risk of brain injury, liver damage, heart attacks, and strokes. Mixing depressants increases risk of organ damage, overdose, and death (Centers for Disease Control and Prevention 2022). Presentations of commonly used substances and combinations are described in Table 2–1. A physical examination can yield clues to substance use, including the following:

- Poor personal hygiene
- Significant weight loss or weight gain
- Signs of injection drug use, including scars from intravenous use (i.e., track marks) or healed scars of subcutaneous use (skin popping)
- Signs of drug inhalation, including atrophy of the nasal mucosa and perforation of the nasal septum
- Evidence of acute intoxication or withdrawal: slurred speech, unsteady gait, pinpoint pupils, bizarre or atypical behavior, changes in level of arousal

Table 2–1.    Effects of commonly used substances and combinations

| Substance | Intoxication | Withdrawal | Management |
|---|---|---|---|
| Tobacco/Nicotine | Euphoria, alertness, decreased appetite, weight loss<br><br>Toxicity: nausea, vomiting, dizziness, tremors, sweating, tachycardia, hypertension | Irritability, restlessness, and agitation, anxiety, depressed mood, difficulty concentrating, increased appetite, weight gain, insomnia, headaches, fatigue | Intoxication: supportive care. For nicotine poisoning (e.g., children), activated charcoal can be used within 1 hour of ingestion.<br><br>Withdrawal: nicotine replacement products (patch and gum/lozenge) |
| Cannabinoids | Altered mental status, conjunctival injection, nystagmus, tachycardia, slurred speech, incoordination, appetite stimulation, altered perception of time (e.g., time feels slow)<br><br>Toxicity: delusions, hallucinations, paranoia | Irritability, anxiety, depression, nervousness, insomnia, nightmares or vivid dreams, loss of appetite, depressed mood, tremor | Intoxication: supportive care, rest in a quiet environment. Benzodiazepines may be used for agitation. Antipsychotics may be used for psychosis.<br><br>Withdrawal: supportive care. Symptomatic treatment for insomnia, gabapentin 1,200 mg/day in divided doses has evidence for withdrawal and craving (Substance Abuse and Mental Health Services Administration 2021). |

**Table 2–1.** Effects of commonly used substances and combinations *(continued)*

| Substance | Intoxication | Withdrawal | Management |
|---|---|---|---|
| CNS depressants: alcohol, barbiturates, benzodiazepines | Sedation, confusion, disorientation, slurred speech, ataxia, disinhibition, dizziness, impaired psychomotor performance, poor memory, emotional lability, irritability, depression, and suicidal gestures or attempts<br><br>Toxicity: can cause respiratory depression/arrest, coma, and death | Insomnia, anxiety, panic attacks, tremor, nausea, vomiting, elevated blood pressure and pulse rate, irritability, agitation, sweating, hyperactive reflexes, grand mal seizures, confusion, hallucinations, delirium | Intoxication: supportive care, intubation if needed. Flumazenil can precipitate seizures and thus has a limited role in management.<br><br>Withdrawal from sedatives/alcohol: transition to equivalent dose of long-acting benzodiazepines, then taper (e.g., diazepam, chlordiazepoxide, clonazepam). Monitor withdrawal using CIWA-Ar. |
| CNS stimulants: cocaine, methamphetamines, amphetamines, ecstasy (MDMA) | Euphoria, increased energy, hypersexuality, decreased appetite, insomnia, weight loss, sympathetic nervous system activation<br><br>Toxicity: psychosis, hypertension, tachycardia, hyperthermia, cardiac arrest, stroke, seizures | Depression, anxiety, irritability, suicidal ideation, impaired concentration, sleep disturbances, increased appetite, aches and pains, tremors, sweating, and headaches | Intoxication: supportive care for dehydration and hyperthermia, phentolamine for hypertensive crisis (avoid β-blockers), benzodiazepines for agitation and seizures. Antipsychotics may be used if benzodiazepines are insufficient or there is severe psychosis, but it increases risk of neuroleptic malignant syndrome.<br><br>Withdrawal: supportive care |

**Table 2–1.    Effects of commonly used substances and combinations** (*continued*)

| Substance | Intoxication | Withdrawal | Management |
|---|---|---|---|
| Combining stimulants with depressants (Attaran et al. 2005) | Gives conflicting symptoms of both substances, leading user to have false sense of less intoxication, and further continued use with accumulating levels of both substances, leading to high potential of overdose. Atypical presentation may lead to missed diagnoses. For example, in the combination of injectable cocaine and heroin known as "speedballing," heroin can mask common cocaine toxicity symptoms such as chest pain. | Mixed withdrawal symptoms give user perception of less severe withdrawal symptoms initially, but as levels of substances decrease, exaggerated withdrawal of the combination ensues. | Intoxication: supportive care and symptomatic management Withdrawal: supportive care and symptomatic management depending on primary syndrome. For example, if opioid withdrawal is prominent, then manage using opioid withdrawal protocol. |
| Hallucinogens: LSD, psilocybin, ayahuasca, others | Visual hallucinations, flushed face, pupillary dilation, increased blood pressure and pulse rate, anxiety Toxicity: hyperthermia, hyperreflexia, muscle weakness, tremor, dizziness, weakness, nausea, vomiting, paresthesia, panic attacks | Some patients may experience flashbacks to intoxication long after use and develop hallucinogen persisting perception disorder. | Intoxication: reassurance, supportive care; benzodiazepines for severe agitation |

**Table 2–1.** Effects of commonly used substances and combinations *(continued)*

| Substance | Intoxication | Withdrawal | Management |
|---|---|---|---|
| Inhalants: household items such as toluene, benzene, xylene; nitrous oxide | Euphoria, excitement, slurred speech, drowsiness, irritability, cognitive impairment, tremors, emotional lability, nystagmus, ataxia, weakness, mucus membrane irritation, nausea, vomiting, gastritis, anorexia, hepatomegaly, urinary dysfunction (renal tubular necrosis, renal failure), cardiovascular (irregular heartbeat, increased pulse rate), eye irritation, rash around mouth or nose, cough, pneumonia<br><br>Toxicity: Confusion, disorientation, seizures, cardiac arrhythmias, hypokalemia, methemoglobinemia, respiratory depression, coma, death | Irritability, dysphoria, sleep disturbance, headache, dry mouth, and lacrimation | Intoxication: supportive care, oxygen, intubation with severe respiratory depression.<br><br>Hypokalemia and acidosis: potassium and sodium bicarbonate<br><br>Methemoglobinemia: oxygen and methylene blue<br><br>Neurotoxicity from nitrous oxide: vitamin $B_{12}$<br><br>Ventricular fibrillation: amiodarone and lidocaine preferred over epinephrine if medications needed<br><br>Psychosis/agitation: antipsychotic (e.g., Haldol)<br><br>Seizures: benzodiazepines<br><br>Withdrawal: supportive care; limited literature on temporary use of long-acting benzodiazepines such as clonazepam |

**Table 2–1.    Effects of commonly used substances and combinations** (*continued*)

| Substance | Intoxication | Withdrawal | Management |
|---|---|---|---|
| Opioids | Analgesia, euphoria, drowsiness, nausea, vomiting, pupillary constriction or pinpoint pupils (may be dilated with meperidine), constipation, suppression of cough reflex<br><br>Toxicity: grand mal seizures (particularly with tramadol), hypotension, respiratory depression, pulmonary edema, respiratory arrest, coma, death | Lacrimation, rhinorrhea, yawning, irritability, sweating, restlessness, tremor, insomnia, piloerection, abdominal cramps, nausea, vomiting, diarrhea, muscle and bone pain, tachycardia and hypertension | Intoxication: supportive care, naloxone (multiple doses may be needed for fentanyl overdose)<br><br>Withdrawal: use COWS to assess severity and guide management; long-acting opioids such as buprenorphine and methadone. Symptomatic treatment may include clonidine for anxiety or hypertension, NSAIDs for muscle aches, sedating medications for sleep (e.g., trazodone, benzodiazepine, hypnotics, mirtazapine). |
| Phencyclidines | Agitation, tachycardia, hypertension, ataxia, slurred speech, vertical and horizontal nystagmus, delusions, hallucinations, aggression<br><br>Toxicity: hyperthermia, rigidity, rhabdomyolysis and acute renal failure, grand mal seizures, death | Depression, anxiety, fatigue, hypersomnia | Intoxication: supportive care, phentolamine for hypertensive crisis, benzodiazepines for agitation and seizures. Antipsychotics may be used if benzodiazepines are insufficient or there is severe psychosis. |

*Note.*    CIWA-Ar = Clinical Institute Withdrawal Assessment Alcohol Scale Revised; COWS = Clinical Opiate Withdrawal Scale; LSD = lysergic acid diethylamide; MDMA = 3,4-methylenedioxymethamphetamine; NSAIDs = nonsteroidal anti-inflammatory drugs.

(agitation or sedation), tachycardia, conjunctival injection, sweating, watery eyes, and/or runny nose

Medical conditions that can result from and serve as indicators of substance use include the following:

- Cardiovascular problems such as hypertension, cardiomyopathy, endocarditis, and heart failure
- Serious gastrointestinal and renal problems such as pancreatitis, cirrhosis, chronic liver disease, kidney failure, hepatitis B, and hepatitis C
- CNS issues such as dementia, memory and attention impairments, intraparenchymal hemorrhage, cerebral vasculitis, ischemic events and strokes, and traumatic brain injury
- Pulmonary problems such as bronchospasm, chronic obstructive lung disease, pulmonary edema, pneumonia, hypersensitivity pneumonitis, barotrauma, undifferentiated hemoptysis, and tuberculosis
- Anemia and bone marrow hypofunction
- Sexually transmitted infections such as HIV, syphilis, gonorrhea, and genital warts
- Bacterial infections, including methicillin-resistant *Staphylococcus aureus*
- Pregnancy and birth complications

# Laboratory Testing

Laboratory testing to detect substance use is not sufficient to diagnose SUDs or MSUD but is a valuable tool to guide and monitor treatment. In the acute setting, with a nonverbal patient, toxicology detection might help guide the process of managing withdrawal or identifying an accident's cause. Laboratory tests also provide information about the extent of substance use over time in patients frequently presenting to primary care or psychiatric care. For patients already in treatment, the tests allow monitoring of abstinence or agonist therapy adherence in inpatient and outpatient treatment programs. Laboratory tests and biomarkers of chronic use are discussed in more detail in Chapter 4, "Laboratory Testing." If the patient's history does not indicate any specific medical issue, then a comprehensive metabolic panel, complete blood count, electrocardiogram, and chest X-ray are complementary to the initial evaluation. Results can inform clinicians about complications and guide them toward the right level of care.

# Intoxication and Withdrawal States

The prevalence of any substance use among the general population in the past month is about 57.8% (Substance Abuse and Mental Health Services Administration 2021). The percentage of MSUD varies significantly depending on the combination of substances used. For example, among people diagnosed with cocaine use disorder, 59.8% also have alcohol use disorder, whereas only 13.4% have co-occurring heroin use disorder (National Institute on Drug Abuse 2020). Therefore, encountering intoxication and withdrawal is relatively common in a medical setting. Primary care physicians should be aware of MSUD when planning treatment, especially among adults who are male, younger, less educated, or unemployed (John et al. 2018). Combining patient history and laboratory testing results is essential to assess for the degree of risk associated with symptoms of intoxication or withdrawal. The assessment may include the following:

- Substances used
- Frequency and amount used most recently
- Route of administration
- Exact time of last use
- Any history of complicated alcohol or sedative withdrawal

Laboratory tests can verify recent use, involvement of more than one substance, and current levels of intoxication. A high level found with toxicology testing without obvious physical impairment is a strong indicator of tolerance and physical dependence. Depending on the substance in question, the severity of the withdrawal symptoms can be assessed using clinical tools. For alcohol withdrawal, the Clinical Institute Withdrawal Assessment for Alcohol–Revised (CIWA-Ar) is a brief 10-item scale that quantifies the severity of the alcohol withdrawal syndrome and can be used to monitor progress over time. It has been adjusted for the assessment of benzodiazepine withdrawal (Sullivan et al. 1989). The Clinical Institute Narcotic Assessment (CINA) Scale and the Clinical Opiate Withdrawal Scale (COWS) are validated tools for quantifying opioid withdrawal symptoms (Tompkins et al. 2009).

# Approach to the Psychiatric Evaluation

Distinguishing between psychiatric symptoms resulting from substance use and those from a co-occurring psychiatric disorder can be challenging. Various substances can induce anxiety, depression, mania, and psychosis. These symptoms may be observable with chronic use and during specific substance-induced states, including intoxication and withdrawal. In order to differentiate between substance-induced and co-occurring disorders, the clinician may consider drawing a timeline of substances used, psychiatric symptoms, and prior treatments. This approach can help the clinician determine the chronology of symptom development and the presence or absence of symptoms during extended substance-free periods. Another way to determine whether the symptoms stem from a primary psychiatric disorder or a substance is by performing repeated longitudinal psychiatric assessments. This method enables the clinician to evaluate psychiatric symptoms and their relationship to abstinence or ongoing substance use over time. The probability that someone with an SUD has a co-occurring psychiatric disorder and not a substance-induced psychiatric disorder increases if 1) at least one first-degree relative has a history of a similar disorder, 2) the symptoms are observed independently of substance use, 3) the psychiatric symptoms preceded the onset of the SUD, and/or 4) the symptoms are evident during extended substance-free periods.

People who use multiple substances are vulnerable to increased frequency and severity of both substance-induced disorders and co-occurring psychiatric disorders. Depending on the mixture of substances used, most substance-induced symptoms improve hours or days after use is stopped. In those with heavy and long-term MSUD, psychotic and neurocognitive disorders can become chronic, especially with substances that are directly toxic to the brain, such as amphetamines, alcohol, inhalants such as gasoline, and hallucinogens.

# Making a Diagnosis

DSM-5 (American Psychiatric Association 2022) defines SUD as a problematic pattern of substance use leading to clinically significant impairment or distress, manifested by at least 2 of the 10–11 diagnostic criteria occurring within a 12-month period. DSM-5 does not categorize MSUD as a distinct diagnosis but instead has 10 separate classes of SUD: alcohol use; cannabis use; opioid use; sedative, hypnotic, or anxiolytic use; stimulant use; tobacco use; other (or unknown) substance use; hallucinogen use (phencyclidine and other hallucinogens); inhalant use; and caffeine use. There are 11 criteria for most of these SUDs; phencyclidine, hallucinogen, and inhalant use disorders only have 10 criteria because they lack a distinct withdrawal syndrome. The criteria are further grouped under four main subgroups considered to be the hallmarks of pathological substance use. The first subgroup has symptoms and signs of loss of control over use:

1. The substance is often taken in larger amounts or over a longer period than was intended.
2. There is a persistent desire or have been unsuccessful efforts to cut down or control use.
3. A great deal of time is spent in activities necessary to obtain the substance, use the substance, or recover from its effects.
4. There is a craving or a strong desire or urge to use the substance.

The second subgroup includes indications of continued use despite knowing and/or experiencing adverse and negative consequences:

1. Recurrent use results in a failure to fulfill major role obligations at work, school, or home.
2. Use continues despite persistent or recurrent social or interpersonal problems caused or exacerbated by the effects of substance.
3. Important social, occupational, or recreational activities are given up or reduced because of use.

The third subgroup includes risky use:

1. There is recurrent use in situations in which it is physically hazardous.
2. Substance use continues despite knowledge of having a persistent or recurrent physical or psychological problem likely to have been caused or exacerbated by use.

The fourth subgroup specifies tolerance and withdrawal:

1. Tolerance, as defined by either of the following:
   - A need for markedly increased amounts of substance to achieve intoxication or desired effect.
   - A markedly diminished effect with continued use of the same amount of substance.
2. Withdrawal, as manifested by either of the following:
   - The characteristic withdrawal syndrome for the substance.
   - The substance is taken to relieve or avoid withdrawal symptoms.

DSM-5 makes a special provision for the fourth subgroup under indicated medical treatment with prescription opioids, sedatives, and stimulants. Tolerance and withdrawal symptoms under these circumstances are not counted when diagnosing an SUD. However, clinicians should still diagnose a use disorder for those receiving medical treatment who meet two or more criteria in the first three subgroups but not for those who meet criteria in the fourth subgroup alone.

Because DSM-5 (American Psychiatric Association 2013) steered away from the categorical approach adopted in DSM-IV (American Psychiatric Association 1994) and followed a dimensional approach, severity in DSM-5 is estimated by the number of criteria present. The presence of two or three criteria indicates a mild SUD, four or five indicate a moderate SUD, and six or more indicate a severe SUD. This change also eliminated the need for the polysubstance dependence diagnosis used in DSM-IV because this diagnosis was meant to include individuals who met the "abuse" criteria for several substances but not the "dependence" criteria for any single substance. Table 2–2 shows the differences between DSM-IV and DSM-5 criteria.

When a patient has stopped use for an extended period, DSM-5 adds specifiers for SUDs that aid in determining where that patient is in their recovery. The specifiers "in early remission" and "in sustained remission" apply when a patient no longer meets criteria (except for craving) for 3–12 months and for 12 months or longer, respectively. The specifier "in a controlled environment" also helps to capture recovery because it indicates whether the patient is abstinent in an environment in which the substance is available. For opioid and tobacco use disorders, for which maintenance therapies are available, the specifier "on maintenance therapy" can be added.

## Conclusion

Evaluation and treatment of individuals who use multiple substances must be multifaceted and include physical, social, and psychiatric factors and an interpersonal view of the patient's disorder. A nonjudgmental, collaborative approach facilitates the therapeutic alliance essential for recovery.

**Table 2–2.** Comparison between DSM-IV and DSM-5 criteria for substance-related disorders

| DSM-IV | Criteria number | DSM-5 | Criteria number |
|---|---|---|---|
| **Substance dependence (three criteria required)** | | **Substance use disorder** | |
| Tolerance | 1 | Substance is often taken in larger amounts or over a longer period than was intended | 1 |
| Withdrawal | 2 | Persistent desire or unsuccessful efforts to cut down or control use | 2 |
| Substance is often taken in larger amounts or over a longer period than was intended | 3 | A great deal of time is spent in activities necessary to obtain the substance, use the substance, or recover from its effects | 3 |
| Persistent desire or unsuccessful efforts to cut down or control use | 4 | Craving, or a strong desire or urge to use | 4 |
| A great deal of time is spent in activities necessary to obtain the substance, use the substance, or recover from its effects | 5 | Recurrent use resulting in a failure to fulfill major role obligations at work, school, or home | 5 |
| Important activities are given up or reduced because of use | 6 | Continued use despite physical and/or psychological problems | 6 |
| Continued use despite physical and/or psychological problems | 7 | Important activities are given up or reduced because of use | 7 |

**Table 2–2.** Comparison between DSM-IV and DSM-5 criteria for substance-related disorders (*continued*)

| DSM-IV | Criteria number | DSM-5 | Criteria number |
|---|---|---|---|
| **Substance abuse (one criterion required)** | | **Substance use disorder** (*continued*) | |
| Recurrent use resulting in a failure to fulfill major role obligations at work, school, or home | 1 | Recurrent use in physically hazardous situations | 8 |
| Recurrent use in physically hazardous situations | 2 | Continued use despite having persistent or recurrent social or interpersonal problems caused or exacerbated by the effects of substance | 9 |
| Recurrent substance-related legal problems | 3 | Tolerance | 10 |
| Continued use despite having persistent or recurrent social or interpersonal problems caused or exacerbated by the effects of substance | 4 | Withdrawal | 11 |

# References

American Psychiatric Association: Diagnostic and Statistical Manual of Mental Disorders, 4th Edition. Washington, DC, American Psychiatric Association, 1994

American Psychiatric Association: Diagnostic and Statistical Manual of Mental Disorders, 5th Edition. Arlington, VA, American Psychiatric Association, 2013

American Psychiatric Association: Diagnostic and Statistical Manual of Mental Disorders, 5th Edition Text Revision. Washington, DC, American Psychiatric Association, 2022

Attaran R, Ragavan D, Probst A: Cocaine-related myocardial infarction: concomitant heroin use can cloud the picture. Eur J Emerg Med 12(4):199–201, 2005 16034268

Basu D, Ghosh A, Sarkar S, et al: Initial treatment dropout in patients with substance use disorders attending a tertiary care de-addiction centre in north India. Indian J Med Res 146(Suppl):S77–S84, 2017 29578199

Bhalla IP, Stefanovics EA, Rosenheck RA: Clinical epidemiology of single versus multiple substance use disorders: polysubstance use disorder. Med Care 55(55):S24–S32, 2017 28806363

Centers for Disease Control and Prevention: Polysubstance Use Facts. Atlanta, GA, Centers for Disease Control and Prevention, 2022. Available at: https://www.cdc.gov/stopoverdose/polysubstance-use/index.html. Accessed September 20, 2022.

Coffin PO, Galea S, Ahern J, et al: Opiates, cocaine and alcohol combinations in accidental drug overdose deaths in New York City, 1990–98. Addiction 98(6):739–747, 2003 12780362

John WS, Zhu H, Mannelli P, et al: Prevalence, patterns, and correlates of multiple substance use disorders among adult primary care patients. Drug Alcohol Depend 187(June):79–87, 2018 29635217

Johnson SD, Striley C, Cottler LB: The association of substance use disorders with trauma exposure and PTSD among African American drug users. Addict Behav 31(11):2063–2073, 2006 16580784

Morgen K: Substance Use Disorders and Addictions. Thousand Oaks, CA, Sage, 2017

National Institute on Drug Abuse: Common Comorbidities With Substance Use Disorders Research Report. Bethesda, MD, National Institute on Drug Abuse, 2020

Schaper E, Padwa H, Urada D, et al: Substance use disorder patient privacy and comprehensive care in integrated health care settings. Psychol Serv 13(1):105–109, 2016 26845493

Shaffer HJ, LaPlante DA, LaBrie RA, et al: Toward a syndrome model of addiction: multiple expressions, common etiology. Harv Rev Psychiatry 12(6):367–374, 2004 15764471

Substance Abuse and Mental Health Services Administration: Key Substance Use and Mental Health Indicators in the United States: Results From the 2020 National Survey on Drug Use and Health. Rockville, MD, Substance Abuse and Mental Health Services Administration, 2021, p 156. Available at: https://www.samhsa.gov/data/sites/default/files/reports/rpt35325/NSDUHFFRPDFWHTMLFiles2020/2020NSDUHFFR1PDFW102121.pdf. Accessed February 15, 2023.

Sullivan JT, Sykora K, Schneiderman J, et al: Assessment of alcohol withdrawal: the revised Clinical Institute Withdrawal Assessment for Alcohol scale (CIWA-Ar). Br J Addict 84(11):1353–1357, 1989 2597811

Tompkins DA, Bigelow GE, Harrison JA, et al: Concurrent validation of the Clinical Opiate Withdrawal Scale (COWS) and single-item indices against the Clinical Institute Narcotic Assessment (CINA) opioid withdrawal instrument. Drug Alcohol Depend 105(1–2):154–159, 2009 19647958

Vendetti J, Gmyrek A, Damon D, et al: Screening, brief intervention and referral to treatment (SBIRT): implementation barriers, facilitators and model migration. Addiction 112(Suppl 2):23–33, 2017

# 3

# Neurobiology of Addiction and Principles of Pharmacology

Tabark Altai, M.D.
Nidal Moukaddam, M.D., Ph.D.

*In this chapter,* we discuss the neurobiological principles that underlie addictive processes. The biology of addiction is complex and entails pharmacological and genetic variations and acute and chronic neurocircuitry alterations, as well as substance-specific effects. We cover the circuits involved in addiction, the phases of the process, how it translates into real-life personality and psychological factors, and pharmacodynamic and pharmacokinetic principles affecting brain responses to substance use.

## Case Example

MB is a 22-year-old female who presents to the psychiatry clinic to ask for help with an "addictive personality." She reports that since her teenage years, she has always wanted to live her life "to the max," gets bored easily, and tries new things to have more excitement in her life. This led her to experiment with cannabis at about age 13; various stimulants between the ages of 16 and 18; and uncommon substances such as 2C-I, kratom, and pills with unknown content. MB is aware of the risks of unlabeled substances but enjoys the excitement of trying new things. She has experienced unpleasant physical symptoms when using but generally dismisses them as inconsequential. Some consequences of her substance use that she regrets include achieving low grades in college and experiencing negative effects in her relationships because she has had mood swings and has been verbally hurtful to her loved ones. However, when MB tries to abstain from substance use, she becomes anxious, sad, and anhedonic. She tries to resist for a few days but eventually gives in to relieve negative feelings. She describes herself as "mean" when intoxicated. She has trouble limiting her use once she starts.

This case example illustrates the following points:

- Binge and intoxication stages are characterized by loss of control over use and behavioral and/or physiological manifestations.
- Withdrawal stages carry the risk of negative affect and cravings.
- Personality factors make people more likely to engage in risky behaviors.

# Neurobiology of Addictive Disorders

Addictive processes entail impaired interactions between three functional systems of the brain: *motivation-reward, affect regulation,* and *behavioral inhibition.* For decades, addiction has been considered a dysregulation of reward circuitry; the steep increase of dopamine release into the ventral striatum in states of drug intoxication is well known and thought to be instrumental in the development of any addiction. Substances (including alcohol) with abuse and reinforcing potential are known to activate the brain reward systems; reward is the event that increases positive hedonic response (Koob and Volkow 2016; Tambour and Quertemont 2007). However, although activation of reward circuitry is a cornerstone of getting a "high," many neurochemical substrates have been identified as the cause of impairment in the three functional systems, going beyond the dopaminergic system (Feldman et al. 2011).

The neurobiology of addiction involves brain structures associated with the addictive process and how they affect learning and behaviors. Many models have been proposed to identify these brain structures. The model proposed by Volkow et al. (2003) identified four brain circuits involved in the development of drug abuse and addiction (Table 3–1): 1) the *reward circuit* in the nucleus accumbens and the ventral pallidum, 2) the *motivation/drive circuit* in the orbitofrontal cortex (OFC) and the subcallosal cortex, 3) the *memory and learning circuit* in the amygdala and the hippocampus, and 4) the *control circuit* in the prefrontal cortex (PFC) and the anterior cingulate gyrus. Dopamine neurons directly innervate these circuits and interconnect with each other directly and indirectly via glutamatergic projections. The circuits'

**Table 3–1.** Circuits involved in addiction neurobiology

| Circuit | Elements | Role | Main neurotransmitters |
|---|---|---|---|
| Reward circuit | Nucleus accumbens | Reward and motivation | Dopamine |
| | Ventral pallidum and ventral tegmental area | | |
| Motivation/drive circuit | Orbitofrontal cortex | Impulse regulation | Dopamine, serotonin |
| | Subcallosal cortex | | |
| Memory and learning circuit | Amygdala | Emotion processing | Serotonin, dopamine, glutamate, GABA |
| | Hippocampus | Memory conversion | Serotonin, dopamine, glutamate, GABA |
| | Thalamus | Relaying information | Serotonin, dopamine, glutamate, GABA |
| | Hypothalamus | Homeostasis | Serotonin, dopamine, glutamate, GABA |
| Control circuit | Prefrontal cortex and anterior cingulate gyrus | Cognitive control function | Dopamine, serotonin, norepinephrine |

responses to stimuli differ depending on the saliency value of the substance (or reward) at hand and the individual's experience. The stronger the value of the positive stimuli from a previous experience is, the stronger the activation of the motivational circuit that is controlled by the PFC and cingulate gyrus. In individuals with substance use disorder (SUD), the saliency value of the drug is thought to be enhanced in the motivation/drive circuit. This enhancement is due to the higher intrinsic reward of the drug, which increases dopamine in the nucleus accumbens three- to fivefold compared with natural reinforcers (Volkow et al. 2003).

Evolutionarily, the reward circuit is thought to provide the body information and motivation to acquire essentials (e.g., food, water, love) to sustain body functions and maintain homeostatic balance. Any deviation from that homeostatic balance will generate the need to look for these essentials in the environment. The human brain evolved two systems to maintain homeostasis: the hypothalamic centers responsible for feeding and drinking and the reward centers responsible for reinforcement of behaviors needed to obtain the essentials (Blum et al. 2018). The balance between these two systems plays a functional survival value. Drugs create short- and long-term changes in these systems, influencing how the individual experiences reward, learning, and drug-seeking behavior.

# Intoxication and Conditioned Reinforcement

Drug intoxication causes a steep increase in dopamine release into the ventral striatum; any drug that becomes addictive activates the dopaminergic system, and the high associated with a drug is related to the levels of dopamine release. Studies have identified other neurotransmitters that have indirect effects on dopamine release, such as GABA, glutamate, serotonin, and endocannabinoids. Repeated use of a substance has profound effects on the balance between neurotransmitter levels and homeostasis between brain areas. Behaviorally, the substance is then associated with a specific environment, individuals, and methods of use. These conditions (people, places, things) then become associated with reward and memories of drug use. This process of *conditioned reinforcement* and *incentive salience* ("wanting") occurs when a previously neutral stimulus becomes reinforcing because it has been associated with drug-induced reward. Indeed, individuals with addiction have increases in dopamine levels in response to drug-condition cues even before using the drug (Koob and Volkow 2016). Conditioned reinforcement is an essential step in the formation of habitual substance use and is used in animal models to assess the reinforcing potential of a substance. During a cue-induced recurrence, many report a seemingly automatic drug-seeking behavior on exposure to the cue. Therefore, breaking established patterns in everyday life is essential to achieve abstinence and recovery from substance use.

Chronic drug exposure causes neurochemical adaptations in the brain system responsible for how a person experiences the drug reward (within-system neuroadaptations). It also activates other systems, such as the recruitment of anti-reward systems that neutralize the drug's effects and are involved in the unpleasant symptoms experienced during drug withdrawal. Such adaptations can include (but are not limited to) decreased dopamine and serotonin release in the nucleus accumbens, which leads to needing higher drug doses to achieve the same euphoric effects. Human functional brain imaging studies in amphetamine and methamphetamine users show that dopamine release in the nucleus accumbens is decreased by up to 50% in those who have recently stopped using and up to 80% in active users compared with nonusers. These individuals also report lower drug-rewarding effects compared with nonusers.

In opioid withdrawal, an increase in μ opioid receptor activity, a decrease in GABAergic transmission, and an increase in norepinephrine and N-methyl-D-aspartate (NMDA) glutamatergic transmission in the nucleus accumbens have been observed (Koob and Volkow 2016).

# Brain Disease Model of Addiction

The brain disease model of addiction (BDMA) posits that drugs of addiction can alter important areas in the brain needed for healthy social interaction and daily life functions, such that the user develops compulsive drug-seeking and drug-using behavior. Addiction as explained by the BDMA involves a repeating cycle of three stages (Figure 3–1): 1) the *binge/intoxication* stage associated with the basal ganglia, in which the use of drugs gives the individual the rewarding and pleasuring effect; 2) the *withdrawal/negative affect* stage associated with the amygdala, manifesting as negative emotions in the absence of the drug; and 3) the *preoccupation/anticipation stage* associated with the PFC, in which the individual seeks the substance again after a period of abstinence. The BDMA identifies other factors that increase the person's vulnerability to engaging in risky substance use behaviors and addiction, including genetics and environmental and social factors (Hazelden Betty Ford Foundation 2021).

# Genetics and Personality Factors

Several studies have investigated the role of heritable factors and genetics in the development of addiction. People have genetic variations in their drug response, metabolism, drug toxicity, and neurochemical transmission (Moran et al. 2021). Thus, genetic factors affect the mental and emotional states preceding substance use, the processes by which substances are metabolized, and how the brain reacts acutely and long term to the substance use. Genetics can also influence endophenotypes, or personality traits, of addiction use, such as low-avoidance, high-novelty-seeking, and high-impulsivity traits.

Studies of twins who grew up in similar compared with different environments (e.g., separated at birth for adoption) indicate that genetic factors play an important role in the development of an addiction. It is estimated that 33%–71% of nicotine addiction, 48%–66% of alcohol addiction, 51%–59% of cannabis addiction, 42%–79% of opioid addiction, and 49% of disordered gambling can be attributed to genetics. However, risk varies widely depending on the stage of addiction and the developmental course of the patient. Environ-

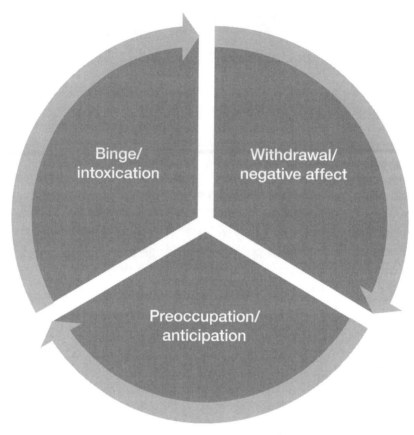

Figure 3–1.  Stages of addiction.

mental factors may have a greater influence at an early age, such that traumatic experiences and early-life adversity may increase vulnerability to later-life addiction. The early stages of addiction are less attributable to genetics than the later stages. In adolescence, shared environmental factors such as neighborhood, peer influence, socioeconomic status, and abuse have a greater impact on addiction liability. However, genetic factors may contribute to addiction up to 75% in adults. Multiple genes have been identified in addiction-related phenotypes, many increasing or decreasing the risk for a specific substance. Some examples include *GABRA2* (rs279858, rs279826, rs279871), which is associated with alcohol use disorder and binge drinking, and the dopamine single nucleotide polymorphisms in the *CHRNA5-CHRNA3-CHRNB4* cluster on chromosome 15, which is associated with cocaine use disorder (Agrawal et al. 2012).

It is estimated that 40%–60% of addiction risk is due to genetics (Dingel et al. 2015; Koob and Volkow 2016), but the scope of each gene and its impact on the development of addiction varies. In addition to the biological factors that contribute to a patient's vulnerability to addiction, these genes can influence the response to psychosocial environments, such as socioeconomic situation, family structure, peer influence, and community support. Taken together, genetic factors influence the person's biological and psychological responses to their environment and to substances, which affects their risk of developing an addictive disorder (Dingel et al. 2015). Genetics can also influence broad personality and coping traits involved in the maintenance of addictive behaviors that generalize across substances. High impulsivity is a trait shared among individuals with addiction. Other personality traits associated with addiction include high neuroticism, low conscientiousness, low agreeableness, and disinhibition (Zilberman et al. 2018). Feldman et al. (2011) revealed a correlation between the type of drug and personality traits. Higher-sociability individuals seem to prefer heroin and opiates, whereas those with lower sociability preferred stimulants such as cocaine.

These personality traits are shared within family systems. A study that examined impulsivity in drug users using the Barratt Impulsivity Scale (BIS-11) found that impulsivity was increased not only in drug users but also in their siblings. Higher BIS-11 scores were associated with brain neurochemical and structural variations linked to the development of addiction. At-risk participants had reduced striatal dopamine receptor availability and gray matter volume in their OFC (Ersche et al. 2010). Novelty seeking and low harm avoidance combined with impulsivity increase the chance that a person will experiment with new substances and experiences.

# Psychological Theories and Link to Neurobiology

The American Psychological Association (2023) defined SUD as "a cluster of cognitive, behavioral, and psychological symptoms indicating continued use of a substance despite significant substance-related problems." Psychological models developed to explain the cause and maintenance of addictions can be grouped under three broad categories: 1) learning theory–based models, 2) psychodynamic theories, and 3) transtheoretical models. Learning theory–based models explain addictive behaviors as overlearned habits, such that a person begins with experimental and recreational use and gradually transitions to excessive use, loss of control, and then use disorder. Psychodynamic theories cover a range of viewpoints from psychoanalytic thinking to transactional analysis. Hopper (1995) linked substance misuse and personality disorders to posttraumatic syndrome, whereas Khantzian (1997) emphasized the role of substance use as self-medication to relieve self-deficits. Transtheoretical models of addiction include the stages of change model, the excessive appetite model, and the PRIME (plans, responses, impulses, motives, and evaluations) theory, which attributes addiction to malfunctioning of any of the five levels of human motivation (Wanigaratne 2006). Understanding these models may help the clinician customize a treatment program that uniquely resonates with each patient.

# Pharmacology

## Pharmacokinetics

*Pharmacokinetics* refers to how the body processes a substance, including absorption, distribution, metabolism, and excretion. These processes are influenced by genetic, biological, environmental, and behavioral factors (Allain et al. 2015). *Drug absorption* is the process of the drug entering the body and reaching systemic circulation. *Bioavailability* is the fraction of the administered drug that reaches the systemic circulation, largely affected by the drug's route of administration (e.g., oral, sublingual, injection). *Drug distribution* refers to the movement of a drug to and from systemic circulation to the various tissues of the body and the proportion of that drug in each tissue; it is determined by factors such as diffusion, plasma or tissue protein binding, body weight, muscle mass, fat composition, and total body water. In circulation, drugs are either protein bound or free; the latter form allows for binding to receptors and has a greater potential for toxicity. *Drug metabolism* is the chemical alteration of the drug by the body, which may either make it more water soluble for renal clearance or metabolize and convert it into its active form. Most drug metabolism occurs in the liver via the cytochrome P450 (CYP) enzyme system and in the gastrointestinal tract. Drug excretion is the process of drug elimination from the body, which is conducted by the kidneys for most drugs (Grogan and Preuss 2022). Any disruption in these processes can cause significant health consequences, which is commonly seen in chronic severe SUDs. Liver and kidney diseases can have critical effects on pharmacokinetics. Liver disease can lead to changes in drug intestinal absorption, plasma protein binding, hepatic extraction, biliary excretion, and enterohepatic circulation. These changes can alter drug concentration and bioavailability. Patients with liver cirrhosis, for instance, have slower metabolism of opioids and thus are at higher risk for overdose. Renal diseases that lower the glomerular filtration rate result in decreased clearance and accumulation of the drug. For individuals who use multiple substances, the combined effects often produce a complicated toxidrome.

The route of drug administration determines how fast and how much of the drug reaches systemic circulation and the brain. How fast a drug reaches the brain plays an important role in addiction progression. Smoking and injection are the most efficient methods of getting a drug into the bloodstream, whereas the oral route is slower and therefore has less addiction liability. Addiction is usually more severe in those who use rapid routes of delivery. Generally, individuals who smoke or inject are likely to use drugs more frequently and for longer periods and to spend more money on drugs, and they are more likely to overdose. They also experience more health-threatening conditions such as blood-borne diseases (i.e., hepatitis C, HIV), drug-induced mental health conditions, and all-cause mortality (Allain et al. 2015). Smoking and injection bypass the first-pass effect in the gut and liver, allowing for a higher drug concentration.

## Pharmacogenomics

*Pharmacogenomics* (or *pharmacogenetics*) is a field of research that examines how a person's genes influence their response to substances or medications. Common approaches to identifying genetic causes include genetic linkage and genome-wide association studies (GWASs). Genetic linkage studies identify risk genes within a family. GWASs query the genome to assess for alleles that are commonly seen among individuals with a given disorder. GWASs have identified genetic biomarkers responsible for variations in cell adhesion, enzyme activities, transcriptional regulation, and other processes associated with SUD phenotypes. Polymorphisms identified by GWASs include enzymes in the CYP system, dopamine β-hydroxylase (DβH) and monoamine oxidase (MAO) enzymes, receptors such as those for dopamine (*DRD2*) and μ opioid (*OPRM1*), and the serotonin (*5-HTT*) and dopamine (*DAT1*) transporters (Mroziewicz and Tyndale 2010). Pharmacogenetics is useful in drug development and to guide treatment.

## Pharmacodynamics

*Pharmacodynamics* is an area in pharmacology that studies a substance's effects on the body and its mechanisms of action. In general, each drug produces a unique physiological and emotional response based on its action on different neurochemicals and receptors. The following is a brief overview of the mechanisms of common substances.

- *Alcohol* exerts its effects by directly activating GABA receptors (inhibitory) and inhibiting NMDA receptors (excitatory). Alcohol also indirectly increases dopamine release and activates the opioid system. Its effect on the opioid system is thought to explain why the opioid receptor antagonist naltrexone is effective for the treatment of alcohol use disorder (Tambour and Quertemont 2007).
- *Stimulants* increase the activity of dopamine, norepinephrine, and serotonin in the CNS and the peripheral nervous system. Cocaine blocks the activity of reuptake transporters, allowing a higher concentration of catecholamines to stay active in the synapse. Amphetamines inhibit vesicular monoamine transport and induce the release of catecholamines. Cocaine and amphetamines transiently increase extracellular dopamine concentrations in the dorsal striatum (Ciccarone 2011).
- *Opioids* are associated with three types of receptors in the human body (δ, κ, μ), all of which are G-protein-coupled receptors. Stimulation of the different opioid receptors produces a wide range of clinical effects depending on the location of the receptor. Opioid receptors are widely distributed in the CNS, the peripheral nervous system, and the nonneural tissues. In the CNS, opioid receptors are found in high concentrations in the periaqueductal gray (PAG), locus coeruleus, rostral ventral medulla, and substantia gelatinosa of the dorsal horn. Activation of μ opioid receptors produces euphoria, analgesia, sedation, bradycardia, nausea, and vomiting. Pain control stems from stimulation of μ opioid receptors in midbrain, leading to indirect stimulation of the descending inhibitory pathways to the PAG and the nucleus reticularis paragigantocellularis. The PAG projects to the nucleus raphe magnus, leading to downstream release of serotonin and enkephalin in the substantia gelatinosa of the dorsal horn. Activation of the δ opioid receptors produces spinal and supraspinal analgesia and reduction in gastric motility. Activation of κ opioid receptors produces dysphoria, spinal analgesia, and diuresis. Opioids with addictive potential all act on the μ opioid receptors. In contrast, the hallucinogen *Salvia divinorum* is a κ opioid receptor agonist and produces disturbing altered realities. Buprenorphine is a partial agonist at the μ opioid receptor and antagonist at the κ opioid receptor; the latter mechanism is thought to underly its antidepressant effects (Pathan and Williams 2012).

- *Nicotine* activates nicotinic acetylcholine receptors (nAChRs). Brain imaging studies show that nicotine increases activity in the PFC, thalamus, and visual system, consistent with the cortico-striatal-thalamic loop circuits. Activation of central nAChRs by nicotine leads to a release of various neurotransmitters in the brain, most importantly, dopamine in the mesolimbic area, the corpus striatum, and the frontal cortex. Nicotine activation of the dopamine neurons in the ventral tegmental area and downstream dopamine release in the nucleus accumbens is critical in drug-induced reward. Nicotine also modulates the activity of other neurotransmitters, including norepinephrine, acetylcholine, serotonin, GABA, glutamate, and endorphins. Chronic exposure to nicotine downregulates brain MAO-A and MAO-B, further increasing monoamine concentrations in synapses (Benowitz 2009).

- *Cannabinoids* act on cannabinoid type 1 ($CB_1$) and type 2 ($CB_2$) receptors; $CB_1$ is the main receptor found in the CNS, with the highest density in the cerebellum, basal ganglia, hippocampus, and cerebral cortex. The distribution of the $CB_1$ receptors in those regions correlates with cannabinoid effects on motor and cognitive impairment. $CB_2$ receptors are found mostly in immune cells, where they are thought to have a regulatory role in immune function and inflammation (Hosking and Zajicek 2014). The primary psychoactive component in the cannabis plant is Δ-9-tetrahydrocannabinol (Δ-9 THC). THC stimulates the dopamine release in the nucleus accumbens and PFC, likely contributing to its reinforcing properties and the individual's risk of developing cannabis use disorder (Ashton 2001).

## Conclusion

In this chapter, we covered the basic neurobiological underpinnings of how addictive processes develop and highlighted the influence of genetics on personality traits, developmental stage, and pharmacokinetics in the development and maintenance of SUDs. In the treatment of SUDs, clinicians may help patients understand the unique interplay of biological, psychological, and environmental processes, which may enhance collaboration between clinician and patient in designing a personalized recovery plan.

## References

Agrawal A, Verweij KJH, Gillespie NA, et al: The genetics of addiction—a translational perspective. Transl Psychiatry 2(7):e140, 2012 22806211

Allain F, Minogianis E-A, Roberts DCS, et al: How fast and how often: the pharmacokinetics of drug use are decisive in addiction. Neurosci Biobehav Rev 56(Sept):166–179, 2015 26116543

American Psychological Association: APA Dictionary of Psychology. Washington, DC, American Psychological Association, 2023. Available at: https://dictionary.apa.org. Accessed January 30, 2023.

Ashton CH: Pharmacology and effects of cannabis: a brief review. Br J Psychiatry 178(Feb):101–106, 2001 11157422

Benowitz NL: Pharmacology of nicotine: addiction, smoking-induced disease, and therapeutics. Annu Rev Pharmacol Toxicol 49:57–71, 2009 18834313

Blum K, Gondré-Lewis M, Steinberg B, et al: Our evolved unique pleasure circuit makes humans different from apes: reconsideration of data derived from animal studies. J Syst Integr Neurosci 4(1):10.15761/JSIN.1000191, 2018 30956812

Ciccarone D: Stimulant abuse: pharmacology, cocaine, methamphetamine, treatment, attempts at pharmacotherapy. Prim Care 38(1):41–58, 2011 21356420

Dingel MJ, Ostergren J, McCormick JB, et al: The media and behavioral genetics: alternatives coexisting with addiction genetics. Sci Technol Human Values 40(4):459–486, 2015 26392644

Ersche KD, Turton AJ, Pradhan S, et al: Drug addiction endophenotypes: impulsive versus sensation-seeking personality traits. Biol Psychiatry 68(8):770–773, 2010 20678754

Feldman M, Boyer B, Kumar VK, et al: Personality, drug preference, drug use, and drug availability. J Drug Educ 41(1):45–63, 2011 21675324

Grogan S, Preuss CV: Pharmacokinetics, in StatPearls. Treasure Island, FL, StatPearls Publishing, 2022. Available at: https://www.ncbi.nlm.nih.gov/books/NBK557744/. Accessed December 2022.

Hazelden Betty Ford Foundation: The Brain Disease Model of Addiction. Center City, MN, Hazelden Betty Ford Foundation, May 2021. Available at: https://www.hazeldenbettyford.org/research-studies/addiction-research/brain-disease-model. Accessed January 30, 2023.

Hopper E: A psychoanalytical theory of "drug addiction": unconscious fantasies of homosexuality, compulsions and masturbation within the context of traumatogenic processes. Int J Psychoanal 76(Pt 6)(December):1121–1142, 1995

Hosking R, Zajicek J: Pharmacology: cannabis in neurology: a potted review. Nat Rev Neurol 10(8):429–430, 2014 25002109

Khantzian EJ: The self-medication hypothesis of substance use disorders: a reconsideration and recent applications. Harv Rev Psychiatry 4(5):231–244, 1997

Koob GF, Volkow ND: Neurobiology of addiction: a neurocircuitry analysis. Lancet Psychiatry 3(8):760–773, 2016 27475769

Moran M, Blum K, Ponce JV, et al: High Genetic Addiction Risk Score (GARS) in chronically prescribed severe chronic opioid probands attending multi-pain clinics: an open clinical pilot trial. Mol Neurobiol 58(7):3335–3346, 2021 33683627

Mroziewicz M, Tyndale RF: Pharmacogenetics: a tool for identifying genetic factors in drug dependence and response to treatment. Addict Sci Clin Pract 5(2):17–29, 2010 22002450

Pathan H, Williams J: Basic opioid pharmacology: an update. Br J Pain 6(1):11–16, 2012 26516461

Tambour S, Quertemont E: Preclinical and clinical pharmacology of alcohol dependence. Fundam Clin Pharmacol 21(1):9–28, 2007 17227441

Volkow ND, Fowler JS, Wang G-J: The addicted human brain: insights from imaging studies. J Clin Invest 111(10):1444–1451, 2003 12750391

Wanigaratne S: Psychology of addiction. Psychiatry 5(12):455–460, 2006

Zilberman N, Yadid G, Efrati Y, et al: Personality profiles of substance and behavioral addictions. Addict Behav 82(July):174–181, 2018 29547799

# 4

# Laboratory Testing

Benjamin Li, M.D.

*Laboratory* testing for substances has an important role in the evaluation of patients with suspected or diagnosed substance use disorders (SUDs). However, to effectively use drug screening in clinical practice, clinicians must be aware of the scope of those tests, the causes of false positives, the rates of false negatives, the metabolites of various substances that would be detected by these screens, and the specific metabolites detected by each confirmatory test. Different laboratory companies may also vary in detection accuracy for individual substances. Even with expertly interpreted laboratory results, the clinician must determine how those results affect the overall treatment plan. Although the urine drug screen (UDS) is one objective tool, it should not solely dictate the treatment plan. Instead, it should be used as a part of a comprehensive evaluation to gauge a patient's progress toward meeting treatment goals. Patients may still have improved quality of life and meet their treatment goals even in the presence of positive drug testing results. Such an outcome would be expected in a harm reduction approach, in which reduction in substance use or risky behavior—as opposed to complete abstinence from substances—is the patient's goal.

## Interpreting Positive Screening Results

An isolated positive result for a UDS is not enough for the presumption of an SUD diagnosis. A person may use a substance with no significant impairment and without meeting at least 2 of the 11 DSM-5 criteria for most SUDs (American Psychiatric Association 2022; see also Chapter 2, "General Approach to Patients With Multi-substance Use Disorders"). On the other hand, recurrent use corroborated by multiple drug screen findings may be more indicative of an SUD if other clinical evidence or history supports additional criteria.

Discussing a positive result with a patient who denies use has an inherent set of challenges. First, doing so could erode the rapport if the patient truly has maintained abstinence, but the clinician conveys mistrust by putting too much weight on the drug screen result without awareness of the potential for false positives. At the same time, denial or minimization is a defense mechanism commonly seen in patients with SUD; in particular, shame is a common reason why someone may not be ready to disclose or discuss specific results. A preferred method is to transparently explain the UDS results and objectively discuss them while asking the patient for feedback or an explanation. If the patient denies all possibilities, the clinician can first give them the benefit of the doubt and follow-up with a review of prescribed and over-the-counter medications to identify possible causes of false positives. The patient can also be asked about any other substances they have used that may have been adulterated ("laced") or counterfeit medication. Figure 4–1 provides a suggested algorithm for such a discussion. One study found that among opioid-related overdose deaths in 2016, 79.7% were involved with alcohol or another drug (Jones et al. 2018). With the increase in synthetic opioids being mixed with cocaine, heroin, methamphetamine, and counterfeit pills, clinicians must consider the possibility that a patient is not intentionally or knowingly ingesting a specific substance (Cheng et al. 2019). They should also consider the possibility that a normally used substance was received from a different dealer and adulterated. If no obvious causes are seen after exploring all of the above, a confirmation test can be ordered to reevaluate the existing urine sample.

A consensus on routine drug screening may not exist in a primary care setting or general psychiatry clinic. A UDS should be included in routine laboratory tests, provided the patient is informed that it will be ordered. As long as the clinician reflects the results nonjudgmentally to the patient, the UDS can be a powerful tool to shape treatment planning and help diagnostically clarify whether psychiatric symptoms are exacerbated or induced by substance use. This knowledge is crucial because patients with comorbid major depressive disorder and SUD (lifetime prevalence 5.82%) have more frequent and more severe depressive episodes and higher suicide rates than those who have depression without SUD. Although substance-induced depressive disorder has a lower lifetime prevalence (0.26%), it is associated with high clinical severity, low rates of medication treatment, and high rates of substance use to self-treat depressive symptoms (Blanco et al. 2012).

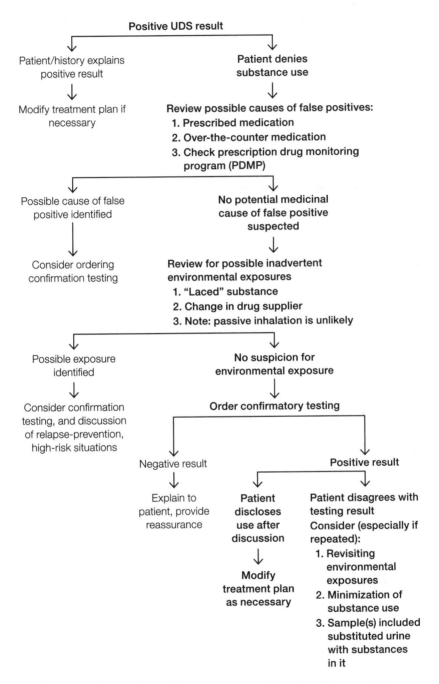

**Figure 4–1.** Approach to exploring and managing positive results on a urine drug screen (UDS).

Particularly with co-occurring SUDs, the presence of multiple substances in testing may help predict the prognosis, risk of overdose death due to the combined effects of multiple substances, and safety profile for a patient who may be prescribed narcotic medications. Laboratory testing should always be combined with evaluating for other prescribed medication using a prescription drug monitoring program (PDMP). Although the implementation of PDMPs has effectively led to reductions in opioid overdoses and mortality related to benzodiazepines and psychostimulants, these programs exclude documentation of any nonprescribed narcotics (Vuolo et al. 2022). Laboratory testing can help address this limitation.

# Types and Sources of Testing

The most common source of drug testing performed in offices is urine (Martini et al. 2020). Urine immunoassay tests have the advantage of being quick and easy to obtain within the same appointment. However, they have the disadvantage of more frequent false positives and false negatives due to the nature of the assay. Furthermore, when a collection is not monitored, it is more susceptible to urine tampering, substitution, and dilution. In these cases, analyzing urine creatinine, specific gravity, or pH may help identify tampering. A positive screen may be followed by confirmatory testing (or testing to identify a false-negative result) using gas chromatography–mass spectrometry (GC-MS) or liquid chromatography–mass spectrometry (LC-MS) (Tamama 2021). Although confirmatory testing often involves higher cost and a longer processing time, it is worthwhile to order tests to confirm or refute the initial result. The resultant findings could change the course of treatment. Although an observed urine collection may reduce the risk of tampering or substitution, it does not eliminate the risk. Various apparatuses, such as prosthetic body parts designed to create an illusion of compliance with observed testing, are sold online. Moreover, implementation is complicated by cost and time for staff and the perceived intrusiveness of observed testing by patients.

Rapid dipstick tests can be used for even faster results. Results inconsistent with a patient's report can be followed by submitting the urine sample for confirmatory testing. Saliva testing is another rapid option for those who decline or cannot complete urine testing. However, most substances are undetectable in saliva 12–24 hours after use; on average, illicit drugs can be detected within 5 to 48 hours. Although saliva allows for more immediate detection of Δ-9-tetrahydrocannabinol (Δ-9 THC), cocaine, and methamphetamine, it is not as helpful for late detection because urine retains a higher level of drug metabolites in comparison (Martini et al. 2020). Although blood testing may be significantly harder to adulterate because it involves direct collection, the detection windows of substances in blood may be shorter than that in urine. Blood tests are also more invasive than other sources of detection. Finally, hair testing may be used in forensic settings and may detect metabolites of substances for significantly more extended periods than other types of drug testing. It may detect cocaine and opiates for 3–4 months and methamphetamine for 6 months after use (Suwannachom et al. 2015). Although hair testing is not routinely done in office-based treatment, its long range of detection provides a complete picture of substance use that may have evaded standard UDSs obtained at regular intervals. However, hair testing may also be affected by treatments such as bleaching and perming (He et al. 2021). A comparison of the different types of testing available is summarized in Table 4–1.

# False Positives

Table 4–2 lists the most common false positives encountered with a standard UDS (immunoassay). The number of false positives among different drug classes differs widely; amphetamines have the largest range of other medications that can cause a false positive, whereas cocaine has very few, if any, causes for false positives. Being mindful of potential false-positive results may help even before prescribing certain medications if there are concerns that these medications could lead to false-positive results in a forensic setting. Some commonly prescribed psychiatric medications can cause false positives; for example, sertraline may appear as a benzodiazepine and trazodone and bupropion as amphetamines.

Sometimes, a patient may explain that a positive result was from secondhand exposure, such as being around others using cocaine or cannabis. Several studies, however, suggest that secondhand exposure causing a positive result in urine testing is unlikely at typical and plausible exposure levels (Cone et al. 1995; Niedbala et al. 2004; Westin and Slørdal 2009). Most of the discussion of false positives has been in case literature, so actual false-positives rates for each substance and whether they are dose related remain unclear.

# False Negatives

In some cases, a UDS may not detect a particular drug in a specified class. For example, a standard UDS may not detect benzodiazepines such as clonazepam, lorazepam, and alprazolam (Mikel et al. 2012). Opioid screens may not

Table 4–1.　Summary of strengths and limitations of types of drug testing

| Test type | Strengths | Limitations | Other considerations |
|---|---|---|---|
| Immunoassay, urine | Quick<br>Easily available<br>Noninvasive<br>Easy to collect in sufficient quantities to retest or send confirmation | Prone to false positives and false negatives and urine tampering<br>Limited correlation to serum concentrations<br>Shorter detection window compared with those for hair and sweat<br>Some patients have difficulty providing urine when requested (hemodialysis, urinary retention) | Most widely used screening tool for substance use |
| GC-MS/LC-MS, urine | Accuracy | Often takes days for results<br>Significantly higher cost | Very helpful to check for false positive or false negative from screening tests |
| Dipstick (POC) | Very quick | Accuracy | |
| Saliva | Not invasive<br>Can be monitored fully<br>Quick results<br>Decent correlation with serum concentrations<br>Parent drug usually present in higher concentrations compared with urine | Smoking and mouthwash may interfere with results<br>More expensive than urine analysis<br>Smaller detection windows compared with those for urine, hair, and sweat | |

**Table 4–1.** Summary of strengths and limitations of types of drug testing (*continued*)

| Test type | Strengths | Limitations | Other considerations |
|---|---|---|---|
| Hair | Long detection range<br>Easy to collect | May not be feasible in many office-based settings<br>Cannot evaluate recent drug exposures<br>Results may be affected by certain hair treatments | May be considered in forensic settings, CPS cases |
| Blood | Harder to tamper with or adulterate results | May be difficult to obtain from some patients with damaged vasculature<br>Shorter duration of detection | More helpful in evaluating biomarkers for alcohol use disorder (CDT, GGT, LFT, MCV, PeTH) |

*Note.*  CDT=carbohydrate-deficient transferrin; CPS=child protective services; GC=gas chromatography; GGT=γ-glutamyltransferase; LC=liquid chromatography; LFT=liver function tests; MCV=mean corpuscular volume; MS=mass spectrometry; PeTH=phosphatidyl ethanol; POC=point of care.

Table 4–2.    Drug classes and documented false positives on urine testing (immunoassay)

| Substance class | Potential causes of false positives |
| --- | --- |
| Cannabis | Dronabinol, efavirenz, nabiximols, nonsteroidal anti-inflammatory drugs, pantoprazole, quinacrine |
| Cocaine | Coca leaf, topicals with cocaine |
| Amphetamines | Amantadine, aripiprazole, atomoxetine, benzphetamine, bupropion, chloroquine, chlorpromazine, desipramine, dextroamphetamine, dimethylamylamine, ephedrine, fenfluramine, fluoxetine, isometheptene, isoxsuprine, labetalol, MDMA, metformin, methylphenidate, mexiletine, N-acetylprocainamide, ofloxacin, oxymetazoline, phentermine, phenylephrine, phenylpropanolamine, promethazine, propranolol, pseudoephedrine, quinacrine, ranitidine, selegiline, thioridazine, trazodone, trimethobenzamide, trimipramine, tyramine, vapor inhaler containing levomethamphetamine (e.g., Vicks inhaler) |
| Benzodiazepines | Efavirenz, oxaprozin, sertraline |
| Opiates | Dextromethorphan, naloxone, papaverine, pefloxacin, poppy seeds, quinolones, rifampicin |
| Methadone | Chlorpromazine, diphenhydramine, doxylamine, quetiapine, tramadol, verapamil |
| Phencyclidine | Dextromethorphan, diphenhydramine, doxylamine, ibuprofen, imipramine, ketamine, lamotrigine, thioridazine, tramadol, venlafaxine |
| Barbiturates | Ibuprofen, naproxen, phenytoin |

*Note.*    MDMA=3,4-methylenedioxymethamphetamine.
*Source.*    Based on data from Moeller et al. 2017 and Saitman et al. 2014.

detect synthetic or semisynthetic opioids such as hydrocodone or oxycodone. A false negative could have important implications in situations in which the detection of a substance is needed to verify compliance with prescribed medication. A patient who is taking prescribed hydrocodone as directed but tests negative on a UDS should not be seen as breaking a pain treatment contract. This scenario is another example of why UDS alone should not determine treatment planning. On the other hand, a patient with a negative UDS result who displays other concerning clinical signs, such as slurring of speech or unstable gait, should raise concern for a possible false negative. It may also be

Table 4–3.    Drug classes and false negatives on standard
              urine drug screen

| Substance class | Drug prone to false negative | Notes |
|---|---|---|
| Amphetamines | | False negatives are rare; methylphenidate does not cross-react with amphetamines and requires separate testing |
| Benzodiazepine | Clonazepam | One study cited 50% false-negative rate (Mikel et al. 2012) |
| | Alprazolam | False-negative rates are not available |
| | Lorazepam | One study cited 50% false-negative rate (Mikel et al. 2012) |
| Cannabinoids | Synthetic cannabinoids | Too heterogeneous to detect reliably |
| Opiates | Fentanyl | Requires fentanyl screen |
| | Methadone | Requires methadone screen |
| | Buprenorphine | Requires buprenorphine screen |
| | Hydrocodone | One study found 72.3% false-negative rate (Bertholf et al. 2015) |
| | Oxycodone | False-negative rate can be $\geq 88\%$ (Tenore 2010) |
| | Hydromorphone | Requires hydromorphone screen |
| | Oxymorphone | Requires oxymorphone screen |
| | Tramadol | Requires tramadol screen |
| | Kratom | Requires mitragynine screen |
| | Propoxyphene | Requires propoxyphene screen |
| Barbiturates | | False negatives are rare |

possible that the patient is actively using a substance but the substance has been metabolized or excreted to a concentration that is no longer detected or is detected but is below the reporting threshold. Thus, knowing the specific detection cutoffs of a screening test can be very important because increasing the threshold cutoff for detection would lead to higher rates of false negatives. False-negative results can also be created artificially and intentionally by a patient who tampers with the urine sample or substitutes fake urine. Examining creatinine levels and specific gravity may be helpful in identifying tampering (Table 4–3).

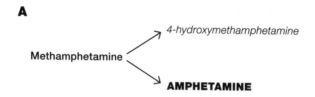

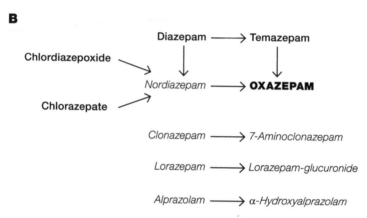

## Figure 4–2. Metabolism of different drugs.

Metabolites in **bold** are those most often detected on routine urine drug screens. (**A**) Methamphetamine. (**B**) Benzodiazepines.

# Metabolites of Various Substances

UDSs are designed to detect the drug metabolites for which they are specifically calibrated (Figure 4–2). For example, a standard immunoassay UDS detects opioids if they break down into morphine. Thus, morphine itself or any substance that eventually metabolizes to morphine will have a higher rate of detection than substances that do not metabolize to morphine. Substances that metabolize to morphine include, but are not limited to, heroin, codeine, and poppy seeds. One study determined that healthy volunteers eating a single poppy seed muffin (with poppy seed content estimated to be 7.6 g) was adequate to cause them to screen positive for opiates by urine enzyme immunoassay at 4 and 6 hours after consumption (Lewis et al. 2021). Therefore, a clinician can have more confidence that if a patient is actively using heroin, it would likely be detected in a UDS if at least some amount has metabolized to morphine.

C

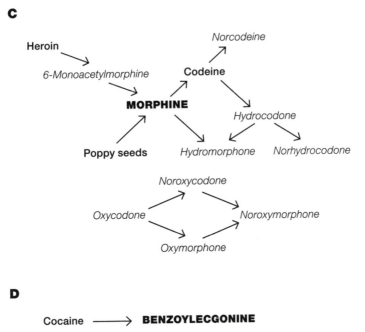

D

Cocaine ⟶ **BENZOYLECGONINE**

Figure 4–2. Metabolism of different drugs (*continued*).

Metabolites in **bold** are those most often detected on routine urine drug screens. (**C**) Opiates. (**D**) Cocaine.

# Duration of Detection

Understanding typical detection times is helpful in determining active use. In rarer cases with very heavy use of a substance, the substance can be detected beyond the typical window. Other factors affecting urinary detection time include hepatic status and medication interactions (cytochrome inducers or inhibitors). Ranges of substance detection time is summarized in Table 4–4 (Moeller et al. 2017; Standridge et al. 2010).

# Laboratory Testing in Agonist Therapy

Stimulant replacement therapy is not yet widely adopted in many practices and institutions, and its adoption may require more intensive laboratory testing options and greater knowledge of metabolite detection. For example, if methylphenidate is prescribed off-label for cocaine or methamphetamine use disorder, a standard UDS may not detect methylphenidate; thus, an amphet-

Table 4–4.     Duration of detection of substances on standard immunoassay urine drug screen

| Substance class | Duration of detection | Other considerations |
| --- | --- | --- |
| Amphetamines | 1–3 days | |
| Methamphetamines | 2–3 days | |
| Cannabis | Single use: 2–3 days<br>Chronic heavy use: >30 days | Knowing frequency, duration, and amount is crucial |
| Cocaine | 2–5 days<br>Heavy use: 8 days | |
| Barbiturates | Short acting: 1–4 days<br>Long acting: 3 weeks | Long-acting barbiturates (phenobarbital) may be used in some withdrawal regimens and may be detected for several weeks |
| Opioids | 1–4 days | |
| Phencyclidine (PCP) | 7–14 days | |
| Benzodiazepines | Short acting: 3 days<br>Long acting: 30 days | Benzodiazepines with long half-lives such as diazepam may be detected for weeks |

amine-positive UDS should be followed by confirmatory testing to evaluate for amphetamine or methamphetamine use. However, if another amphetamine-based stimulant is prescribed as part of treatment (i.e., lisdexamfetamine or D-amphetamine), patients who are compliant with treatment would be expected to have a positive amphetamine UDS. Additional confirmatory testing would need to be available in this case to distinguish between the consumption of the prescribed agonist medication and illicit methamphetamine use. Providers must be aware that, in addition to illicit methamphetamines, a number of other prescription medications can lead to a positive result for methamphetamine in a confirmation test: selegiline patch, benzphetamine, methamphetamine hydrochloride (Desoxyn), and vapor inhalers containing levomethamphetamine (e.g., Vicks inhaler). There are two enantiomers to methamphetamine: D-methamphetamine and L-methamphetamine. Vicks inhaler should metabolize to L-methamphetamine, whereas illicit methamphet-

Table 4–5.  Example laboratory results for different substances when urine drug screen is positive for amphetamines

| Substance used | Confirmation results: *ng/mL* |
|---|---|
| Prescribed mixed amphetamine salts | Amphetamines: 800 |
| | Methamphetamine: 0 |
| Illicit methamphetamine[a] | Amphetamines: 730 |
| | Methamphetamine: 3,211 |
| | L-Methamphetamine: 12 |
| | D-Methamphetamine: 2,999 |
| Vicks inhaler[b] | Amphetamine: 203 |
| | Methamphetamine: 300 |
| | L-Methamphetamine: 270 |
| | D-Methamphetamine: 30 |

[a]Illicit methamphetamine has a higher ratio of D- to L-methamphetamine.
[b]Vicks inhaler is primarily L-methamphetamine.

amine tends to be detected as the more centrally acting D-methamphetamine (Saitman et al. 2014). Additional laboratory testing can distinguish the levels of D- and L-methamphetamine isomers in a sample. Table 4–5 depicts example interpretations of urine toxicology results.

# Opioid Use Disorder Treatment and Buprenorphine Ratios

Using buprenorphine and norbuprenorphine levels can be very helpful for gauging compliance with buprenorphine therapy. Although buprenorphine therapy helps increase treatment retention, reduce the risks of overdose and blood-borne illness, and improve recidivism, diversion of medication and suboptimal compliance are treatment limitations. Urine buprenorphine confirmation testing can detect both the parent compound (buprenorphine) and the metabolite norbuprenorphine. Quantitative buprenorphine testing is preferred over qualitative testing. A qualitative buprenorphine screen will detect only whether buprenorphine is in the urine (typically reported as positive or negative); it does not allow differentiation from a urine sample that has been substituted or subjected to tampering, in which a buprenorphine product is submerged directly into the sample, a process referred to as *spiking* (Accurso et al. 2017). Patients may spike the urine to feign compliance with their medication or conceal their use of other substances by using substituted, synthetic, or tampered urine. Spiking a sample would not result in the expected amounts of the metabolite norbuprenorphine produced through hepatic metabolism. Although the frequency of this practice may vary among treatment programs, spiking estimates based on several studies range from 0.35% to 29% (Accurso et al. 2017; Suzuki et al. 2017; Warrington et al. 2020).

A growing number of studies have explored the interpretation of buprenorphine to norbuprenorphine ratios to identify urine samples with suspected tampering. Because norbuprenorphine has a longer half-life, steady-state levels of buprenorphine from consistent medication adherence would be expected to have a higher concentration of norbuprenorphine than buprenorphine. The tendency toward higher norbuprenorphine level versus buprenorphine levels is supported by several studies (Mariottini et al. 2021; Suzuki et al. 2017). The mean ratio of norbuprenorphine to buprenorphine may be between 2 and 4. If buprenorphine levels exceed norbuprenorphine, the patient may have missed some doses and resumed shortly prior to the specimen collection. Notably, most studies show that buprenorphine and norbuprenorphine levels do not correlate well with buprenorphine dose; thus, urine drug levels alone are insufficient to determine medication adherence. Evidence also indicates that the timing of urine testing in relation to the last dose may influence drug levels (Donroe et al. 2017). For the most part, in healthy control subjects, even low doses of buprenorphine and norbuprenorphine are present in the urine within hours of a single 0.4-mg dose (Kronstrand et al. 2008). A patient who reports dosing about 6 hours before testing but has negative buprenorphine or norbuprenorphine levels would raise concern about adherence.

Drug interactions and hepatic impairment could affect concentrations. Buprenorphine is metabolized in the liver primarily through cytochrome P450 (CYP) 3A4 and secondarily by CYP2C8, CYP3A5, and CYP3A7. Low buprenorphine levels could be related to the patient also taking a P450 inducer. Genetic polymorphisms of CYP3A4 and pregnancy may also affect levels (Donroe et al. 2017; Holt et al. 2018; Mariottini et al. 2021). Urine diluted through either sample tampering or the consumption of large amounts of water may be reflected by low creatinine levels in the results. Creatinine levels below 20 mg/dL should raise concern. One author suggested using buprenorphine-to-creatinine ratios and norbuprenorphine-to-creatinine ratios to help standardize varying concentrations of urines (Furo et al. 2021). Naloxone levels are also helpful to determine misuse. Although naloxone should have limited bioavailability when taken as part of sublingual buprenorphine/naloxone, a study showed that most of the urine samples taken from patients in maintenance treatment have median naloxone levels less than 200 ng/mL (Heikman et al. 2014). A much higher naloxone-to-buprenorphine ratio may indicate parenteral use of buprenorphine/naloxone. In general, lower ratios may make a specimen suspect for tampering. The literature documents cutoff ratios ranging from 0.02 to 0.26. Samples below the cutoff ratio are considered positive, which suggests that as the ratio increases, the sensitivity of detecting tampered urine increases, but the specificity decreases (Table 4–6) (Furo et al. 2021; Heikman et al. 2014).

Discordant urine results, particularly if they occur repeatedly, can lead to fruitful discussions about the patient's motivation to spike their urine samples. These discussions may lead to meaningful changes in treatment planning, such as increased frequency of visits (to increase monitoring of compliance or other substance use), referral to a higher level of care, or discontinuation or tapering of buprenorphine treatment. Supervised urine collection could also be considered, although this approach has strengths and limitations. Alternatively, oral saliva testing could be pursued. Table 4–7 provides an example of utilizing buprenorphine levels and ratios in a UDS to gauge treatment progress. For patients who are transitioning from inpatient to outpatient care, it may be helpful to obtain buprenorphine levels during inpatient admission. During an admission, buprenorphine is directly administered to the patient; thus, the likelihood of motivation (or access to materials) to tamper with or substitute urine specimens is much lower. These levels may help establish a baseline pattern for outpatient treatment.

# Blood Biomarkers for Alcohol Use

Use of laboratory testing via blood has limitations in detecting illicit drug use in a clinical context because it is more invasive and has a smaller window of detection. However, serum biomarkers are useful for detecting chronic heavy alcohol consumption (Table 4–8). Indirect markers of consumption are those that reflect alcohol's effects on the body organs, such as liver function tests, γ-glutamyltransferase, mean corpuscular volume, and carbohydrate-deficient transferrin. One disadvantage of indirect biomarkers is their low specificity. They are also not ideal for abstinence monitoring because alcohol intake in small amounts or even binge drinking may not lead to changes. On the other hand, direct biomarkers measure alcohol or its metabolites and can be used

Table 4–6.    Factors to consider in identifying discordant urine buprenorphine testing

| Laboratory test | Study findings | Comments |
| --- | --- | --- |
| Buprenorphine (B) and norbuprenorphine (NB), quantitative | Studies show a range of NB:B ratios between 0.067 and 25, with mean values between 2 and 4. Analysis of 174 undiluted urine samples showed 94% of samples with NB > B (Hull et al. 2008; Pesce 2014). | Generally, with regular compliance, NB level > B level. |
| | One study used an NB:B ratio of <0.02 as cutoff for suspicion for urine tampering (Hull et al. 2008). In another study using the same ratio, patients with ratio <0.02 all had B > 2,000 ng/mL, and mean NB was 11.9 ng/mL (Suzuki et al. 2017). This 0.02 cutoff for tampering has high specificity (rare false positives) but low sensitivity (more frequent false negatives). | |
| | A third study used an NB:B ratio <0.2 (vs. 0.02) to represent suspected spiking (Accurso et al. 2017). | |
| | A fourth study used a further increased NB:B ratio of ≤0.26, which has a sensitivity of 100% and specificity of 58%, to detect adulterated samples. Compared with a ratio of 0.02, this ratio has a higher sensitivity (fewer false negatives) but lower specificity (more false positives). In this study, a total urine B level ≥700 ng/mL had a sensitivity of 77% and specificity of 85% for detecting urine adulteration by spiking (Donroe et al. 2017). | |

**Table 4–6.** Factors to consider in identifying discordant urine buprenorphine testing (*continued*)

| Laboratory test | Study findings | Comments |
|---|---|---|
| Buprenorphine (B) and norbuprenorphine (NB), quantitative (*continued*) | In one study, 18 healthy volunteers received a single 0.4-mg B dose. Mean time for NB level to surpass B level was 7 hours. Both B and NB were detected in the urine via confirmatory testing up to 96 hours later. More than 75% had an NB level >5 ng/mL within 2–5 hours (Kronstrand et al. 2008). | |
| Creatinine (C), quantitative | Urine C samples with a level of 20 mg/dL should be suspected for dilution. A concentration <20 mg/dL is defined as a dilute sample per Substance Abuse and Mental Health Services Administration guidelines (Hull et al. 2008). | |
| | Urine level could be used to standardize for dilution. | |
| | For those taking buprenorphine 8 mg/day, an NB:C ratio consistently <0.5×10⁻⁴ may be suspect for tampering. | |
| | For those taking 12 mg/day, an NB:C ratio consistently <1.5×10⁻⁴ may be suspect for tampering. | |
| Naloxone (N), quantitative | Suspect tampering (spiking) if NB:B ratio is <0.02 and N concentrations are high (>1,000 ng/mL). | |
| | In those receiving B/N maintenance treatment, N was found in urine samples of all patients, although typically below the 100 ng/mL cutoff; 85% of cases had an N concentration of 5–90 ng/mL. | |

**Table 4–6.** Factors to consider in identifying discordant urine buprenorphine testing (*continued*)

| Laboratory test | Study findings | Comments |
|---|---|---|
| Naloxone (N), quantitative (*continued*) | Median N:B ratio of 9,000 specimens (with suspected adulterated samples excluded) tested by one laboratory was 1.15 (Aegis Labs 2021). | Very high N:B ratio may suggest parenteral use. |
| Specific gravity, urine | Specific gravity not consistent with normal physiological levels (1.003–1.030) may imply tampering or dilution. | Specific gravity < 1.003 may indicate diluted urine; > 1.030 may indicate addition of adulterants or additives. |

*Note.*　A limitation in these studies is a lack of clarity about whether the urine drug screens or buprenorphine administration was directly observed. They also do not all include data on how many patients disclosed tampered urine. Future studies incorporating urine levels of both observed buprenorphine administration and urine collection should provide more information. The studies also do not include samples from subjects given extended-release buprenorphine injections.

**Table 4–7.** Clinical example of a theoretical patient with discordant buprenorphine levels

| Date | UDS result | Confirmatory testing, *ng/mL* | Notes |
|---|---|---|---|
| 1/13/2021 | Negative | B: 450 NB: 1,500 | In supervised RTP where medication is administered |
| 2/13/2021 | Negative | B: 562 NB: 1,688 | In supervised RTP where medication is administered |
| 3/14/2021 | Negative | B: 1,892 NB: 11 | 1 week following RTP discharge |
| 3/28/2021 | Negative | B: 5,640 NB: 14 | Results discussed with patient during visit |
| 4/10/2021 | Cocaine + | B: 399 NB: 1,333 | Levels improved; patient admitted to cocaine use |
| 4/17/2021 | Cocaine + | B: 413 NB: 1,288 | Patient working on joining 12-step groups or IOP |
| 4/24/2021 | Negative | B: 512 NB: 1,760 | Patient reports doing well |

*Note.* Laboratory results obtained on 3/14/2021 and 3/28/2021 are likely discordant because NB:B ratio is well below 0.02. Also, these results occurred during a time following discharge from a RTP, when a patient may be at higher risk of return to substance use.

B=buprenorphine; IOP=intensive outpatient program; NB=norbuprenorphine; RTP= residential treatment program; UDS=urine drug screen.

to monitor abstinence. They include, but are not limited to, phosphatidyl ethanol, ethyl glucuronide, ethyl sulfate, and fatty acid ethyl esters. These tests are not often obtained in routine psychiatric evaluations but are helpful when objective evaluations are needed to determine the current level of drinking of a patient receiving treatment for alcohol use disorder. Transparently sharing the results of improved laboratory tests (e.g., normalizing liver function testing trends) can provide great relief to those concerned about their hepatic status and may be a motivating factor toward reducing consumption or abstinence (Andresen-Streichert et al. 2018; Peterson 2004; Tavakoli et al. 2011).

Many factors are involved in determining which markers to test. Cost and availability may be the first and primary barriers to ordering tests for some of them. Generally, the indirect markers are less costly and more widely available. In some instances, a cost-effective option is combining multiple indirect

**Table 4–8.    Summary of biomarkers for alcohol use**

| | Lab test | Detection window | Sens | Spec | Type of drinking | Sources of false positives | Relative cost |
|---|---|---|---|---|---|---|---|
| Indirect markers | LFT | 2–3 weeks | + | + | Chronic heavy drinking | Many, including, but not limited to, diabetes mellitus, liver disease, heart disease | $ |
| | MCV | 2–4 months | + | ++ | Chronic heavy drinking | Chronic liver disease, hypothyroidism, $B_{12}$ or folate deficiency, smoking | $ |
| | GGT | 2–3 weeks | ++ | ++ | Chronic heavy drinking | Fatty liver, obstructive liver disease, antiepileptic drugs, cirrhosis, obesity, pancreatitis, hypertension, hyperlipidemia, smoking | $ |
| | CDT | 2–3 weeks | ++ | +++ | Heavy drinking over 7–10 days | Few; advanced liver disease and genetic variations of transferrin | $$$ |
| Direct markers | PEth | 2–4 weeks | ++++ | ++++ | Heavy drinking for approximately ≤5 days | Not influenced by any liver disease | $$ |
| | EtG (urine) | 2–5 days | +++ | +++ | Recent use | Performance not affected by liver disease severity (Stewart et al. 2013) | $$ |
| | FAEE (serum) | 2–3 days | +++ | +++ | Recent use of at least several drinks | Unknown | $$$$$ |

**Table 4–8.** Summary of biomarkers for alcohol use *(continued)*

| | Lab test | Detection window | Sens | Spec | Type of drinking | Sources of false positives | Relative cost |
|---|---|---|---|---|---|---|---|
| Combination markers | CDT+GGT (Hietala et al. 2006) | | +++ | +++ | Chronic heavy drinking | | $$$$ |
| | CDT+MCV (Tavakoli et al. 2011) | | +++ | +++ | Chronic heavy drinking | | $$$$ |

*Note.* Because the ranges of sensitivity and specificity vary significantly between sources, they are approximated from + (lowest) to ++++ (highest) to help indicate the relative strength and weakness of each biomarker relative to the others. The general cost of each marker is ranked from $ (lowest) to $$$$ (highest). For the combination biomarkers, data are based on *either* of the individual markers being elevated in the combination.

CDT=carbohydrate-deficient transferrin; EtG=ethyl glucuronide; FAEE=fatty acid ethyl esters; GGT=γ-glutamyltransferase; LFT=liver function test; MCV=mean corpuscular volume; PEth=phosphatidyl ethanol; Sens=sensitivity; Spec=specificity.

biomarkers, which may raise the sensitivity of testing compared with that for either marker alone (Hietala et al. 2006). From a clinical standpoint, the window of detection, sensitivity, and specificity may all be considered in deciding the preferred time frame and accuracy of detection. Because false positives are more likely in tests with lower specificity, these results must be interpreted carefully.

# Conclusion

Use of laboratory testing is crucial in addiction treatment as part of screening, progress monitoring, and identifying return to substance use. Using these tests appropriately, however, requires broad knowledge of the strengths and limitations of each test, substance metabolites, causes of false positives and false negatives, and sensitivity and specificity. By expertly interpreting laboratory results, providers can be better equipped to guide their patients toward healthier change.

# Clinical Cases

### Case Example 1

A 30-year-old female with a history of anxiety and methamphetamine use disorder has been in treatment for the past 6 months. For the past two visits, her UDS results have been positive for amphetamine. She states that she is positive for the amphetamine because she used her sister's prescribed stimulant dextroamphetamine for ADHD on the days prior to her urine testing. She has also had some new onset of paranoia over the past few months, feeling that people are talking about her through the vents, and she has lost about 15 lb in the past 3 months.

Given the patient's history, as well as her weight loss and paranoia, an amphetamine confirmation test, which would detect amphetamine and methamphetamine, should be considered to rule out return to methamphetamine use. If the test shows amphetamine but no methamphetamine, that would be consistent with her report of dextroamphetamine use. However, if methamphetamine is present in combination with amphetamine, then methamphetamine use would be higher on the differential.

### Case Example 2

An 18-year-old male with a history of cannabis use presents to outpatient treatment. He reported his last use of cannabis was 2 months ago. Prior to that, he was smoking cannabis about once a week. He submitted a UDS on the day of the visit that was positive for cannabis. A review of his medications includes fluoxetine. Otherwise, he has not used any over-the-counter or prescribed medication.

Cannabis detected in the urine beyond 1 month after last use occurs when a patient has used heavily and chronically prior to cessation. It is possible that the patient may be minimizing cannabis use, either the last date of use or the frequency prior to cessation. If there are concerns about a false-positive result, then confirmation testing can be ordered. If the confirmation test is positive for THC and the patient reports ongoing abstinence, then follow-up confirmation tests should show a declining level of THC concentration.

### Case Example 3

A 50-year-old male is receiving treatment through a pain management clinic under an opioid treatment contract in which he is prescribed hydrocodone regularly. He is expected to submit UDSs on each visit to verify that he has been taking the hydrocodone. Three months into treatment, his first two screens were positive for opioids, but the third was negative despite the patient reporting compliance with the hydrocodone.

With a standard immunoassay UDS, false negatives for hydrocodone are possible. The patient could be taking the hydrocodone appropriately but still have a negative screen. The next best step would be to order a confirmation test that specifically detects hydrocodone. Some opioid confirmation tests will detect only morphine and codeine and thus would not detect hydrocodone because hydrocodone does not metabolize to morphine or codeine.

### Case Example 4

A 25-year-old male with depression and tobacco use disorder is prescribed sertraline and bupropion for depression and smoking cessation. He also occasionally uses cannabidiol for anxiety. A standard UDS from his primary care physician showed a positive result for benzodiazepine, amphetamine, and cannabis. The patient consistently denies use of any of those substances.

Bupropion can cause a false positive for amphetamine, whereas sertraline causes a false positive for benzodiazepines. In addition, cannabidiol products currently can contain up to 0.3% THC content, which may lead to the possibility of detection in a UDS. Therefore, confirmation tests could be ordered if positive results would potentially change the treatment plan.

## Case Example 5

A 32-year-old male with opioid use disorder is currently receiving buprenorphine therapy. His first three buprenorphine levels were as follows:

- Buprenorphine: 568 ng/mL, norbuprenorphine: 1,400 ng/mL
- Buprenorphine: 412 ng/mL, norbuprenorphine: 1,299 ng/mL
- Buprenorphine: 617 ng/mL, norbuprenorphine: 1,388 ng/mL

On his most recent visit, his levels were 627 ng/mL for buprenorphine and 330 ng/mL for norbuprenorphine. He has no new hepatic issues and is not taking any new medications.

The first three buprenorphine and norbuprenorphine levels appear to be consistent with compliance, with norbuprenorphine being at a higher level than buprenorphine. On the patient's most recent visit, his buprenorphine level was higher than his norbuprenorphine level, and the norbuprenorphine was lower than his typical baseline. It is possible that the patient missed some doses of norbuprenorphine for a few days prior to the date of the UDS, which would explain the declining norbuprenorphine levels. In addition, the last dose of buprenorphine may have been taken very close to the time of specimen submission, causing it to remain close to baseline. The patient could be engaged in discussion about medication compliance and whether there were missed doses.

# References

Accurso AJ, Lee JD, McNeely J: High prevalence of urine tampering in an office-based opioid treatment practice detected by evaluating the norbuprenorphine to buprenorphine ratio. J Subst Abuse Treat 83(December):62–67, 2017 29129197

Aegis Labs: Interpretation of buprenorphine and naloxone results: considerations for dosage form and specimen type. Clinical Update, May 12, 2021. Available at: https://www.aegislabs.com/resources/clinical-update/May2021. Accessed March 6, 2022.

American Psychiatric Association: Diagnostic and Statistical Manual of Mental Disorders, 5th Edition, Text Revision. Washington, DC, American Psychiatric Association, 2022

Andresen-Streichert H, Müller A, Glahn A, et al: Alcohol biomarkers in clinical and forensic contexts. Dtsch Arztebl Int 115(18):309–315, 2018 29807559

Bertholf RL, Johannsen LM, Reisfield GM: Sensitivity of an opiate immunoassay for detecting hydrocodone and hydromorphone in urine from a clinical population: analysis of subthreshold results. J Anal Toxicol 39(1):24–28, 2015 25288720

Blanco C, Alegría AA, Liu S-M, et al: Differences among major depressive disorder with and without co-occurring substance use disorders and substance-induced depressive disorder: results from the National Epidemiologic Survey on Alcohol and Related Conditions. J Clin Psychiatry 73(6):865–873, 2012 22480900

Cheng J, Wang S, Lin W, et al: Computational systems pharmacology: target mapping for fentanyl-laced cocaine overdose. ACS Chem Neurosci 10(8):3486–3499, 2019 31257858

Cone EJ, Yousefnejad D, Hillsgrove MJ, et al: Passive inhalation of cocaine. J Anal Toxicol 19(6):399–411, 1995 8926734

Donroe JH, Holt SR, O'Connor PG, et al: Interpreting quantitative urine buprenorphine and norbuprenorphine levels in office-based clinical practice. Drug Alcohol Depend 180(November):46–51, 2017 28866369

Furo H, Schwartz DG, Sullivan RW, et al: Buprenorphine dosage and urine quantitative buprenorphine, norbuprenorphine, and creatinine levels in an office-based opioid treatment program. Subst Abuse 15:11782218211061749, 2021 34898987

He X, Wang JF, Wang Y: Influence of cosmetic hair treatments on hair of methamphetamine abuser: bleaching, perming and coloring. Ecotoxicol Environ Saf 222:112542, 2021 34311424

Heikman P, Häkkinen M, Gergov M, et al: Urine naloxone concentration at different phases of buprenorphine maintenance treatment. Drug Test Anal 6(3):220–225, 2014 23512803

Hietala J, Koivisto H, Anttila P, et al: Comparison of the combined marker GGT-CDT and the conventional laboratory markers of alcohol abuse in heavy drinkers, moderate drinkers and abstainers. Alcohol Alcohol 41(5):528–533, 2006 16799164

Holt SR, Donroe JH, Cavallo DA, et al: Addressing discordant quantitative urine buprenorphine and norbuprenorphine levels: case examples in opioid use disorder. Drug Alcohol Depend 186(May):171–174, 2018 29579725

Hull MJ, Bierer MF, Griggs DA, et al: Urinary buprenorphine concentrations in patients treated with suboxone as determined by liquid chromatography-mass spectrometry and CEDIA immunoassay. J Anal Toxicol 32(7):516–521, 2008 18713521

Jones CM, Einstein EB, Compton WM: Changes in synthetic opioid involvement in drug overdose deaths in the United States, 2010–2016. JAMA 319(17):1819–1821, 2018 29715347

Kronstrand R, Nyström I, Andersson M, et al: Urinary detection times and metabolite/parent compound ratios after a single dose of buprenorphine. J Anal Toxicol 32(8):586–593, 2008 19007507

Lewis J, De Monnin K, Smith J, et al: Interpreting urine drug test results in the context of chronic opioid analgesic therapy and poppy seed consumption. Pain Med 22(11):2776–2778, 2021 33710300

Mariottini C, Gergov M, Ojanperä I: Determination of buprenorphine, norbu-prenorphine, naloxone, and their glucuronides in urine by liquid chromatography-tandem mass spectrometry. Drug Test Anal 13(9):1658–1667, 2021 34047070

Martini MBA, Batista TBD, Henn IW, et al: Whether drug detection in urine and oral fluid is similar? A systematic review. Crit Rev Toxicol 50(4):348–358, 2020 32343161

Mikel C, Pesce AJ, Rosenthal M, et al: Therapeutic monitoring of benzodiazepines in the management of pain: current limitations of point of care immunoassays suggest testing by mass spectrometry to assure accuracy and improve patient safety. Clin Chim Acta 413(15–16):1199–1202, 2012 22484396

Moeller KE, Kissack JC, Atayee RS, et al: Clinical interpretation of urine drug tests: what clinicians need to know about urine drug screens. Mayo Clin Proc 92(5):774–796, 2017 28325505

Niedbala S, Kardos K, Salamone S, et al: Passive cannabis smoke exposure and oral fluid testing. J Anal Toxicol 28(7):546–552, 2004 15516313

Pesce A: Analytical considerations when monitoring pain medications by LC-MS/MS. Journal of Analytical and Bioanalytical Techniques s5(01):003, 2014

Peterson K: Biomarkers for alcohol use and abuse: a summary. Alcohol Res Health 28(1):30–37, 2004 19006989

Saitman A, Park H-D, Fitzgerald RL: False-positive interferences of common urine drug screen immunoassays: a review. J Anal Toxicol 38(7):387–396, 2014 24986836

Standridge JB, Adams SM, Zotos AP: Urine drug screening: a valuable office procedure. Am Fam Physician 81(5):635–640, 2010 20187600

Stewart SH, Koch DG, Burgess DM, et al: Sensitivity and specificity of urinary ethyl glucuronide and ethyl sulfate in liver disease patients. Alcohol Clin Exp Res 37(1):150–155, 2013 22725265

Suwannachom N, Thananchai T, Junkuy A, et al: Duration of detection of methamphetamine in hair after abstinence. Forensic Sci Int 254(September):80–86, 2015 26197350

Suzuki J, Zinser J, Issa M, et al: Quantitative testing of buprenorphine and norbu-prenorphine to identify urine sample spiking during office-based opioid treatment. Subst Abus 38(4):504–507, 2017 28723256

Tamama K: Advances in drugs of abuse testing. Clin Chim Acta 514(March):40–47, 2021 33333045

Tavakoli HR, Hull M, Michael Okasinski L: Review of current clinical biomarkers for the detection of alcohol dependence. Innov Clin Neurosci 8(3):26–33, 2011 21487543

Tenore PL: Advanced urine toxicology testing. J Addict Dis 29(4):436–448, 2010 20924879

Vuolo M, Frizzell LC, Kelly BC: Surveillance, self-governance, and mortality: the impact of prescription drug monitoring programs on U.S. overdose mortality, 2000–2016. J Health Soc Behav 63(3):337–356, 2022 35001700

Warrington JS, Warrington GS, Francis-Fath S, et al: Urinary buprenorphine, norbuprenorphine and naloxone concentrations and ratios: review and potential clinical implications. J Addict Med 14(6):e344–e349, 2020 32530884

Westin AA, Slørdal L: Passive inhalation of cannabis smoke: is it detectable? [in Norwegian]. Tidsskr Nor Laegeforen 129(2):109–113, 2009 19151803

# 5

# Alcohol and Co-occurring Substance Use

Benjamin Li, M.D.

*Alcohol* is a widely misused substance causing significant physical and psychological comorbidities. Hundreds of studies have investigated pharmacotherapy trials to treat alcohol use disorder (AUD) with varying success. In this chapter, we pay special attention to other co-occurring use disorders.

Although the FDA-approved medications for AUD have been well studied, off-label medications may have less related literature, placing an even more significant burden of risk-benefit analysis on clinicians when considering these medications. In addition, much of the literature includes secondary analysis to ascertain any moderators that may improve treatment response to a medication. Moderators may include, but are not limited to, the intensity of the use disorder, preexisting psychiatric symptoms, genetic polymorphisms, and age at onset of use. Because many off-label options do not significantly apply to all populations with a substance use disorder (SUD), targeting some medications toward a specific subpopulation may yield better results. Moreover, a pharmacological option that can also treat a comorbid medical illness (e.g., migraines) may receive higher consideration for treating a co-occurring use disorder. Treatment refractoriness may be expected in use disorders, just as in major depression and other psychiatric illnesses. Although some patients may benefit from combination treatments, an important consideration is compounding side effects of polypharmacy. The benefits must outweigh

73

the risks in these situations. Finally, even if evidence has shown that a medication has benefits for separately occurring classes of use disorders, it may not be efficacious for co-occurring disorders. Theoretically, ongoing substance use in one class may impair an person's ability to abstain from the other substance, or the combination of substances may have a synergistic or additive effect that may render both use disorders treatment refractory.

To identify the treatment of co-occurring SUDs, we reviewed the literature for specific agents that were used to treat co-occurring use disorders in the same trial. If no such trials were available, we conjectured about using a specific agent based on the literature supporting consideration of its use in each separate use disorder. More weight was given to meta-analyses, systematic reviews, and high-quality blinded, randomized, placebo-controlled trials. Smaller trials and open-label or case studies were less likely to influence recommendations. The pharmacological options explored in this chapter are for treating specific use disorders outside of the acute intoxication and withdrawal stages. Pharmacotherapy is also only part of a holistic, well-rounded treatment plan and should be used in conjunction with evidence-based therapies for each use disorder.

# Pharmacotherapy for Alcohol Use Disorder

## FDA-Approved Medications

### Naltrexone

Naltrexone is one of three FDA-approved medications for treatment of AUD and is available in both oral and extended-release intramuscular forms. Although intramuscular naltrexone has been used at many clinical sites for AUD, controlled interventions directly comparing the oral and injectable naltrexone formulations are still relatively lacking. Only four studies performed in various settings (Veterans Affairs, inpatient, outpatient) provided data that favored injectable naltrexone over oral naltrexone for medication adherence or for treatment retention. However, the cost-benefit analysis was mixed, and drinking outcomes were not directly studied in three of the four studies (Beatty and Stock 2018; Bryson et al. 2011; Busch et al. 2017; Stewart et al. 2021). Currently, no prospective randomized controlled trials (RCTs) have compared oral naltrexone directly with intramuscular naltrexone in the previously mentioned outcome measures. A study of this type by Malone and colleagues to explore the two forms in a primary care setting in New York was under way, but outcomes have not been posted (Malone et al. 2019). Nevertheless, because low adherence and low treatment retention undermine treatment outcomes, intramuscular naltrexone should be considered in those who are particularly vulnerable to noncompliance with oral medication. Of note, some patients report feeling the effects of naltrexone "wearing off" at around 3 weeks after injection (Knopf 2019).

The use and tolerability of injections of the extended-release formulation, naltrexone XR, every 3 weeks were documented in a clinical trial for methamphetamine use disorder (Trivedi et al. 2021). Studies have attempted to identify moderators to naltrexone response, including alleles of opioid receptor gene *OPRM1* (mixed evidence), abstinence early in treatment (also mixed evidence), cue-induced activation in the ventral striatum, and smoking. A study by Schacht et al. (2017) found that smoking moderated effects such that naltrexone was superior to placebo only in those who smoked. The same study found that the magnitude of reduction in cue-elicited brain activation also predicted treatment response to naltrexone. Unfortunately, in a busy clinical practice with limited resources, obtaining genotype testing or brain imaging may not be feasible.

### Disulfiram

Disulfiram is another FDA-approved medication for the treatment of AUD. It has had utility in patients by creating the expectation that drinking while taking disulfiram will lead to an aversive reaction. This expectation is thought to underly disulfiram's effectiveness, as opposed to a direct pharmacophysiological effect of the medication. This leaves room for interpretation of whether blinded studies provide an accurate representation of the medication's efficacy because blinded studies would acknowledge the psychological aversion present in both medication *and* placebo arms. However, the most recent meta-analysis by Skinner et al. (2014), after removing blinded studies, found that disulfiram had a positive effect on maintaining abstinence or preventing return to use that was even more significant in studies with supervised dosing. Perhaps patients who are highly motivated and receiving supervised medication administration are more likely to benefit from treatment with disulfiram.

### Acamprosate

Acamprosate is an FDA-approved medication that may be more beneficial for those who recently completed withdrawal or are already abstinent from alcohol. The most recent meta-analyses in 2020 in a primary care population in the United Kingdom found supporting evidence that acamprosate may be beneficial in maintaining abstinence for up to 12 months. In contrast, naltrexone, topiramate, and disulfiram did not show the same quality of evidence (Cheng et al. 2020). Other systematic reviews support acamprosate's efficacy in reducing the risk of any drinking and increasing the cumulative duration of abstinence (Rösner et al. 2010). Although 4%–45% of those who received the placebo remained abstinent through various studies, about 18%–61% of participants who received acamprosate remained abstinent (Boothby and Doering 2005). In addition, acamprosate's effect on improving abstinence may not differ between depressed and nondepressed patients, but the effect of maintaining abstinence may lead to improvement in depression (Lejoyeux and Lehert 2011). In this sense, whereas acamprosate may be more effective in promoting and maintaining abstinence, naltrexone is more effective in reducing heavy drinking and craving (Soyka 2013).

The optimal duration of abstinence prior to a trial with acamprosate is unclear. One analysis of the COMBINE study showed that the acamprosate-treated subgroup with shorter abstinence (≤1 week) combined with a low or normal BMI had double the rate of abstinence of the placebo group (Gueorguieva et al. 2015). On the other hand, another COMBINE study analysis suggested that those who were abstinent for 14 days or more and had consistent, daily drinking had worse prognosis on acamprosate (Gueorguieva et al. 2011). These two COMBINE analyses seem to contradict the findings of an analysis of the PREDICT study, which is that those who were able to maintain abstinence for more than 2 weeks were more likely to have a good outcome in treatment (Schacht et al. 2017).

## Off-Label, Second-Line Interventions

### Topiramate

Topiramate is an off-label treatment for AUD, although its efficacy in many trials as well as its evidence for comorbid conditions may make it a strong consideration for a first-line treatment according to a review by Guglielmo et al. (2015). A systematic review by Palpacuer et al. (2018) concluded that for total alcohol consumption, topiramate was superior to the FDA-approved options naltrexone and acamprosate and had medium to large effect sizes for most consumption outcomes. A third systematic review of seven RCTs found the largest effect on abstinence, followed by heavy drinking and then by craving, and topiramate was actually superior to naltrexone and acamprosate in these same outcomes (Blodgett et al. 2014). However, a more recent review of the literature by Morley et al. (2021) concluded that although several meta-analyses of RCTs showed medium effect sizes for topiramate in AUD treatment, potential side effects may limit its use, and further studies are needed before recommendation as first-line treatment.

Although not contraindicated in hepatic impairment because of its only partial hepatic metabolism, topiramate must be used with caution in hepatic encephalopathy because of its potential for exacerbating cognitive side effects and confounding the treatment of hepatic encephalopathy (Leggio and Lee 2017). Overall, although topiramate is not FDA approved for AUD and has some side effects to monitor, it could be considered as a first-line option for those with comorbidities that may also benefit, such as binge-eating disorder, migraines, and antipsychotic-induced weight gain. Topiramate also has efficacy for cocaine use disorder, as detailed in Chapter 6, "Stimulants and Co-occurring Substance Use."

### Gabapentin

Gabapentin is used off-label for AUD and is FDA approved for treating neuropathic pain. It is also frequently prescribed off-label for anxiety. The first meta-analysis of gabapentin use in treating AUD was published in 2019 and covered data from seven RCTs; the authors concluded that the only examined outcome measure that showed reasonable evidence of benefit from gabapentin was a lower percentage of heavy-drinking days (Kranzler et al. 2019). This study asked whether individuals with a history of alcohol withdrawal may be more responsive to gabapentin. To shed more light on this question, a more recent RCT by Anton et al. (2020) found that gabapentin might be most effective after initiation of abstinence and in those with a pretreatment history of more severe alcohol withdrawal symptoms. Whereas only 1% of the placebo group had total abstinence, 41% of participants with high alcohol withdrawal symptoms had total abstinence with gabapentin therapy. While no clinical trials exist specifically on the use of gabapentin in comorbid AUD and hepatic impairment, it could be considered to be hepatically safe if there is no hepatorenal syndrome.

### Baclofen

The evidence for the muscle relaxer baclofen is, in general, mixed. A 2018 meta-analysis comparing this medication with placebo found that it provided no benefit in maintaining abstinence or in reducing drinking frequency or amount, indicating it is not a first-choice recommendation for treatment of

AUD (Minozzi et al. 2018). However, subgroup analysis may help identify candidates for baclofen. A meta-analysis by Agabio et al. (2021) looking at 13 trials on the effect of baclofen on alcohol consumption and anxiety after 12 weeks of treatment found that individuals with higher baseline anxiety or a co-occurring anxiety disorder may have a better response. This subgroup had more abstinent days than those who had lower baseline anxiety (Morley et al. 2014). Also, those with alcohol-induced liver disease may have a larger treatment effect with baclofen in delaying time to lapse or return to use compared with subgroups without alcohol-induced liver disease (Morley et al. 2018). Because baclofen is renally metabolized, it may be preferred in populations with liver disease. A review of the existing studies showed a positive correlation between the efficacy of baclofen and the severity of AUD, even in patients with alcohol-induced liver disease and cirrhosis (Mosoni et al. 2018). Although the United States has not approved this medication for treatment of AUD, it has been approved in France for dosages up to 80 mg/day for patients who did not respond to other AUD treatments (Rolland et al. 2020). In summary, baclofen may be considered in those with hepatic impairment or preexisting anxiety or for whom first-line interventions have not been successful.

## Off-Label Third-Line Interventions

Third-line options include those agents that either have weak evidence or lack a consistent body of higher-quality trials to justify more immediate use before the first- and second-line agents. However, if more acute psychiatric or medical comorbidities may benefit from use of these medications, they could be considered. These third-line options include ondansetron, prazosin, doxazosin, and varenicline.

### Ondansetron

Ondansetron, through its serotonin type 3 receptor ($5\text{-}HT_3$) antagonist effects, has been studied in treatment of AUD and has garnered interest related to the identification of various predictors of response (including genetic polymorphisms, age at onset, and severity of drinking pretreatment). Although many of the studies involving ondansetron are small, open-label, and heterogeneous, the highest-quality RCT by Johnson et al. (2000) corroborated findings from other trials that those with early-onset AUD tend to respond better to ondansetron (Dawes et al. 2005; Johnson et al. 2013; Kenna et al. 2009, 2014; Kranzler et al. 2003; Sellers et al. 1994).

### Prazosin and Doxazosin

Prazosin was found in a double-blind RCT to reduce the number of drinks consumed and number of heavy-drinking days (Simpson et al. 2018). Another double-blind RCT in 2021 corroborated similar effects for reducing the amount of drinking. In groups with high alcohol withdrawal symptom severity, prazosin had greater benefit relative to placebo to reduce heavy drinking, number of drinking days, and average drinks per day (Sinha et al. 2021).

Doxazosin has a longer half-life than prazosin and may have similar benefits. A 2017 double-blind RCT found on post hoc analysis that participants with higher standing diastolic blood pressure who were given doxazosin had significantly reduced heavy-drinking days and drinks per week compared with their counterparts who were given placebo (Haass-Koffler et al. 2017). An earlier study found no benefit of doxazosin in drinking outcomes for the general AUD population but found a significant reduction in heavy-drinking days and drinks per week in those with a high "family history density of alcoholism" (Kenna et al. 2016). Thus, the use of doxazosin for AUD may be better suited to patients with a strong family history of AUD or those with high baseline diastolic blood pressure. Doxazosin tends to be well tolerated, with a low risk of side effects. Given the high prevalence of AUDs among patients with PTSD, these two medications may be considered for patients with nightmares who may use alcohol as self-medication.

### Varenicline

Compared with that for ondansetron and prazosin, a larger body of literature explores the effect of varenicline on drinking. A meta-analysis by Gandhi et al. (2020) on using varenicline to treat AUD did not show improvements in drinking-related outcomes even though varenicline reduced alcohol cravings. Two RCTs, including a newer RCT published more than a year after the previous meta-analysis, concluded that treatment response to varenicline may be moderated by alcohol severity, such that treatment response to varenicline may be greater with less severe AUD (Donato et al. 2021; Falk et al. 2015).

## Combination Treatment

Combination therapy has been explored for patients who may have an inadequate response to monotherapy or who may benefit from a presumed synergistic effect of combining medications for AUD. A systematic review by Naglich et al. (2018) found that naltrexone was the medication most often combined with others in dual therapy for alcohol consumption. Although the highest-quality studies were those analyzing a naltrexone-acamprosate combination, the authors concluded that no significant benefit over monotherapy occurred for any combination. The landmark COMBINE trial also did not find a benefit to adding acamprosate to naltrexone (Anton et al. 2006).

One trial examined the combination of gabapentin and naltrexone and found that adding gabapentin was beneficial, with participants reporting a longer delay to heavy drinking, fewer heavy-drinking days, and fewer drinks per drinking day compared with those receiving naltrexone monotherapy. In addition, a history of alcohol withdrawal correlated with a better response in the combination group (Anton et al. 2011). This potential added synergy is not surprising, given that another study published 9 years later concluded that those with a strong history of alcohol withdrawal may receive more benefits from gabapentin compared with placebo on outcomes of no heavy-drinking days and total abstinence (Anton et al. 2020). Sertraline used in combination with naltrexone in comorbid AUD and depression led to a significantly higher abstinence rate (53.7%) and a longer delay in returning to heavy drinking compared with placebo (23.1%), naltrexone (21.3%), or sertraline (27.5%) monotherapy (Pettinati et al. 2010). Overall, the evidence for combination therapy is weak at best; thus, monotherapy should be used first to minimize the risk of side effect burden prior to adding additional agents for specific subpopulations.

# Smoking and Alcohol

It is important to address the use of nicotine products in patients with AUD because rates of smoking are estimated to be as high as 80% for such patients in treatment (Kalman et al. 2010). Furthermore, tobacco users tend to have increased binge drinking because they experience alcohol as more reinforcing than alcohol alone, and they can consume alcohol for longer periods (McKee and Weinberger 2013). At the same time, alcohol can potentiate the positive effects of nicotine (Roberts et al. 2018). Thus, treating both use disorders simultaneously may lead to better outcomes. Treatment of tobacco use disorder (TUD) is discussed in the paragraphs that follow, with additional information given in Chapter 6.

## Varenicline

Varenicline is an FDA-approved option for treatment of TUD. In the Evaluating Adverse Events in a Global Smoking Cessation Study (EAGLES) trial, a landmark study that was the largest smoking cessation clinical trial ever conducted, varenicline had superior outcomes compared with other options, such as nicotine replacement therapy (NRT), bupropion, and placebo (Anthenelli et al. 2016). Varenicline may be considered the first-line treatment for individuals seeking treatment for TUD who also drink. In particular, studies show varenicline reduces ethanol self-administration in rats; in human studies, it reduced alcohol craving and consumption compared with placebo (Yardley et al. 2015). Several RCTs have shown evidence that varenicline can increase rates of prolonged abstinence from smoking (Bold et al. 2019; Hurt et al. 2018). Interestingly, one study found that varenicline delayed escalation in smoking and decreased smoking after an alcohol prime. These data support considering varenicline in individuals who want to stop smoking but may intend to continue drinking (Roberts et al. 2018). However, another study suggested that varenicline did not lead to differential treatment outcomes for smoking abstinence compared with NRT among those who binge drink, indicating a potential limitation for that subgroup (Kaye et al. 2020). Overall, varenicline is an option to consider in those whose primary goal is smoking cessation, with or without a secondary goal of reducing drinking.

The range of studies on the effect of varenicline on alcohol consumption reflects its potential to reduce alcohol consumption rather than promote abstinence. Other studies found varenicline to be efficacious in reducing drinking and alcohol cravings, independent of smoking status (Litten et al. 2013). One RCT found that people who smoked and also drink heavily had reduced alcohol consumption (but not increased rates of abstinence) while receiving varenicline (Mitchell et al. 2012). However, a systematic review of nine randomized, double-blind, placebo-controlled trials published in 2019 showed that varenicline was effective for decreasing alcohol consumption but was not effective for reducing heavy-drinking days (Oon-Arom et al. 2019). Similarly, in another systematic review and meta-analysis published a year later, varenicline was shown to reduce alcohol craving but not improve drinking-related outcomes in participants with AUD. A limitation of this study was that it did not consider moderating patient factors (e.g., sex, severity of AUD) in the analysis (Gandhi et al. 2020).

Other studies have attempted to evaluate some of these moderating factors. According to Donato et al. (2021), varenicline improved drinking outcomes with regard to percentage of heavy-drinking days, number of drinks per day, and number of drinks per drinking day in only the low-severity AUD group (compared with a high-severity AUD group). Similarly, another RCT found that varenicline appeared to have greater efficacy than placebo among less severely alcohol-dependent patients (Falk et al. 2015). In a longitudinal RCT of varenicline for treatment of AUD with comorbid smoking published in 2019, the authors determined that male participants had higher rates of non-heavy-drinking days while taking varenicline versus placebo but that female participants did not (Bold et al. 2019). Perhaps the dosage of varenicline is related to its effectiveness, because a randomized trial that compared various dosages of varenicline found that only dosages of 2 mg/day (compared with a lower dosage of 1 mg/day) reduced craving for alcohol, and reductions in drinking and heavy drinking were associated with higher plasma varenicline levels (Verplaetse et al. 2016). In summary, varenicline in comorbid alcohol use and TUD may have more effect on a patient's smoking, with a lesser effect on alcohol consumption (Erwin and Slaton 2014; Gandhi et al. 2020). If varenicline is to be used strictly for its effects on alcohol consumption, using a higher dosage or using it only in those with lower-severity AUD may produce better outcomes, although one should expect reduced consumption as opposed to complete abstinence.

Combination treatment has been studied, but results have been mixed. Varenicline combined with naltrexone, for example, was more effective at reducing post-alcohol euphoria and cigarette cravings than varenicline alone, naltrexone alone, or placebo. The same combination also decreased the number of drinks per drinking day compared with placebo and the number of cigarettes per day compared with naltrexone alone and placebo (Yardley et al. 2015). When the treatment outcome was smoking abstinence in participants who smoke and who drink heavily, a 2021 RCT did not show a benefit of adding naltrexone to varenicline (Ray et al. 2021). An alternative combination is naltrexone plus NRT, which has had mixed results for reducing smoking compared with placebo plus NRT (Yardley et al. 2015).

## Bupropion

Bupropion is another FDA-approved medication for smoking cessation, although the clinical evidence to support its use in reducing drinking in patients who smoke is much more limited than that for varenicline. One small open-label trial found that bupropion in combination with naltrexone reduced the number of binge-drinking days per month (Walter et al. 2020). Otherwise, much of the work related to bupropion in comorbid alcohol use and smoking involves evaluating the reduction in smoking. Although bupropion has shown promising evidence of reducing smoking in the general population, it is not clear based on the limited trials available whether bupropion has the same effect on people with AUD. One open-label study found that those who were taking sustained-release bupropion were more likely to abstain from smoking in a population with early remission from alcohol use (Karam-Hage et al. 2014). However, another study did not find a benefit with sustained-release bupropion for preventing relapse tobacco relapse in patients recovering from alcoholism (Hays et al. 2009). Based the results of two clinical trials that examined individuals who smoked and had a history of AUD (Kalman et al. 2011; McGeary et al. 2012), there is no clear evidence that use of combination therapy with bupropion and NRT would improve outcomes compared with NRT monotherapy.

## Topiramate

Topiramate is another interesting option as an off-label, but effective, treatment for AUD that has also shown positive evidence for reducing smoking in those who drink, with multiple studies focusing on male subjects (Anthenelli et al. 2017; Baltieri et al. 2009; Isgro et al. 2017; Johnson et al. 2005). However, a 2020 systematic review and meta-analysis of five studies did not find topiramate helpful for smoking cessation in the general population (Lotfy et al. 2020), and another meta-analysis of studies on smoking cessation in participants with comorbid AUD also did not find a benefit with topiramate for smoking cessation (Guo et al. 2021).

## Naltrexone

Naltrexone is also FDA-approved for the treatment of AUD but has weak evidence for use in smoking cessation. A systematic review did not find naltrexone to be helpful for long-term smoking abstinence in the general smoking population either as monotherapy or in combination with NRT (David et al. 2013). Guo et al. (2021) arrived at the same conclusions about using naltrexone for smoking cessation in the AUD population. Despite these negative results, some clinical trials found that naltrexone may be more helpful for individuals who drink heavily but do not necessarily have a diagnosis of AUD (Fridberg et al. 2014; King et al. 2009). In searching for combination treatments, a 26-week RCT published in 2021 surprisingly discovered that adding naltrexone to varenicline led to poorer outcomes compared with varenicline monotherapy in terms of rates of smoking abstinence among individuals who drink heavily. However, adding naltrexone to standard tobacco treatment may improve drinking-related outcomes (Ray et al. 2021).

# Cannabis and Alcohol

Unfortunately, no medications have yet been FDA-approved to treat cannabis use disorder (CaUD), which has made finding treatments for comorbid CaUD and AUD even more challenging. Overall, no clinical trials have been completed using FDA-approved medications for AUD (e.g., acamprosate, naltrexone, disulfiram) or the second-line, off-label options (e.g., topiramate, baclofen, gabapentin) for the treatment of comorbid AUD and CaUD.

## Potential Pharmacotherapy for Cannabis Use Disorder and Alcohol Use Disorder

In studying potential pharmacotherapy for CaUD in the general population, a 2020 analysis of multiple studies of different medication classes concluded that buspirone, selective serotonin reuptake inhibitors, and cannabinoids are ineffective. This analysis was also unable to draw conclusions regarding other drug classes, such as glutamatergic modulators, antipsychotics, and mood stabilizers (Kondo et al. 2020). Regarding naltrexone, a very small open-label pilot study with 12 participants receiving naltrexone XR found that the number of cannabis use days per week significantly decreased, although this decrease was not observed in participants with AUD (Notzon et al. 2018). A slightly larger study using oral naltrexone 50 mg/day in patients who smoked cannabis daily determined that, relative to placebo, naltrexone reduced active cannabis self-administration and its positive subjective effects (Haney et al. 2015). No trials available to date have examined the effect of disulfiram or acamprosate on CaUD.

## Cannabis Withdrawal

A 2018 systematic review of the treatment of insomnia from cannabis withdrawal demonstrated that many trials had limitations due to small size, short duration, and heterogeneous methodology. However, the authors found that mirtazapine, gabapentin, lofexidine, quetiapine, and zolpidem had positive effects on sleep (Zhand and Milin 2018). Of these options, only mirtazapine and gabapentin have evidence for treating AUD. Mirtazapine has some mixed evidence for use in treating AUD; although two open-label trials in comorbid depression and AUD found it had benefit in reducing either craving or drinking, a more recent RCT found no significant reduction in drinking in the same population (Cornelius et al. 2012, 2016; Yoon et al. 2006). Anecdotally and theoretically, mirtazapine could be considered for its anxiolytic, sedative, anti-nausea, and appetite effects in cannabis users who are self-medicating anxiety, insomnia, nausea, or low appetite. However, no RCTs were identified that examined mirtazapine for treatment of CaUD.

Gabapentin has been used to help with AUD and alcohol withdrawal. According to a 2020 Cochrane review that found no clear treatments for CaUD, gabapentin was one of the three options (in addition to *N*-acetylcysteine [NAC] and oxytocin) with weak positive evidence worth further investigation (Nielsen et al. 2019). This conclusion was based on a 12-week, double-blind RCT in 2012 by Mason and colleagues in which 50 participants were randomly assigned to placebo or to a fixed dosage of 1,200 mg of gabapentin daily. Compared with the placebo group, the gabapentin group had less cannabis use, reduced craving and withdrawal symptoms, and greater overall improvement in marijuana-related problems (Mason et al. 2012).

NAC had one positive double-blind RCT to reduce cannabis use in adolescents, but this result was not replicated in a similar trial in adults that was published 5 years later (Gray et al. 2012, 2017). A secondary analysis of the adult trial showed that, compared with the placebo group, participants in the NAC group consumed less alcohol (Squeglia et al. 2018). Unfortunately, no trials to date directly assess NAC as a treatment for AUD with alcohol use as a primary outcome.

# Alcohol and Benzodiazepines

Managing co-occurring AUD and benzodiazepine use disorder is challenging, mainly because benzodiazepines are typically used in the treatment of alcohol withdrawal syndrome. For example, they are generally avoided during the maintenance phase of AUD treatment, which presents a dilemma when the patient has both disorders.

No FDA-approved treatment exists for benzodiazepine use disorder. Unfortunately, off-label options to prevent a return to use or to assist a patient during a benzodiazepine taper are limited. Although earlier studies showed promise in using carbamazepine for benzodiazepine withdrawal or discontinuation, a 2018 Cochrane review examined various agents for chronic benzodiazepine use or benzodiazepine use disorder and showed that the evidence was very low quality in identifying candidates with a potential benefit for benzodiazepine discontinuation or withdrawal, reducing risk to return to benzodiazepine use, or reducing anxiety at the end of intervention (Rickels et al. 1999; Roy-Byrne et al. 1993; Schweizer et al. 1991). Notably, valproate had very low quality evidence for reducing risk of return to benzodiazepine use as well as for benzodiazepine discontinuation. Flumazenil, paroxetine, and pregabalin all had very low quality evidence of efficacy for benzodiazepine withdrawal symptoms and for reduction of anxiety at the end of the intervention (Baandrup et al. 2018). Unfortunately, none of these options is used routinely for the treatment of AUD; in addition, pregabalin must be used with caution because it also carries misuse liability. Flumazenil has limitations in administration (it is given intravenously), and clinicians must be very cautious to not precipitate withdrawal and seizures in a benzodiazepine-dependent patient.

With a lack of reliable pharmacological options for this population, treatment has focused on motivational interviewing, harm reduction, and a flexible taper schedule. We meet with patients frequently, give a limited supply of benzodiazepines until the next appointment, and conduct a very gradual taper to increase the likelihood of tolerability and comfort. Maintaining rapport while also communicating appropriate and consistent boundaries regarding treatment structure is crucial. Referral to a higher level of care or residential treatment is indicated if safety issues arise. In some cases, patients may have been maintained on a benzodiazepine long term without an additional anxiolytic from a previous provider. Judicious and cautious titration of an antidepressant or adjunct medication (e.g., hydroxyzine, trazodone, propranolol) may provide some relief during the tapering process for these patients. Propranolol should be used with caution because it can mask withdrawal symptoms via β-blockade.

# Alcohol and Methamphetamine

No medications have been FDA-approved for the treatment of methamphetamine use disorder (MUD). In addition, except for one naltrexone trial, no trials of the FDA-approved medications for AUD (e.g., naltrexone, disulfiram, acamprosate) were found that addressed comorbid AUD and MUD. Thus, we make inferences about which medications may be helpful for comorbid AUD and MUD. A systematic review by Siefried et al. (2020) on treatment of MUD and amphetamine use disorder found the most consistent positive findings for stimulant agonist treatment (e.g., dexamphetamine and methylphenidate), naltrexone, and topiramate. Bupropion and mirtazapine showed benefits to a less consistent degree. This result is promising, given that naltrexone and topiramate are both medications that also happen to be used for AUD and may be considered for those with comorbid AUD and MUD. Pharmacotherapy for stimulant use disorders is discussed in Chapter 6.

## Topiramate

Topiramate in dosages up to 200 mg/day was shown in a multicenter randomized, double-blind, placebo-controlled trial published in 2012 to reduce the amount of methamphetamine use and recurrence rates, even though it did not appear to promote abstinence in methamphetamine users (Elkashef et al. 2012). Another double-blind RCT, albeit with a smaller sample size and only in males, found that topiramate 200 mg/day reduced the proportion of methamphetamine-positive urine tests at week 6 compared with placebo, but this effect was not sustained through the rest of the study (week 10) (Rezaei et al. 2016). No other studies exploring the effect of topiramate directly on comorbid AUD and MUD were found. Although many clinicians have raised concerns about topiramate's potential to cause cognitive side effects, particularly in those with MUD, a study on topiramate use in recently abstinent methamphetamine-dependent individuals concluded that there were no negative interactions between topiramate and methamphetamine in terms of cognitive performance, attention, and concentration (Johnson et al. 2007).

## Naltrexone

A systematic review by Lam et al. (2019) of the four available RCTs on the use of naltrexone for MUD and amphetamine use disorder did not find sufficient evidence to support the use of naltrexone. Two of these RCTs included oral naltrexone, and the other two utilized naltrexone XR. The authors concluded that naltrexone demonstrates a modest ability to attenuate subjective effects of amphetamine but shows minimal to no impact on methamphetamine use. However, this systematic review was conducted prior to a multisite, randomized, double-blind, two-stage placebo-controlled trial published in 2021 that found that the response in patients who received naltrexone XR 380 mg every 3 weeks in combination with extended-release bupropion (bupropion XL) 450 mg was greater than that in patients who received placebo (Trivedi et al. 2021). An earlier study by Walter et al. (2020)—albeit a small, open-label study—of using oral naltrexone 50 mg/day and bupropion XL 300 mg/day to treat binge drinking showed a reduction in the average number of drinks per binge-drinking day and the percentage of binge-drinking days per month. Combined, these studies strengthen the consideration for naltrexone in the treatment of MUD, although the naltrexone XR formulation seems more promising for both MUD and AUD. Because bupropion is not specifically used to treat AUD, the naltrexone-bupropion combination may be preferred for AUD with comorbid MUD when MUD is dominant. If AUD is the pre-dominant condition (as opposed to MUD), naltrexone monotherapy should be tried first because adding bupropion to treatment for AUD may have limited benefit due to the lack of human studies exploring alcohol reduction as a primary outcome. In addition, bupropion may lower the seizure threshold in individuals at risk of alcohol withdrawal.

## Stimulant Agonist Treatment

Stimulant replacement therapy has some benefit in the treatment of MUD, but it is not recommended for individuals with more dominant AUD because ingestion of alcohol with amphetamines may potentiate cardiovascular side effects. Additionally, methylphenidate combined with alcohol can increase methylphenidate concentrations, leading to side effects (Traccis et al. 2022).

## Mirtazapine

Mirtazapine may have some benefit for treating MUD in men who have sex with men (MSM) and in transgender women who have sex with men. Two double-blind RCTs showed that mirtazapine titrated to a 30-mg/day dosage reduced both methamphetamine use and risky sexual behavior despite suboptimal medication compliance (Coffin et al. 2020; Colfax et al. 2011). A study of naltrexone for methamphetamine-using and binge-drinking MSM who did not have MUD did not lead to differences in methamphetamine use or drinking (Santos et al. 2016). In the same study, only participants with better compliance with naltrexone had reduced binge drinking, and only those with more frequent methamphetamine use (at least weekly use at baseline) had reduced methamphetamine use. Thus, in the MSM population, the use of both mirtazapine and naltrexone could be beneficial in combating MUD and AUD. However, mirtazapine may prove to be more beneficial for those individuals who face challenges in maintaining medication adherence.

## Baclofen and Gabapentin

Baclofen and gabapentin, both of which have a role in the treatment of AUD, were studied against placebo in a small double-blind RCT for treatment of MUD. The study did not find statistically significant differences between either baclofen or gabapentin and placebo for methamphetamine use, treatment retention, medication adherence, craving, or urine drug screen results (Heinzerling et al. 2006).

# Alcohol and Cocaine

Several studies have attempted to find helpful therapeutic agents for comorbid AUD and cocaine use disorder (CUD). Unfortunately, these turned out to be negative trials, which is not surprising given the documented literature about poorer outcomes for those who have both use disorders, with no improvements in use with trials of naltrexone 50 mg/day (Schmitz et al. 2009). One possible explanation for treatment refractoriness is that in the presence of alcohol, cocaine is converted to cocaethylene, which has a plasma half-life 3–5 times that of cocaine and 30% greater toxicity than either cocaine or alcohol. Furthermore, individuals using the combination may experience a prolonged effect of euphoria from cocaine with a concomitant reduction in the negative withdrawal symptoms (Tamargo et al. 2022).

## Naltrexone

Trials with a higher dose of naltrexone (>50 mg) have also shown weak evidence of effectiveness or effectiveness only in specific subgroups. A small open-label trial (N=15) showed some reduction in cocaine and alcohol use with naltrexone 100 mg/day, but in this study, the participants were already at least 5 days abstinent (Oslin et al. 1999). A larger randomized, double-blind, placebo-controlled trial evaluated naltrexone 150 mg/day in patients with co-occurring CUD and AUD and found that reductions occurred in cocaine and alcohol use in males but not in females (Pettinati et al. 2008b). One trial examined dual therapy with participants randomly assigned to naltrexone 100 mg/day, disulfiram 250 mg/day, a combination of both medications, or placebo. The authors concluded that participants in the group receiving combination therapy with both disulfiram and naltrexone were more likely than the other groups to achieve 3 consecutive weeks of abstinence from both cocaine and alcohol (Pettinati et al. 2008a). Finally, another randomized, double-blind, placebo-controlled trial concluded that 100 mg/day of naltrexone showed low treatment retention and low medication compliance versus placebo, with no improvements in cocaine use or drinking in either treatment group (Schmitz et al. 2009). An 8-week trial using naltrexone XR 380 mg every 30 days attempted to reduce medication noncompliance in subjects with comorbid CUD and AUD but failed to show any reduction in either cocaine or alcohol use (Pettinati et al. 2014).

## Disulfiram

Disulfiram has also attracted attention for use in treating CUD (see discussion in Chapter 6). A study by Carroll et al. (1998) found that use of disulfiram up to 500 mg/day in a cocaine-dependent population who also met the criteria for alcohol dependence or alcohol abuse was associated with a longer duration of abstinence from alcohol and cocaine use. These results were supported by another study in a similar population in which disulfiram led to continued reduction in cocaine use after treatment ended and less alcohol use throughout the follow-up period (Carroll et al. 2000).

## Acamprosate

Acamprosate, another FDA-approved medication for AUD, was studied in only one trial for CUD and failed to show a reduction in cocaine cravings or cocaine use (Kampman et al. 2011). Thus, acamprosate seems unlikely to be a candidate for comorbid AUD and CUD.

## Topiramate

Finally, a randomized, double-blind, placebo-controlled trial by Kampman et al. (2013) explored whether topiramate was effective for comorbid AUD and CUD in participants who had been abstinent for at least 3 days. Topiramate was found to not reduce cocaine use or alcohol use compared with placebo, although the subgroup with higher cocaine withdrawal tended to respond better to topiramate in regard to cocaine use.

## Other Agents Requiring Further Study

No human trials using baclofen, mirtazapine, or ondansetron for the treatment of comorbid AUD and CUD are available. Even for the trials evaluating gabapentin in CUD alone, research thus far does not support its use (Berger et al. 2005; Bisaga et al. 2006; Minozzi et al. 2015). A 2003 RCT showed benefit with baclofen over placebo in reducing cocaine use on the basis of urine drug screen results; however, an expanded multisite trial by Kahn et al. (2009) found no benefit of baclofen at 60 mg/day for those actively using cocaine (Shoptaw et al. 2003). Furthermore, Kahn and colleagues included patients with a history of AUD in their study as long as the patients did not require withdrawal management services. This highlights the difficulty of treating comorbid CUD and AUD. On the other hand, doxazosin has shown some positive signs for treating CUD and AUD separately. Several studies have supported the benefit of doxazosin in reducing cocaine use compared with placebo when the medication was titrated quickly to a dosage of 8 mg/day. The response to doxazosin in CUD may be moderated by dopamine β-hydroxylase and $\alpha_1$-adrenoreceptor polymorphisms (Shorter et al. 2013, 2020; Zhang et al. 2019).

# Conclusion

A summary of pharmacotherapy for AUD is highlighted in Figure 5–1 and Table 5–1. Pharmacotherapy for co-occurring AUD and other substance use is summarized in Table 5–2. Treatment options should be selected based on moderators, medical comorbidities, and a review of medications that have and have not been beneficial for the patient in the past, along with their side effects. Additional studies are urgently needed to clarify treatments that are the most likely to improve the quality of life of patients with multi-substance use disorders.

# Clinical Cases

## Case Example 1

A 30-year-old male with a history of depression and liver cirrhosis is seeking treatment for AUD. He started drinking at age 18, with the longest period of abstinence being about 1 week, when he had a brief incarceration following a charge of driving while intoxicated. His last drink was about 6 days ago, and he is currently not in active alcohol withdrawal. He also denies any history of significant alcohol withdrawal. Before he ceased drinking, he consumed about 12 canned beers daily (12 oz each). He desires to stay abstinent from alcohol. A laboratory review shows normal blood urea nitrogen and creatinine levels, with no signs of hepatorenal syndrome. He has never received any pharmacotherapy for AUD before.

This patient may benefit from acamprosate. Given his cirrhosis, the other FDA-approved medications (e.g., disulfiram, naltrexone) would not be first-line options. Acamprosate is a first-line FDA-approved medication for AUD that bypasses hepatic metabolism, making it the safest option for a patient with severe hepatic disease. Furthermore, studies show that patients with recent abstinence are more likely to respond to acamprosate. No dosing change would be needed from the standard 666 mg three times a day, because the patient has no signs of hepatorenal syndrome, and his blood urea nitrogen and creatinine levels are normal.

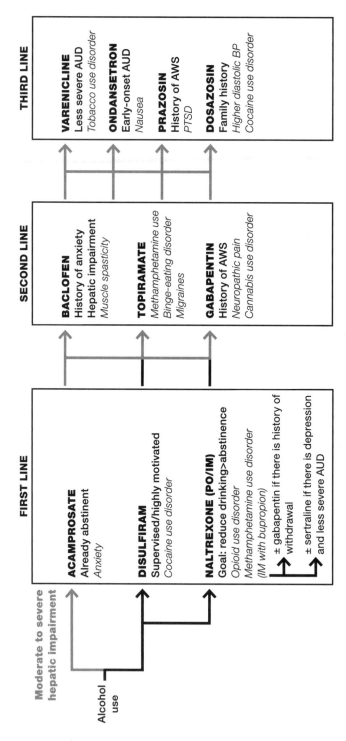

Figure 5–1.  Treatment algorithm for alcohol use disorder (AUD).

When significant hepatic impairment exists, consider the options following the hepatic impairment pathway (*gray*). Moderators for positive treatment response are *bold*, and additional targeted comorbidities are *italicized*. Table 5–1 also provides information on recommended dosages based on studies and side effects of greatest interest. AWS=alcohol withdrawal syndrome; BP=blood pressure; IM=intramuscular; PO=oral (by mouth).

**Table 5–1.** Summary of pharmacotherapy for alcohol use disorder (AUD)

| Medication | Dosage | Moderators | Medical comorbidities | Notes |
|---|---|---|---|---|
| **First line** | | | | |
| Naltrexone (FDA-approved) | 380 mg IM q 4 weeks; or 50 mg+ PO daily | Goal to reduce heavy drinking | Opioid use disorder | Caution with hepatic impairment; benefit should outweigh risk if used in setting of elevated LFTs |
| Acamprosate (FDA-approved) | 666 mg tid | Already abstinent | Anxiety | Safe with hepatic impairment |
| Disulfiram (FDA-approved) | 250–500 mg/day | Supervision bolsters compliance | Cocaine use disorder | Avoid in patients with hepatic impairment, psychosis, significant cardiovascular disease |
| **Second line** | | | | |
| Topiramate | Up to 300 mg/day | GRIK1 may moderate adverse effects | Migraines Binge-eating disorder Seizures | Monitor for cognitive impairment |
| Baclofen | Start 10 mg tid | History of anxiety Hepatic impairment | Muscle spasticity | Risk of withdrawal delirium |
| Gabapentin | Start 300–400 mg tid | History of alcohol withdrawal | Neuropathic pain Vasomotor hot flashes | Monitor cognition |

**Table 5–1.** Summary of pharmacotherapy for alcohol use disorder (AUD) *(continued)*

| Medication | Dosage | Moderators | Medical comorbidities | Notes |
|---|---|---|---|---|
| **Third line** | | | | |
| Varenicline | At least 2 mg/day | Less severe alcohol use disorder | Tobacco use disorder | |
| Ondansetron | Up to 2 mg bid | Early-onset AUD (before age 22) | Nausea | |
| Prazosin | Up to 16 mg/day | History of alcohol withdrawal syndrome | PTSD-related nightmares BPH | Monitor for orthostasis |
| Doxazosin | Up to 16 mg/day | Family history Higher diastolic blood pressure | PTSD-related nightmares Cocaine use disorder | Monitor for orthostasis |

*Note.* LFT = liver function test.

**Table 5–2.** Options for multi-substance use disorders in which alcohol is a secondary substance

| SUD combination | Pharmacological considerations | Dosing recommendation | Notes |
|---|---|---|---|
| Tobacco + alcohol | Varenicline ± naltrexone | At least 2 mg/day varenicline if also treating AUD ± naltrexone 50 mg/day | Adding naltrexone to varenicline may help to further reduce smoking and drinking (but not necessarily lead to smoking cessation) compared with varenicline monotherapy |
| | Bupropion | 150–450 mg/day | Caution if patient has a history of alcohol withdrawal seizures |
| | NRT | As indicated per formulation | |
| Cannabis + alcohol | Gabapentin | Start 300–400 mg tid for most patients; adjust if reduced creatinine clearance | |
| | N-acetylcysteine | 1,200 mg bid | Positive results in adolescent trials not replicated in adults |
| | Naltrexone | 50 mg/day | |
| | Mirtazapine | Titrate to effect | Consider in patients with insomnia, low appetite, anxiety leading to substance use |
| Benzodiazepine + alcohol | Carbamazepine | | Low-quality evidence; monitor for drug-drug interactions |
| | Valproate | | Low-quality evidence |

**Table 5–2.    Options for multi-substance use disorders in which alcohol is a secondary substance (*continued*)**

| SUD combination | Pharmacological considerations | Dosing recommendation | Notes |
|---|---|---|---|
| Methamphetamine + alcohol | Naltrexone XR + bupropion | Naltrexone XR 380 mg IM q 3 weeks + bupropion 450 mg/day | Use with caution in patient with history of alcohol withdrawal seizures |
| | Topiramate | Can titrate up to 200 mg/day | |
| | Bupropion monotherapy | Titrate up to maximum 450 mg/day | Use with caution in patient with history of alcohol withdrawal seizures |
| | Mirtazapine | Titrate up to 30 mg/day | Consider in MSM population, which the studies targeted |
| Cocaine + alcohol | High-dose naltrexone ± disulfiram | Naltrexone 100–150 mg | |
| | Disulfiram | Up to 500 mg/day | |
| | Doxazosin | Can titrate up to 8 mg/day as fast as within 4 weeks | Doxazosin studies for AUD alone used dosages as high as 16 mg/day |
| | Topiramate | | |

*Note.*    The more dominant substance (e.g., stronger cravings, greater frequency and/or intensity of use) is listed first in the paired SUDs. Dosing recommendations assume normal hepatic and renal function.

AUD=alcohol use disorder; MSM=men who have sex with men; NRT=nicotine replacement therapy; SUD=substance use disorder; XR=extended release.

## Case Example 2

A 45-year-old female has been in treatment for AUD for the past year. She has found naltrexone 50 mg/day to be helpful and does not want intramuscular naltrexone. With oral naltrexone, her drinking has reduced from a pint of vodka daily to two shots daily. She has had difficulty obtaining her goal of complete abstinence because of experiences with sweating, tremor, and elevated pulse whenever she reduces consumption further. She has no hepatic or renal conditions but has diabetic neuropathy.

Addition of gabapentin could be considered for this patient. In a patient-centered treatment plan, naltrexone could continue because of patient preference, and adding gabapentin may help alleviate some of the alcohol-related withdrawal symptoms that likely drive the negative reinforcement process of drinking. A dosage of 300 mg or 400 mg three times a day could be started while the patient is monitored patient for sedation. Gabapentin may also help the comorbid medical condition of diabetic neuropathy.

## Case Example 3

A 27-year-old female with morbid obesity presents for her first-ever psychiatric treatment. She states she has multiple "addictions," including alcohol and food. She has been drinking around 11 beers daily and meets the criteria for AUD. Her last drink was about 8 hours ago. She also reports episodes of eating large amounts of food, often so quickly that she vomits and then feels ashamed afterward. A review of laboratory results shows normal hepatic and renal functioning. After discussing some initial options for AUD, she says, "I heard about the one that makes you really sick if you drink on top of it. I don't want that one!" She also does not want naltrexone because she is concerned about the potential need to take opioid pain medication in the future, although she is currently not taking any opioids.

This patient meets criteria for AUD and likely binge-eating disorder. She has no interest in disulfiram or naltrexone, and the third FDA-approved first-line option, acamprosate, may not be as helpful because it may have more benefit if the patient is already abstinent. In reviewing the second-line options, topiramate may be a good option given that it also has some success in treating binge-eating disorder.

## Case Example 4

A 60-year-old male with AUD, TUD, and borderline personality disorder has a 20-pack-per-year smoking history as well as a history of 10 years of heavy drinking. He occasionally engages in self-injurious behavior (cutting himself on the forearms) because of stress. He would like to cut down and eventually quit both substances. He notes that he usually has a cigarette "like a habit" after drinking alcohol and believes that if he quit drinking, he would likely smoke less as well. He has no medical conditions, and a review of his laboratory results shows no hepatic or renal abnormalities. He declines any psychotherapy or pharmacological treatment for anxiety or depression.

A reasonable starting consideration would be naltrexone. This patient has no hepatic issues, and naltrexone is an FDA-approved first-line treatment for AUD. It also may help reduce self-injurious behaviors in some patients. Although starting with monotherapy is the most recommended course to reduce the risk of side effects, if the patient has an inadequate response in terms of alcohol or smoking, adding varenicline (Chantix) to the naltrexone could also be considered.

## Case Example 5

A 30-year-old male with AUD and co-occurring MUD presents for treatment. He lives 2 hours away from the clinic and has no insurance, so he wants "a medication to help me stop using" and prefers to do outpatient treatment instead of residential treatment. He has no comorbid medical conditions but has a history of seizures during alcohol withdrawal. He identifies the cravings to be strong for both alcohol and methamphetamine. A combination of naltrexone XR and bupropion is considered; however, he is unable to come to the clinic and says, "I don't like needles."

The patient already declined the combination of naltrexone XR and bupropion for MUD, an off-label combination that showed promise in treating MUD in a rather large clinical trial. Bupropion monotherapy has some weak evidence in treating males with low-level methamphetamine use (Siefried et al. 2020). However, given that this patient has a history of alcohol-related seizures, there may be a significant amount of risk involved with bupropion. Mirtazapine may help in co-occurring AUD and MUD, but the available studies, as discussed earlier (see "Alcohol and Methamphetamine" section), were performed primarily in the MSM population. Topiramate could be considered in this case. Although there are no known trials directly assessing its use in comorbid AUD and MUD, topiramate is a second-line off-label option for AUD. It has also shown some possible benefit in the treatment of MUD. Provided that a patient has no contraindications to topiramate, it may be worthwhile to consider.

## Case Example 6

A 48-year-old female with AUD, CUD, and PTSD presents for outpatient treatment. She is currently taking naltrexone 50 mg/day for AUD and finds it helpful because she has reduced her drinking to about two beers daily. She cites no desire to achieve complete abstinence, stating that "I'm controlling the drinking just fine at this level." She has no current life dysfunction or health issues from drinking. However, her ongoing cocaine use has been excessively costly, and she wants to quit using cocaine.

This patient may have more difficulty quitting both substances due to her comorbid alcohol and cocaine use, which creates cocaethylene. Because she also continues to drink, it may thus help to provide more aggressive treatment of CUD. Some studies, as discussed earlier (see "Alcohol and Cocaine" section), demonstrated lower evidence for combining naltrexone and disulfiram to help reduce cocaine use. However, disulfiram would be contraindicated in this patient because her goal is not complete alcohol abstinence. Topiramate has some potential benefit for CUD, but the only trial using topiramate for both CUD and AUD found no benefit in reducing either substance. Doxazosin could be added to naltrexone because it has shown some promise in treating either AUD or CUD; in addition, the patient has a history of PTSD, and doxazosin may help with any PTSD-related nightmares and hyperarousal. Rapid titration to a dosage of 8 mg (within 1 month or less) would be recommended on the basis of the findings from previous trials.

# References

Agabio R, Baldwin DS, Amaro H, et al: The influence of anxiety symptoms on clinical outcomes during baclofen treatment of alcohol use disorder: a systematic review and meta-analysis. Neurosci Biobehav Rev 125(June):296–313, 2021 33454289

Anthenelli RM, Benowitz NL, West R, et al: Neuropsychiatric safety and efficacy of varenicline, bupropion, and nicotine patch in smokers with and without psychiatric disorders (EAGLES): a double-blind, randomised, placebo-controlled clinical trial. Lancet 387(10037):2507–2520, 2016 27116918

Anthenelli RM, Heffner JL, Wong E, et al: A randomized trial evaluating whether topiramate aids smoking cessation and prevents alcohol relapse in recovering alcohol-dependent men. Alcohol Clin Exp Res 41(1):197–206, 2017 28029173

Anton RF, O'Malley SS, Ciraulo DA, et al: Combined pharmacotherapies and behavioral interventions for alcohol dependence: the COMBINE study: a randomized controlled trial. JAMA 295(17):2003–2017, 2006 16670409

Anton RF, Myrick H, Wright TM, et al: Gabapentin combined with naltrexone for the treatment of alcohol dependence. Am J Psychiatry 168(7):709–717, 2011 21454917

Anton RF, Latham P, Voronin K, et al: Efficacy of gabapentin for the treatment of alcohol use disorder in patients with alcohol withdrawal symptoms: a randomized clinical trial. JAMA Intern Med 180(5):728–736, 2020 32150232

Baandrup L, Ebdrup BH, Rasmussen JØ, et al: Pharmacological interventions for benzodiazepine discontinuation in chronic benzodiazepine users. Cochrane Database Syst Rev 3(3):CD011481, 2018 29543325

Baltieri DA, Daró FR, Ribeiro PL, et al: Effects of topiramate or naltrexone on tobacco use among male alcohol-dependent outpatients. Drug Alcohol Depend 105(1–2):33–41, 2009 19595518

Beatty A, Stock C: Efficacy of long-acting, injectable versus oral naltrexone for preventing admissions for alcohol use disorder. Ment Health Clin 7(3):106–110, 2018 29955507

Berger SP, Winhusen TM, Somoza EC, et al: A medication screening trial evaluation of reserpine, gabapentin and lamotrigine pharmacotherapy of cocaine dependence. Addiction 100(Suppl 1):58–67, 2005 15730350

Bisaga A, Aharonovich E, Garawi F, et al: A randomized placebo-controlled trial of gabapentin for cocaine dependence. Drug Alcohol Depend 81(3):267–274, 2006 16169160

Blodgett JC, Del Re AC, Maisel NC, et al: A meta-analysis of topiramate's effects for individuals with alcohol use disorders. Alcohol Clin Exp Res 38(6):1481–1488, 2014 24796492

Bold KW, Zweben A, Fucito LM, et al: Longitudinal findings from a randomized clinical trial of varenicline for alcohol use disorder with comorbid cigarette smoking. Alcohol Clin Exp Res 43(5):937–944, 2019 30817018

Boothby LA, Doering PL: Acamprosate for the treatment of alcohol dependence. Clin Ther 27(6):695–714, 2005 16117977

Bryson WC, McConnell J, Korthius PT, et al: Extended-release naltrexone for alcohol dependence: persistence and healthcare costs and utilization. Am J Manag Care 17(Suppl 8):S222–S234, 2011 21761949

Busch AC, Denduluri M, Glass J, et al: Predischarge injectable versus oral naltrexone to improve postdischarge treatment engagement among hospitalized veterans with alcohol use disorder: a randomized pilot proof-of-concept study. Alcohol Clin Exp Res 41(7):1352–1360, 2017 28605827

Carroll KM, Nich C, Ball SA, et al: Treatment of cocaine and alcohol dependence with psychotherapy and disulfiram. Addiction 93(5):713–727, 1998 9692270

Carroll KM, Nich C, Ball SA, et al: One-year follow-up of disulfiram and psychotherapy for cocaine-alcohol users: sustained effects of treatment. Addiction 95(9):1335–1349, 2000 11048353

Cheng HY, McGuinness LA, Elbers RG, et al: Treatment interventions to maintain abstinence from alcohol in primary care: systematic review and network meta-analysis. BMJ 371(November):m3934, 2020 33239318

Coffin PO, Santos G-M, Hern J, et al: Effects of mirtazapine for methamphetamine use disorder among cisgender men and transgender women who have sex with men: a placebo-controlled randomized clinical trial. JAMA Psychiatry 77(3):246–255, 2020 31825466

Colfax GN, Santos GM, Das M, et al: Mirtazapine to reduce methamphetamine use: a randomized controlled trial. Arch Gen Psychiatry 68(11):1168–1175, 2011 22065532

Cornelius JR, Douaihy AB, Clark DB, et al: Mirtazapine in comorbid major depression and alcohol dependence: an open-label trial. J Dual Diagn 8(3):200–204, 2012 23230395

Cornelius JR, Chung T, Douaihy AB, et al: Mirtazapine in comorbid major depression and an alcohol use disorder: a double-blind placebo-controlled pilot trial. Psychiatry Res 242(Aug):326–330, 2016 27327217

David SP, Lancaster T, Stead LF, et al: Opioid antagonists for smoking cessation. Cochrane Database Syst Rev (3):CD003086, 2013 23744347

Dawes MA, Johnson BA, Ait-Daoud N, et al: A prospective, open-label trial of ondansetron in adolescents with alcohol dependence. Addict Behav 30(6):1077–1085, 2005 15925118

Donato S, Green R, Ray LA: Alcohol use disorder severity moderates clinical response to varenicline. Alcohol Clin Exp Res 45(9):1877–1887, 2021 34486130

Elkashef A, Kahn R, Yu E, et al: Topiramate for the treatment of methamphetamine addiction: a multi-center placebo-controlled trial. Addiction 107(7):1297–1306, 2012 22221594

Erwin BL, Slaton RM: Varenicline in the treatment of alcohol use disorders. Ann Pharmacother 48(11):1445–1455, 2014 25095786

Falk DE, Castle IJ, Ryan M, et al: Moderators of varenicline treatment effects in a double-blind, placebo-controlled trial for alcohol dependence: an exploratory analysis. J Addict Med 9(4):296–303, 2015 26083958

Fridberg DJ, Cao D, Grant JE, et al: Naltrexone improves quit rates, attenuates smoking urge, and reduces alcohol use in heavy drinking smokers attempting to quit smoking. Alcohol Clin Exp Res 38(10):2622–2629, 2014 25335648

Gandhi KD, Mansukhani MP, Karpyak VM, et al: The impact of varenicline on alcohol consumption in subjects with alcohol use disorders: systematic review and meta-analyses. J Clin Psychiatry 81(2):19r12924, 2020 32097546

Gray KM, Carpenter MJ, Baker NL, et al: A double-blind randomized controlled trial of N-acetylcysteine in cannabis-dependent adolescents. Am J Psychiatry 169(8):805–812, 2012 22706327

Gray KM, Sonne SC, McClure EA, et al: A randomized placebo-controlled trial of N-acetylcysteine for cannabis use disorder in adults. Drug Alcohol Depend 177(Aug):249–257, 2017 28623823

Gueorguieva R, Wu R, Donovan D, et al: Baseline trajectories of drinking moderate acamprosate and naltrexone effects in the COMBINE study. Alcohol Clin Exp Res 35(3):523–531, 2011 21143249

Gueorguieva R, Wu R, Tsai W-M, et al: An analysis of moderators in the COMBINE study: identifying subgroups of patients who benefit from acamprosate. Eur Neuropsychopharmacol 25(10):1586–1599, 2015 26141511

Guglielmo R, Martinotti G, Quatrale M, et al: Topiramate in alcohol use disorders: review and update. CNS Drugs 29(5):383–395, 2015 25899459

Guo K, Li J, Li J, et al: The effects of pharmacological interventions on smoking cessation in people with alcohol dependence: a systematic review and meta-analysis of nine randomized controlled trials. Int J Clin Pract 75(11):e14594, 2021 34228852

Haass-Koffler CL, Goodyear K, Zywiak WH, et al: Higher pretreatment blood pressure is associated with greater alcohol drinking reduction in alcohol-dependent individuals treated with doxazosin. Drug Alcohol Depend 177(Aug):23–28, 2017 28551590

Haney M, Ramesh D, Glass A, et al: Naltrexone maintenance decreases cannabis self-administration and subjective effects in daily cannabis smokers. Neuropsychopharmacology 40(11):2489–2498, 2015 25881117

Hays JT, Hurt RD, Decker PA, et al: A randomized, controlled trial of bupropion sustained-release for preventing tobacco relapse in recovering alcoholics. Nicotine Tob Res 11(7):859–867, 2009 19483180

Heinzerling KG, Shoptaw S, Peck JA, et al: Randomized, placebo-controlled trial of baclofen and gabapentin for the treatment of methamphetamine dependence. Drug Alcohol Depend 85(3):177–184, 2006 16740370

Hurt RT, Ebbert JO, Croghan IT, et al: Varenicline for tobacco-dependence treatment in alcohol-dependent smokers: a randomized controlled trial. Drug Alcohol Depend 184(Mar):12–17, 2018 29324248

Isgro M, Doran N, Heffner JL, et al: Type A/type B alcoholism predicts differential response to topiramate in a smoking cessation trial in dually diagnosed men. J Stud Alcohol Drugs 78(2):232–240, 2017 28317503

Johnson BA, Roache JD, Javors MA, et al: Ondansetron for reduction of drinking among biologically predisposed alcoholic patients: a randomized controlled trial. JAMA 284(8):963–971, 2000 10944641

Johnson BA, Ait-Daoud N, Akhtar FZ, et al: Use of oral topiramate to promote smoking abstinence among alcohol-dependent smokers: a randomized controlled trial. Arch Intern Med 165(14):1600–1605, 2005 16043677

Johnson BA, Roache JD, Ait-Daoud N, et al: Effects of topiramate on methamphetamine-induced changes in attentional and perceptual-motor skills of cognition in recently abstinent methamphetamine-dependent individuals. Prog Neuropsychopharmacol Biol Psychiatry 31(1):123–130, 2007 16978753

Johnson BA, Seneviratne C, Wang X-Q, et al: Determination of genotype combinations that can predict the outcome of the treatment of alcohol dependence using the 5-HT(3) antagonist ondansetron. Am J Psychiatry 170(9):1020–1031, 2013 23897038

Kahn R, Biswas K, Childress A-R, et al: Multi-center trial of baclofen for abstinence initiation in severe cocaine-dependent individuals. Drug Alcohol Depend 103(1–2):59–64, 2009 19414226

Kalman D, Kim S, DiGirolamo G, et al: Addressing tobacco use disorder in smokers in early remission from alcohol dependence: the case for integrating smoking cessation services in substance use disorder treatment programs. Clin Psychol Rev 30(1):12–24, 2010 19748166

Kalman D, Herz L, Monti P, et al: Incremental efficacy of adding bupropion to the nicotine patch for smoking cessation in smokers with a recent history of alcohol dependence: results from a randomized, double-blind, placebo-controlled study. Drug Alcohol Depend 118(2–3):111–118, 2011 21507585

Kampman KM, Dackis C, Pettinati HM, et al: A double-blind, placebo-controlled pilot trial of acamprosate for the treatment of cocaine dependence. Addict Behav 36(3):217–221, 2011 21112155

Kampman KM, Pettinati HM, Lynch KG, et al: A double-blind, placebo-controlled trial of topiramate for the treatment of comorbid cocaine and alcohol dependence. Drug Alcohol Depend 133(1):94–99, 2013 23810644

Karam-Hage M, Robinson JD, Lodhi A, et al: Bupropion-SR for smoking reduction and cessation in alcohol-dependent outpatients: a naturalistic, open-label study. Curr Clin Pharmacol 9(2):123–129, 2014 24218993

Kaye JT, Johnson AL, Baker TB, et al: Searching for personalized medicine for binge drinking smokers: smoking cessation using varenicline, nicotine patch, or combination nicotine replacement therapy. J Stud Alcohol Drugs 81(4):426–435, 2020 32800078

Kenna GA, Zywiak WH, McGeary JE, et al: A within-group design of nontreatment seeking 5-HTTLPR genotyped alcohol-dependent subjects receiving ondansetron and sertraline. Alcohol Clin Exp Res 33(2):315–323, 2009 19032576

Kenna GA, Zywiak WH, Swift RM, et al: Ondansetron and sertraline may interact with 5-HTTLPR and DRD4 polymorphisms to reduce drinking in non-treatment seeking alcohol-dependent women: exploratory findings. Alcohol 48(6):515–522, 2014 25212749

Kenna GA, Haass-Koffler CL, Zywiak WH, et al: Role of the α1 blocker doxazosin in alcoholism: a proof-of-concept randomized controlled trial. Addict Biol 21(4):904–914, 2016 26037245

King A, Cao D, Vanier C, et al: Naltrexone decreases heavy drinking rates in smoking cessation treatment: an exploratory study. Alcohol Clin Exp Res 33(6):1044–1050, 2009 19302083

Knopf A: Patients report vivitrol decreasing in effectiveness by week 3. Alcohol Drug Abuse Wkly 31(23):4–5, 2019

Kondo KK, Morasco BJ, Nugent SM, et al: Pharmacotherapy for the treatment of cannabis use disorder: a systematic review. Ann Intern Med 172(6):398–412, 2020 32120384

Kranzler HR, Pierucci-Lagha A, Feinn R, et al: Effects of ondansetron in early- versus late-onset alcoholics: a prospective, open-label study. Alcohol Clin Exp Res 27(7):1150–1155, 2003 12878921

Kranzler HR, Feinn R, Morris P, et al: A meta-analysis of the efficacy of gabapentin for treating alcohol use disorder. Addiction 114(9):1547–1555, 2019 31077485

Lam L, Anand S, Li X, et al: Efficacy and safety of naltrexone for amfetamine and methamfetamine use disorder: a systematic review of randomized controlled trials. Clin Toxicol (Phila) 57(4):225–233, 2019 30451013

Leggio L, Lee MR: Treatment of alcohol use disorder in patients with alcoholic liver disease. Am J Med 130(2):124–134, 2017 27984008

Lejoyeux M, Lehert P: Alcohol-use disorders and depression: results from individual patient data meta-analysis of the acamprosate-controlled studies. Alcohol Alcohol 46(1):61–67, 2011 21118900

Litten RZ, Ryan ML, Fertig JB, et al: A double-blind, placebo-controlled trial assessing the efficacy of varenicline tartrate for alcohol dependence. J Addict Med 7(4):277–286, 2013 23728065

Lotfy N, Elsawah H, Hassan M: Topiramate for smoking cessation: systematic review and meta-analysis. Tob Prev Cessat 6(February):14, 2020 32548351

Malone M, McDonald R, Vittitow A, et al: Extended-release vs. oral naltrexone for alcohol dependence treatment in primary care (XON). Contemp Clin Trials 81(June):102–109, 2019 30986535

Mason BJ, Crean R, Goodell V, et al: A proof-of-concept randomized controlled study of gabapentin: effects on cannabis use, withdrawal and executive function deficits in cannabis-dependent adults. Neuropsychopharmacology 37(7):1689–1698, 2012 22373942

McGeary JE, Knopik VS, Hayes JE, et al: Predictors of relapse in a bupropion trial for smoking cessation in recently-abstinent alcoholics: preliminary results using an aggregate genetic risk score. Subst Abuse 6(January):107–114, 2012 23032639

McKee SA, Weinberger AH: How can we use our knowledge of alcohol-tobacco interactions to reduce alcohol use? Annu Rev Clin Psychol 9(1):649–674, 2013 23157448

Minozzi S, Amato L, Davoli M, et al: Anticonvulsants for cocaine dependence. Cochrane Database Syst Rev 2015(4):CD006754, 2015 25882271

Minozzi S, Saulle R, Rösner S: Baclofen for alcohol use disorder. Cochrane Database Syst Rev 11(11):CD012557, 2018 30484285

Mitchell JM, Teague CH, Kayser AS, et al: Varenicline decreases alcohol consumption in heavy-drinking smokers. Psychopharmacology (Berl) 223(3):299–306, 2012 22547331

Morley KC, Baillie A, Leung S, et al: Baclofen for the treatment of alcohol dependence and possible role of comorbid anxiety. Alcohol Alcohol 49(6):654–660, 2014 25246489

Morley KC, Baillie A, Fraser I, et al: Baclofen in the treatment of alcohol dependence with or without liver disease: multisite, randomised, double-blind, placebo-controlled trial. Br J Psychiatry 212(6):362–369, 2018 29716670

Morley KC, Perry CJ, Watt J, et al: New approved and emerging pharmacological approaches to alcohol use disorder: a review of clinical studies. Expert Opin Pharmacother 22(10):1291–1303, 2021 33615945

Mosoni C, Dionisi T, Vassallo GA, et al: Baclofen for the treatment of alcohol use disorder in patients with liver cirrhosis: 10 years after the first evidence. Front Psychiatry 9(Oct):474, 2018 30327620

Naglich AC, Lin A, Wakhlu S, et al: Systematic review of combined pharmacotherapy for the treatment of alcohol use disorder in patients without comorbid conditions. CNS Drugs 32(1):13–31, 2018 29273901

Nielsen S, Gowing L, Sabioni P, et al: Pharmacotherapies for cannabis dependence. Cochrane Database Syst Rev 1(1):CD008940, 2019 30687936

Notzon DP, Kelly MA, Choi CJ, et al: Open-label pilot study of injectable naltrexone for cannabis dependence. Am J Drug Alcohol Abuse 44(6):619–627, 2018 29420073

Oon-Arom A, Likhitsathain S, Srisurapanont M: Efficacy and acceptability of varenicline for alcoholism: a systematic review and meta-analysis of randomized-controlled trials. Drug Alcohol Depend 205(December):107631, 2019 31678838

Oslin DW, Pettinati HM, Volpicelli JR, et al: The effects of naltrexone on alcohol and cocaine use in dually addicted patients. J Subst Abuse Treat 16(2):163–167, 1999 10023615

Palpacuer C, Duprez R, Huneau A, et al: Pharmacologically controlled drinking in the treatment of alcohol dependence or alcohol use disorders: a systematic review with direct and network meta-analyses on nalmefene, naltrexone, acamprosate, baclofen and topiramate. Addiction 113(2):220–237, 2018 28940866

Pettinati HM, Kampman KM, Lynch KG, et al: A double blind, placebo-controlled trial that combines disulfiram and naltrexone for treating co-occurring cocaine and alcohol dependence. Addict Behav 33(5):651–667, 2008a 18079068

Pettinati HM, Kampman KM, Lynch KG, et al: Gender differences with high-dose naltrexone in patients with co-occurring cocaine and alcohol dependence. J Subst Abuse Treat 34(4):378–390, 2008b 17664051

Pettinati HM, Oslin DW, Kampman KM, et al: A double-blind, placebo-controlled trial combining sertraline and naltrexone for treating co-occurring depression and alcohol dependence. Am J Psychiatry 167(6):668–675, 2010 20231324

Pettinati HM, Kampman KM, Lynch KG, et al: A pilot trial of injectable, extended-release naltrexone for the treatment of co-occurring cocaine and alcohol dependence. Am J Addict 23(6):591–597, 2014 25251201

Ray LA, Green R, Enders C, et al: Efficacy of combining varenicline and naltrexone for smoking cessation and drinking reduction: a randomized clinical trial. Am J Psychiatry 178(9):818–828, 2021 34080890

Rezaei F, Ghaderi E, Mardani R, et al: Topiramate for the management of methamphetamine dependence: a pilot randomized, double-blind, placebo-controlled trial. Fundam Clin Pharmacol 30(3):282–289, 2016 26751259

Rickels K, DeMartinis N, Rynn M, et al: Pharmacologic strategies for discontinuing benzodiazepine treatment. J Clin Psychopharmacol 19(6)(Suppl 2):12S–16S, 1999 10587279

Roberts W, Shi JM, Tetrault JM, et al: Effects of varenicline alone and in combination with low-dose naltrexone on alcohol-primed smoking in heavy-drinking tobacco users: a preliminary laboratory study. J Addict Med 12(3):227–233, 2018 29438157

Rolland B, Simon N, Franchitto N, et al: France grants an approval to baclofen for alcohol dependence. Alcohol 55(1):44–45, 2020 31761949

Rösner S, Hackl-Herrwerth A, Leucht S, et al: Acamprosate for alcohol dependence. Cochrane Database Syst Rev (9):CD004332, 2010 20824837

Roy-Byrne PP, Sullivan MD, Cowley DS, et al: Adjunctive treatment of benzodiazepine discontinuation syndromes: a review. J Psychiatr Res 27(Suppl 1):143–153, 1993 7908331

Santos GM, Coffin P, Santos D, et al: Feasibility, acceptability, and tolerability of targeted naltrexone for nondependent methamphetamine-using and binge-drinking men who have sex with men. J Acquir Immune Defic Syndr 72(1):21–30, 2016 26674372

Schacht JP, Randall PK, Latham PK, et al: Predictors of naltrexone response in a randomized trial: reward-related brain activation, OPRM1 genotype, and smoking status. Neuropsychopharmacology 42(13):2640–2653, 2017 28409564

Schmitz JM, Lindsay JA, Green CE, et al: High-dose naltrexone therapy for cocaine-alcohol dependence. Am J Addict 18(5):356–362, 2009 19874153

Schweizer E, Rickels K, Case WG, et al: Carbamazepine treatment in patients discontinuing long-term benzodiazepine therapy. Effects on withdrawal severity and outcome. Arch Gen Psychiatry 48(5):448–452, 1991 2021297

Sellers EM, Toneatto T, Romach MK, et al: Clinical efficacy of the 5-HT3 antagonist ondansetron in alcohol abuse and dependence. Alcohol Clin Exp Res 18(4):879–885, 1994 7978099

Shoptaw S, Yang X, Rotheram-Fuller EJ, et al: Randomized placebo-controlled trial of baclofen for cocaine dependence: preliminary effects for individuals with chronic patterns of cocaine use. J Clin Psychiatry 64(12):1440–1448, 2003 14728105

Shorter D, Lindsay JA, Kosten TR: The alpha-1 adrenergic antagonist doxazosin for treatment of cocaine dependence: a pilot study. Drug Alcohol Depend 131(1–2):66–70, 2013 23306096

Shorter DI, Zhang X, Domingo CB, et al: Doxazosin treatment in cocaine use disorder: pharmacogenetic response based on an alpha-1 adrenoreceptor subtype D genetic variant. Am J Drug Alcohol Abuse 46(2):184–193, 2020 31914324

Siefried KJ, Acheson LS, Lintzeris N, et al: Pharmacological treatment of methamphetamine/amphetamine dependence: a systematic review. CNS Drugs 34(4):337–365, 2020 32185696

Simpson TL, Saxon AJ, Stappenbeck C, et al: Double-blind randomized clinical trial of prazosin for alcohol use disorder. Am J Psychiatry 175(12):1216–1224, 2018 30153753

Sinha R, Wemm S, Fogelman N, et al: Moderation of prazosin's efficacy by alcohol withdrawal symptoms. Am J Psychiatry 178(5):447–458, 2021 33207935

Skinner MD, Lahmek P, Pham H, et al: Disulfiram efficacy in the treatment of alcohol dependence: a meta-analysis. PLoS One 9(2):e87366, 2014 24520330

Soyka M: Review: in alcohol use disorders, acamprosate is more effective for inducing abstinence while naltrexone is more effective for reducing heavy drinking and craving. Evid Based Ment Health 16(3):71–71, 2013 23604277

Squeglia LM, Tomko RL, Baker NL, et al: The effect of N-acetylcysteine on alcohol use during a cannabis cessation trial. Drug Alcohol Depend 185(Apr):17–22, 2018 29413434

Stewart H, Mitchell BG, Ayanga D, et al: Veteran adherence to oral versus injectable AUD medication treatment. Ment Health Clin 11(3):194–199, 2021 34026395

Tamargo JA, Sherman KE, Sékaly R-P, et al: Cocaethylene, simultaneous alcohol and cocaine use, and liver fibrosis in people living with and without HIV. Drug Alcohol Depend 232(Mar):109273, 2022 35033954

Traccis F, Presciuttini R, Pani PP, et al: Alcohol-medication interactions: a systematic review and meta-analysis of placebo-controlled trials. Neurosci Biobehav Rev 132(Jan):519–541, 2022 34826511

Trivedi MH, Walker R, Ling W, et al: Bupropion and naltrexone in methamphetamine use disorder. N Engl J Med 384(2):140–153, 2021 33497547

Verplaetse TL, Pittman BP, Shi JM, et al: Effect of lowering the dose of varenicline on alcohol self-administration in drinkers with alcohol use disorders. J Addict Med 10(3):166–173, 2016 27159341

Walter TJ, Navarro M, Thiele TE, et al: A preliminary, open-label study of naltrexone and bupropion combination therapy for treating binge drinking in human subjects. Alcohol 55(1):56–62, 2020 31746964

Yardley MM, Mirbaba MM, Ray LA: Pharmacological options for smoking cessation in heavy-drinking smokers. CNS Drugs 29(10):833–845, 2015 26507831

Yoon S-J, Pae C-U, Kim D-J, et al: Mirtazapine for patients with alcohol dependence and comorbid depressive disorders: a multicentre, open label study. Prog Neuropsychopharmacol Biol Psychiatry 30(7):1196–1201, 2006 16624467

Zhand N, Milin R: What do we know about the pharmacotheraputic management of insomnia in cannabis withdrawal: a systematic review. Am J Addict 27(6):453–464, 2018 30113101

Zhang X, Nielsen DA, Domingo CB, et al: Pharmacogenetics of dopamine β-hydroxylase in cocaine dependence therapy with doxazosin. Addict Biol 24(3):531–538, 2019 29498170

# 6

# Stimulants and Co-occurring Substance Use

Thanh Thuy Truong, M.D.

*Cocaine,* methamphetamine, and other stimulant use disorders are major public health concerns. In 2020, 5.2 million people ages 12 and older used cocaine, and 2.5 million used methamphetamine (Substance Abuse and Mental Health Services Administration 2022). Specifically, methamphetamine use has been steadily rising, increasing by 43% between 2015 and 2019 (Han et al. 2021). Cocaine and methamphetamine use are associated with multiple adverse health outcomes, including cardiovascular and pulmonary disease and psychiatric conditions such as psychosis, depression, and cognitive impairments. When combined with tobacco, cocaine use is associated with an even greater risk for stroke, myocardial infarction, pulmonary disease, and overall mortality (Winhusen et al. 2020). Moreover, overdose deaths involving cocaine and methamphetamine adulterated with synthetic opioids (primarily fentanyl) rose sharply between 2014 and 2020 (National Institute on Drug Abuse 2021).

Although several medications from different classes have been studied, there is no well-established pharmacotherapy or FDA-approved treatment for stimulant use disorder. Pharmacotherapy must be combined with psychosocial interventions, harm reduction strategies, psychotherapy, and contingency management to improve the quality of life for individuals struggling with multi-substance use disorder involving stimulants. The clinical approach involves establishing realistic expectations for pharmacotherapy and engaging patients in behavioral interventions to reduce craving and use. To ensure retention (especially during the early stages of treatment), we collaborate with them to find solutions to barriers such as transportation, scheduling around work, and cognitive impairments. Many patients will need assistance creating organization and structure, so practical strategies such as using a phone calendar, reminders, and daily schedules may be discussed during the appointment. Engagement in peer recovery programs, psychotherapy, and other recovery treatments should be encouraged. When considering pharmacotherapy, clinicians should collaborate with their patients to determine which substance causes the strongest cravings or has led to the most significant consequences. Providing a menu of reasonable options with informed consent and being forthcoming with patients about the role of medications (especially when they are being used off-label) in their overall recovery can empower them and increase their engagement in treatment. Generally, medications for stimulant use disorders exert their effects as substitution treatment (agonism or partial agonism), through antagonism of the stimulant's reinforcing effects, or by altering the pharmacokinetics of dopamine.

Goals of treatment include the following:

- Retention in treatment
- Reduction of harms from stimulant and other drug use
- Reduction of cravings
- Improvement of overall functioning by treating substance-induced and comorbid medical and psychiatric disorders
- Improvement of quality of life by adding psychosocial supports

# Cocaine Use Disorder

Cocaine's reinforcing effects stem from its blockade of norepinephrine and dopamine reuptake pumps, leading to euphoria and sympathetic physiological effects that include increased body temperature, heart rate, and blood pressure. Its anesthetic effects derive from blockade of sodium ion channels in nerve membranes. No medication has been FDA-approved or has demonstrated consistent efficacy for cocaine use disorder (CUD). Numerous clinical studies have examined medications from different classes, so in this section we focus on those that have demonstrated efficacy (Table 6–1).

**Table 6–1. Medications for cocaine use disorder**

| Medication | Dosage | Notes |
|---|---|---|
| Topiramate | 25–150 mg bid | Effective for reducing use and cravings and promoting abstinence. Consider for patients with comorbid AUD and migraines (or BED). May have cognitive side effects even at 50 mg/day. |
| Stimulants | | For methylphenidate and amphetamine stimulants, extended-release formulations may have lower risk of misuse. Strongly consider for patients with comorbid ADHD and CUD. May initiate at higher dosages rather than a slow titration from low dosages. Some patients may need dosing higher than that approved by the FDA for ADHD. |
| Methylphenidate ER | 18 to >72 mg/day | |
| Lisdexamfetamine | 30 to >70 mg/day | |
| Extended-release mixed amphetamine salts | 20–80 mg/day (patients in one study given 80 mg/day did better than those given 60 mg/day) (Levin et al. 2015) | |
| Modafinil | 200–400 mg/day | |
| Bupropion | SR: 150 mg qd for 3 days, then increase to 150 mg bid<br><br>XL: 150–300 mg/day (FDA approves up to 450 mg/day for depression) | Two studies showed efficacy of bupropion for CUD when combined with CBT and contingency management. Consider in patients with comorbid depression or TUD. |
| Doxazosin | Initiate at 2–4 mg/day; dosages up to 8 mg/day have been studied, but consider titrating above 8 mg as tolerated | Consider for patients with nightmares, PTSD, or hypertension. |
| Desipramine | Initiate at 25 mg/day, increase by 25–50 mg as tolerated up to 300 mg/day | May be more effective for patients with milder CUD, comorbid depression, or antisocial personality disorder. Desipramine and cocaine together may increase risk for cardiac arrhythmias. |

**Table 6–1.    Medications for cocaine use disorder** (*continued*)

| Medication | Dosage | Notes |
|---|---|---|
| Disulfiram | 250–500 mg/day | May be helpful for highly motivated patients, those under supervision or who have good social support to promote adherence, or patients with comorbid AUD. Treatment response depends on genetic variations. Alcohol exposure, even small amounts such as in hand sanitizer, causes unpleasant or dangerous physical symptoms. Adherence is generally low. |
| Ondansetron | 4 mg bid | Consider for patients with chronic nausea (e.g., from chemotherapy). Although ondansetron may reduce alcohol use in patients with early-onset AUD (before age 21), it has not been studied in patients with comorbid AUD and CUD. |
| Topiramate + mixed amphetamine salts | See dosing for individual medications | May be more effective for patients with high-frequency cocaine use. |

*Note.*  AUD=alcohol use disorder; BED=binge-eating disorder; CBT=cognitive-behavioral therapy; CUD=cocaine use disorder; ER=extended release; SR=sustained release; TUD=tobacco use disorder; XL=extended release; XR=extended release.

## Antidepressants

Among antidepressants, desipramine and bupropion have demonstrated efficacy for reducing cocaine use, although the therapeutic effect may not be as robust in patients with moderate to severe CUD. Reboxetine (not available in the United States) and maprotiline have shown efficacy in small open-label trials. Mirtazapine reduced cocaine use in patients treated with methadone in a small open-label trial but did not reduce cocaine use in another study with depressed patients. Selective serotonin reuptake inhibitor (SSRI), serotonin-norepinephrine reuptake inhibitor (SNRI), and monoamine oxidase inhibitor (MAOI) classes of antidepressants did not demonstrate greater efficacy than placebo (Chan et al. 2019b).

## Anticonvulsants

A systematic review of 20 clinical trials revealed that anticonvulsants other than topiramate (i.e., carbamazepine, gabapentin, lamotrigine, phenytoin, tiagabine, vigabatrin) did not have significant effects on treatment retention, cocaine use, or cocaine craving. Only topiramate was better than placebo at maintaining 3 weeks of cocaine abstinence (Minozzi et al. 2015).

## Antipsychotics

Antipsychotics as a class may improve retention but were not efficacious for abstinence or reducing use. Aripiprazole increased cocaine cravings in one study (Haney et al. 2011). Risperidone and paliperidone may be helpful for patients who are experiencing substance-induced or -exacerbated psychosis. The long-acting injectable form should be considered for patients struggling with medication adherence. However, antipsychotics increase risk of neuroleptic malignant syndrome when combined with stimulant use.

## Psychostimulants

A meta-analysis of stimulants as a class demonstrated efficacy for promoting 3 weeks of abstinence compared with placebo. Modafinil showed greater efficacy than placebo at reducing cocaine use (Castells et al. 2016). Among specific stimulants, consider using extended-release (ER) or sustained-release (SR) formulations such as methylphenidate ER, lisdexamfetamine, and extended-release mixed amphetamine salts because they generally have a lower risk of misuse compared with their immediate-release counterparts. Stimulants may be preferred for patients who also have comorbid ADHD.

## Other Pharmacotherapies

Disulfiram, doxazosin (Shorter et al. 2013), and ondansetron (Blevins et al. 2021; Johnson et al. 2006) have shown efficacy in small trials for CUD. Varenicline has shown mixed results for CUD. A 2022 randomized controlled trial (RCT) of varenicline plus cognitive-behavioral therapy was not effective (Lynch et al. 2022).

## Combination Treatments

The combination of topiramate plus mixed amphetamine salts has shown efficacy in reducing cocaine use. A combination of bupropion and contingency management was more effective than bupropion alone at reducing cocaine use in patients with opioid use disorder (OUD) who were receiving methadone (Chan et al. 2019b; Poling et al. 2006).

# Cocaine and Tobacco or Nicotine

Research in animal and human studies has established a strong relationship between cocaine and nicotine use, with approximately 80% of individuals who use cocaine also using nicotine/tobacco. Studies in rodents suggest that nicotine's stimulation of the nicotinic acetylcholine receptors (nAChRs) increases dopamine in the mesolimbic system, which potentiates self-administration of cocaine. In humans, the reinforcing effects of either cocaine or nicotine are enhanced by concurrent use of the other drug (Epstein et al. 2010; Morisano et al. 2009). Comorbid tobacco use among those with CUD is associated with earlier onset of cocaine use, more severe use disorders, more legal problems, and use of cocaine by intravenous or smoked methods (Roll et al. 1996). The consequences of this comorbidity also affect recovery, in which the number of cigarettes smoked is associated with cocaine use while in treatment (Harrell et al. 2011; Winhusen et al. 2014). Therefore, treatment of nicotine or tobacco use disorder (TUD) concurrently with CUD is essential to increase the likelihood of sustained recovery.

Data on single medications for treating comorbid CUD and TUD are limited. Therefore, we suggest combining evidence-based and FDA-approved treatments for TUD with those for CUD. Clinicians should ensure that patients know when treatments are being used off-label and should seek informed consent regarding potential treatment risks, benefits, and side effects. Both TUD and CUD are characterized by recurrence and remission; therefore, tailoring the treatment to the patient response and tolerability by adjusting the dosage and combining products is necessary for success (Chaiton et al. 2016). In our experience, combination therapy is the rule rather than the exception in most patients with CUD and TUD. FDA-approved treatments for TUDs include bupropion, varenicline, and nicotine replacement therapy (NRT), which includes the patch, gum, lozenges, vapor inhaler, and nasal spray. Table 6–2 summarizes medications for TUD.

## Nicotine Replacement Therapy

Nicotine gum, patches, and lozenges are available over the counter, whereas the nasal spray and vapor inhaler require a prescription. Combining a long-acting nicotine patch with a short-acting replacement, such as gum, lozenge, inhaler, or nasal spray, has been found to increase the odds of abstinence at 6 months. NRT should be dosed according to the patient's level of dependence. One cigarette is approximately equivalent to 1–2 mg of nicotine. Adequate dosing is assessed based on the relief of withdrawal symptoms. Some patients may need higher than 21 mg/day, up to 44 mg/day; higher dosages appear to be safe for heavy users (Dale et al. 1995). Short-acting therapy with nicotine gum and lozenges is available in 2-mg and 4-mg doses and is used for breakthrough cravings or nicotine withdrawal. The 4-mg dose may be more effective for patients who smoke more than 25 cigarettes per day or who smoke their first cigarette within 30 minutes of awakening (Sachs 1995). The nicotine nasal spray and inhaler are also effective but require a prescription. Combining the nasal spray or inhaler with a nicotine patch results in higher rates of cessation (Blondal et al. 1999; Bohadana et al. 2000).

## Bupropion

Bupropion is an antidepressant that inhibits reuptake of norepinephrine and dopamine, which may attenuate cravings for nicotine and alleviate nicotine withdrawal symptoms. In addition, bupropion's antagonism of the nAChRs likely underlies its efficacy for TUD in patients regardless of depressive symptoms. Although bupropion is available in extended-release, sustained-release, and immediate-release formulations, bupropion SR (150 mg bid) is the only FDA-approved TUD treatment. Bupropion SR increases the abstinence rate by approximately 52%–77% and has demonstrated safety and efficacy in patients with or without comorbid alcohol use disorder (AUD), chronic obstructive pulmonary disease, and cardiovascular disease (Howes et al. 2020; Tashkin et al. 2001; Tonstad et al. 2003). Bupropion may be preferred for patients concerned about weight gain with smoking cessation. The most com-

**Table 6–2. Pharmacotherapy for TUD and nicotine use disorder with or without CUD**

| Medication | Cigarettes per day | Dosage | Notes |
|---|---|---|---|
| Nicotine patch | <10<br>10–20<br>>21 | 7–14 mg/day<br>14–21 mg/day<br>>21 mg/day | OTC; patients with heavier use who respond partially to standard dosing may need multiple patches.<br><br>Side effects: Localized skin reactions. Can be alleviated by moving the patch to different sites or by using topical corticosteroids.<br><br>For sleep disturbance: Patients who have nicotine withdrawal overnight may sleep better with the patch on. If the patch causes vivid dreams, then they can take it off at night. |
| Nicotine gum or lozenge | <25 or first cigarette >30 minutes after rising<br>>25 or first cigarette <30 minutes after rising | 2 mg q 1–2 hours prn<br>4 mg q 1–2 hours prn | OTC; instruct patients to "chew and park" the gum between the gum and cheek rather than chew continuously. Lozenge comes in miniature sizes that dissolve more quickly. |
| Nicotine nasal spray | >1 | One dose (one spray per nostril) = 1 mg nicotine; one or two doses q 1–2 hours prn, up to five doses per hour | Requires prescription; spray has fast absorption and relieves withdrawal symptoms quicker than other NRT. Limited use due to side effects of nasal and throat irritation and higher cost. |

**Table 6–2.** Pharmacotherapy for TUD and nicotine use disorder with or without CUD (continued)

| Medication | Cigarettes per day | Dosage | Notes |
|---|---|---|---|
| Nicotine inhaler | >1 | One cartridge = 4 mg nicotine; 6–16 cartridges per day | Requires prescription; mimics ritual of puffing cigarettes but without rapid rise in nicotine concentrations associated with cigarettes. Side effects include coughing and throat or mouth irritation. Limited use due to cost and frequent puffing needed. |
| Bupropion* | >1 | SR: 150 mg qd for 3 days, then increase to 150 mg bid<br><br>XL: 150–300 mg/day (FDA approves up to 450 mg/day for depression) | Some patients may better tolerate SR 150 mg once daily or other formulations (extended- or immediate-release). May be preferred for patients who are concerned about weight gain with smoking cessation or have comorbid depression. Side effects include insomnia, dry mouth, and headache. Therapy should begin 1 week before target quit date (2–4 weeks after initiation of treatment) and may extend to a minimum of 12 weeks. Treatment duration of 1 year may increase likelihood of sustained abstinence. |

**Table 6–2.** Pharmacotherapy for TUD and nicotine use disorder with or without CUD (*continued*)

| Medication | Cigarettes per day | Dosage | Notes |
| --- | --- | --- | --- |
| Varenicline | >1 | Days 1–3: 0.5 mg qd<br>Days 4–7: 0.5 mg bid<br>Day 8: 1 mg bid | Most common side effects include nausea and sleep disturbance. Nausea often improves within first 2 weeks and can be mitigated by taking it with food. Vivid dreams and insomnia may be mitigated by taking the second dose earlier in the day or skipping the nighttime dose. Sleep disturbance may be due to nicotine withdrawal and not to varenicline. Treatment may extend to a minimum of 12 weeks. Treatment duration of 1 year may increase likelihood of sustained abstinence. |
| Bupropion + NRT* | >10 | See dosing for individual medications | Inconsistent evidence that bupropion + NRT is superior to NRT alone, but it should still be considered in patients who had partial response to bupropion. |
| Varenicline + NRT | >10 | See dosing for individual medications | Greater likelihood of abstinence compared with NRT alone. May be more effective for patients with moderate to severe TUD who did not have an adequate response to monotherapy. |

**Table 6–2.** Pharmacotherapy for TUD and nicotine use disorder with or without CUD *(continued)*

| Medication | Cigarettes per day | Dosage | Notes |
|---|---|---|---|
| Varenicline + bupropion* | >20 | See dosing for individual medications | Greater likelihood of abstinence compared with varenicline alone. May be more effective for patients with moderate to severe TUD who did not have an adequate response to monotherapy. Although combination has not been studied for comorbid TUD and CUD, it is effective in some patients with the comorbidity. |
| Nortriptyline | >10 | Initiate at 25 mg/day, increase every 3 days to weekly as tolerated up to 100 mg/day | Second-line treatment for TUD. Common side effects are dry mouth, sedation, and orthostatic hypotension. Consider in patients with comorbid pain and depression whose TUD did not respond to standard agents. Contraindicated in patients taking an MAOI or those in the acute recovery period from a myocardial infarction. May unmask Brugada syndrome. Monitoring includes heart rate, ECG, and blood pressure in adults who already have existing cardiac disease and in elderly patients. |

Note.   CUD=cocaine use disorder; ECG=electrocardiogram; MAOI=monoamine oxidase inhibitor; NRT=nicotine replacement therapy; OTC=over-the-counter; SR=sustained release; TUD=tobacco use disorder; XL=extended release.
*Possible benefit for CUD.

mon side effects are insomnia, dry mouth, and headache. Patients should be instructed to take the first dose in the early morning and the second dose in the early afternoon to prevent insomnia. Patients who do not tolerate the side effects may take 150 mg once daily. Bupropion XL (extended release) has not been as extensively studied but was efficacious in a small trial with older adolescents (Gray et al. 2012). This formulation may be better tolerated, with improved adherence in some patients. On the other hand, some patients may tolerate only the immediate-release formulation because of the insomnia side effect, which may be related to variations in bupropion metabolism by the enzyme cytochrome P450 (CYP) 2B6 (Tran et al. 2019). Bupropion may lower the seizure threshold and is contraindicated in patients with seizure disorders and eating disorders. Although it may be safely combined with antidepressants such as SSRIs and SNRIs, it is contraindicated in patients taking MAOIs.

## Varenicline

Varenicline (1 mg twice daily) is a partial agonist at the $\alpha_4\beta_2$ nAChR, activating the nAChR at 30%–60% compared with nicotine and blocking nicotine's ability to bind to the receptor. Varenicline more than doubles the rate of abstinence compared with placebo. It has also demonstrated superior efficacy to bupropion and NRT (Cahill et al. 2013; Gonzales et al. 2006). In 2009, the FDA issued a safety warning for suicidal thoughts associated with varenicline use; this was removed in 2016 on the basis of a reanalysis of several studies and a large RCT with 8,144 participants that found no increase in neuropsychiatric events, including depression, suicidal ideation, and suicide attempts (Anthenelli et al. 2016; U.S. Food and Drug Administration 2019).

## Nortriptyline

Nortriptyline (75–100 mg/day) is a tricyclic antidepressant that inhibits the reuptake of serotonin and norepinephrine, thereby increasing the concentration of those neurotransmitters in the synapse. Nortriptyline also antagonizes $H_1$ histaminic, $\alpha_1$-adrenergic, and muscarinic cholinergic receptors. Multiple studies have shown superior efficacy of nortriptyline compared with placebo for smoking cessation, and it may be as efficacious as bupropion. It is considered a second-line medication and is not FDA-approved for TUD (Howes et al. 2020; Wagena et al. 2005). Because it is indicated for use in depression and chronic pain (off-label), nortriptyline may be considered for patients with chronic pain or depression that is unresponsive to standard treatments. The most common side effects are sedation and dry mouth. Nortriptyline is contraindicated in patients taking an MAOI and should be used with caution in patients recovering from a myocardial infarction.

## Combination Therapy

In our experience, most patients with moderate to severe TUD need a combination of products to achieve abstinence. Studies have demonstrated superior efficacy for the combinations of varenicline and NRT or varenicline and bupropion compared with varenicline alone (Koegelenberg et al. 2014; Vogeler et al. 2016). Evidence that bupropion plus NRT is superior to NRT monotherapy is inconsistent, although this combination is still worth considering in patients who have a partial response (Howes et al. 2020). For patients with mild to moderate TUD, a nicotine patch plus gum or lozenge may be adequate. For patients with moderate to severe TUD, consider initiating with bupropion or varenicline with a short-acting NRT and evaluate after 2 weeks for a response. If the patient continues to have significant breakthrough cravings or nicotine withdrawal and is using more than 10 mg of short-acting NRT daily, consider adding a patch. For patients who have a partial response to initial therapy, adding either bupropion or varenicline may be indicated.

## Electronic Nicotine Delivery Systems

Also known as electronic (e-)cigarettes and marketed as safe alternatives to standard tobacco products, nicotine vaping has soared in popularity among youth and adults in recent years. Many patients switched from smoking cigarettes to using e-cigarettes to reduce their use or to achieve abstinence. There is weak evidence that, compared with placebo or behavioral support alone, e-cigarettes are more efficacious for tobacco abstinence and may be as efficacious as NRT (Hartmann-Boyce et al. 2021). Use of e-cigarettes concurrently with conventional cigarettes appears to be associated with more attempts to quit but not with abstinence (Brose et al. 2015). E-cigarettes contain formaldehyde and acetaldehyde and may increase cancer risk, possibly at lower levels than conventional cigarettes. E-cigarette or vaping use associated with lung injury has resulted in thousands of hospitalizations (Kosmider et al. 2020; Triantafyllou et al. 2021). Given the uncertainty of long-term health risks associated with electronic nicotine delivery systems, we do not recommend this option over well-established treatments. In our experience, some patients who switch end up using more nicotine per day than they did with conventional cigarettes. In patients already using nicotine vaping to reduce harm, the clinician may provide psychoeducation on the risks of use, encourage setting a quit date for vaping, and offer medications.

# Cocaine and Alcohol

Among people with CUD, up to 90% also have AUD. Alcohol is often used concurrently with cocaine to enhance and prolong the euphoric effects of cocaine. These effects are partially mediated by the formation of the psychoactive metabolite cocaethylene, a highly cardiotoxic compound with a half-life three times that of cocaine. Concurrent alcohol use also raises plasma cocaine levels by up to 30% compared with cocaine alone. Aside from increased euphorigenic effects, alcohol is used to reduce the discomfort of coming down from cocaine (Pennings et al. 2002).

## Topiramate

Topiramate's (up to 150 mg twice daily) varied mechanism may explain its efficacy in AUD and CUD. It inhibits state-dependent sodium channels and voltage-activated L-type calcium channels, increases GABA concentrations and potentiates GABA transmission, and inhibits glutamatergic activity via α-amino-3-hydroxy-5-methyl-4-isoxazolepropionic acid (AMPA) or kainate receptors. Topiramate has been shown in multiple RCTs to reduce alcohol use and recurrence (Guglielmo et al. 2015). For CUD, topiramate has shown efficacy in some trials in reducing the frequency and amount of cocaine use and in increasing treatment retention (Minozzi et al. 2015). However, in an RCT for comorbid CUD and AUD, topiramate was not more efficacious than placebo in preventing return to either substance (Kampman et al. 2013). Despite reducing alcohol craving, topiramate was not effective at reducing alcohol use. The authors posited that this result was due to the participants having lower severity of alcohol use compared with those of other studies examining topiramate for AUD. The study subjects were mostly African Americans with crack cocaine use, and the results may not be generalizable to other populations. On the other hand, topiramate-treated participants were more likely to achieve 3 weeks of continuous abstinence from cocaine (20% vs. 7%) by the end of the trial, particularly those with more severe cocaine withdrawal symptoms. Results also favored topiramate for treatment retention.

## Naltrexone

For patients who preferentially use alcohol and have low cravings or negative consequences from cocaine use, naltrexone (150 mg/day) should be considered. Naltrexone is a μ opioid antagonist with robust evidence and FDA approval for treatment of AUD. One open-label study demonstrated efficacy at higher dosages (150 mg/day) for combined treatment of cocaine and AUD. Other studies failed to show efficacy at 50 mg/day or 100 mg/day. A placebo-controlled trial of long-acting naltrexone injection did not result in a reduction of cocaine or alcohol use (Oslin et al. 1999; Pettinati et al. 2014; Schmitz et al. 2009).

## Disulfiram

Disulfiram's mechanism for reducing alcohol use involves inhibition of acetaldehyde dehydrogenase, which leads to accumulation of acetaldehyde, causing an adverse reaction on alcohol exposure. Ingesting alcohol, even in small amounts (i.e., hand sanitizer), while taking disulfiram (250 mg/day) may result in flushing, nausea/vomiting, shortness of breath, diaphoresis, chest pain, tachycardia, and hypotension. Severe reactions may involve cardiovascular collapse, acute congestive heart failure, respiratory failure, seizure, and death. For CUD, the mechanism is thought to be disulfiram's inhibition of the enzyme dopamine β-hydroxylase (DβH), which is responsible for converting dopamine into norepinephrine, thereby increasing dopamine concentrations and reducing cocaine craving. A meta-analysis of seven trials showed a trend of superiority to placebo in dropout, frequency of cocaine use, and number of weeks of abstinence, although some of the trials showed no significant difference in the proportion of patients who achieved 3 weeks of abstinence (Pani et al. 2010). The treatment response for CUD may depend on genetic variations of DβH, the dopamine transporter, dopamine $D_2$ receptors, the $\alpha_{1A}$-adrenoceptor gene, ankyrin repeat, or kinase domain-containing protein 1 (ANNK1). Sex may also influence efficacy, with females being less likely to respond than males (Chan et al. 2019b; Kampangkaew et al. 2019). Disulfiram may appeal to highly motivated patients who can adhere to a daily medication schedule. Patients should be warned that this drug may increase plasma cocaine concentrations, blood pressure, and heart rate. Use with caution in patients with cardiovascular disease.

## Disulfiram Plus Naltrexone

Patients receiving a combination of disulfiram 250 mg/day and naltrexone 100 mg/day were more likely to achieve 3 continuous weeks of abstinence from cocaine and alcohol compared with placebo or use of either medication alone. However, medication adherence was low (<50% of patients took 80% of the medications) (Pettinati et al. 2008).

## Other Combinations

Although there has been no clear evidence for use of other combined treatments, we have tried combinations of stimulants plus naltrexone, stimulants plus topiramate, and topiramate plus naltrexone in patients with treatment-refractory CUD and AUD and have had varying success in our complex patient population.

# Cocaine and Methamphetamine

Colloquially termed "croak," the mixture of methamphetamine and crack cocaine constituted 12% of emergency department visits in 2011 (Substance Abuse and Mental Health Services Administration 2014). In our experience, individuals tend to prefer either cocaine or methamphetamine. Cocaine users who have had a negative experience with methamphetamine (i.e., methamphetamine-induced psychosis) may use cocaine unless it becomes unavailable, at which time they would use methamphetamine. Those who transition from cocaine to methamphetamine tend to transition to methamphetamine exclusively. We did not find any investigational treatments for this combination. Thus, clinicians should consider a pharmacotherapeutic approach when treating cocaine-dominant or methamphetamine-dominant use disorders as detailed in other sections of this chapter.

# Methamphetamine or Amphetamine Use Disorder

Amphetamines exert their action by binding to monoamine transporters and inhibiting dopamine and norepinephrine reuptake, as well as serotonin reuptake, although less significantly. Unlike methylphenidate and cocaine, amphetamines also act as monoamine releasers by reversing the direction of transporter efflux and inhibiting vesicular monoamine transporters, which increases the cytoplasmic concentrations of amines available for release (Miller et al. 2019). Methamphetamine is a potent amphetamine that can be snorted, smoked, or injected. It is associated with a number of negative health consequences, including chronic psychosis, cardiovascular disease, hepatitis B and C, and HIV. In 2020, 2.6 million people age 12 or older reported using methamphetamine (Substance Abuse and Mental Health Services Administration 2022). Heralded as the fourth wave of the opioid crisis, drug overdoses from a mixture of opioids and methamphetamine increased more than eightfold between 2012 and 2019 (Han et al. 2021). Most medications tried for CUD have also been tested for methamphetamine use disorder (MUD), but few options have demonstrated efficacy. Therefore, any pharmacotherapy must be combined with psychosocial interventions, psychotherapy, harm reduction, and contingency management if possible to improve quality of life, functioning, and treatment retention.

## Antidepressants

Among antidepressants, mirtazapine showed efficacy in reducing methamphetamine use and risky sexual behaviors in a small study with cisgender men and transgender women who have sex with men. Other antidepressants in the SSRI class and bupropion did not show efficacy (Chan et al. 2019a).

## Anticonvulsants

In a multicenter RCT with 140 participants, topiramate was more effective than placebo at reducing use and recurrence rates. However, it was not effective at promoting abstinence. Baclofen and gabapentin were not more effective than placebo for use, abstinence, craving, or retention. However, in a secondary analysis of participants who were more adherent to the study medication, the baclofen group had a significant reduction in methamphetamine use (Chan et al. 2019a).

## Antipsychotics

Among antipsychotics, risperidone reduced methamphetamine use in two open-label trials (Meredith et al. 2007, 2009). Paliperidone reduces methamphetamine-induced psychotic symptoms and improves treatment retention but does not reduce methamphetamine use (Wang et al. 2019). Aripiprazole is not more effective than placebo at reducing use and is associated with adverse side effects (e.g., fatigue, akathisia). Aripiprazole treatment may also increase the rewarding effects of methamphetamine (Newton et al. 2008). A case series of two patients taking cariprazine showed a reduction of use and cravings and a longer time to return to use. Two other case reports demonstrated the role of cariprazine in improving stimulant-induced psychosis and substance use (Ricci et al. 2022; Rodriguez Cruz et al. 2021; Truong and Li

2022). Treatment with antipsychotics appears to increase retention and reduce psychotic symptoms among patients with methamphetamine-induced psychosis, and we favor using long-acting injectable formulations of risperidone and paliperidone. Once patients can engage in treatment, they may have improved insight into the negative consequences of methamphetamine use.

## Atomoxetine

Atomoxetine is a nonstimulant medication for ADHD that inhibits the norepinephrine transporter, leading to an increase in norepinephrine and, to a lesser extent, dopamine concentration in the prefrontal cortex. A small RCT ($N=69$) in patients receiving buprenorphine/naloxone for OUD showed a significant reduction in methamphetamine cravings and a higher proportion of negative urine drug screens in the group given atomoxetine (80 mg/day) compared with the placebo group. It also reduced depressive symptoms more than placebo (Schottenfeld et al. 2018). Atomoxetine is not a controlled substance and has low misuse potential and thus may be preferred for clinicians and patients, especially patients with comorbid ADHD.

## Psychostimulants

Akin to opioid agonist treatment, stimulants have been studied extensively for amphetamine use disorder or MUD. A meta-analysis of 11 RCTs showed that stimulants as a class (i.e., modafinil, methylphenidate, dexamphetamine) were not more effective than placebo at reducing use or promoting abstinence. However, two individual RCTs favored methylphenidate for the reduction of use (Chan et al. 2019a). Methylphenidate was well tolerated and effective at reducing ADHD symptoms and methamphetamine use in individuals receiving opioid agonist treatment, especially when combined with contingency management. When combined with the Matrix Model treatment, methylphenidate had positive effects on methamphetamine use, craving, addiction severity, mental health, and rates of recurrence (Aryan et al. 2020). The Matrix Model is an evidence-based approach for addiction that combines various therapeutic techniques to address substance use disorders. It integrates individual counseling, group therapy, family education, drug testing, psychoeducation, relapse prevention strategies, and social support.

An RCT of methylphenidate ER doses up to 180 mg/day in criminal offenders with amphetamine use disorder (intravenous amphetamine use) and ADHD showed a reduction of amphetamine and other substance use, better treatment retention, and improvement of ADHD symptoms (Konstenius et al. 2014). A small open-label trial ($N=16$) of high-dose lisdexamfetamine (250 mg/day) reported that it was well tolerated in frequent methamphetamine users and significantly reduced methamphetamine use, with three participants achieving 2 weeks of abstinence (Ezard et al. 2021).

A Swedish cohort study published in *JAMA Psychiatry* in 2022 investigated the association between pharmacotherapies and hospitalization and mortality outcomes in 13,965 participants with amphetamine use disorder or MUD who did not have previous diagnoses of schizophrenia or bipolar disorder. Lisdexamfetamine was the only medication significantly associated with a decreased risk of substance use disorder (SUD) hospitalization, any hospitalization or death, and all-cause mortality. Methylphenidate was also associated with decreased all-cause mortality. In this study, the most beneficial lisdexamfetamine dosages ranged from 45 mg/day to 85 mg/day (Heikkinen et al. 2022). In summary, methylphenidate ER and lisdexamfetamine would be reasonably considered first-line treatment for moderate to severe MUD, particularly for those with comorbid ADHD. The extended-release formulations are less likely to create a "high" due to a slower onset of action.

### Combination Pharmacotherapy

In a trial of bupropion 450 mg plus naltrexone 380 mg extended-release injectable every 3 weeks, 13.6% of participants in the active treatment group compared with 2.5% of those in the placebo group obtained three out of four methamphetamine-negative urine samples in a 6-week period (Trivedi et al. 2021).

# Methamphetamine and Tobacco/Nicotine

Methamphetamine and tobacco/nicotine are often used together, possibly to heighten euphoric effects. In rats, administration of methamphetamine fully substitutes for nicotine, and nicotine partially substitutes for methamphetamine reinforcement. The mechanism of the enhanced euphoria may be due to modulation of dopamine release in the nucleus accumbens by both substances (Gatch et al. 2008). Methamphetamine and tobacco independently have adverse effects on pulmonary and cardiovascular health; thus, concurrent use may compound these risks (Kaye et al. 2007; Tsai et al. 2019). Some methamphetamine users experience an increase in nicotine craving when abstaining from methamphetamine and will need more support for TUD treatment in the initial weeks after they attempt to quit. NRT may reduce the intensity of methamphetamine cravings (Magee et al. 2016). Effective pharmacotherapy for MUD is limited, and recovery should incorporate nonpharmacological interventions. We suggest combining treatments for TUD (see Table 6–2) with medications for MUD (Table 6–3). Weekly assessment of use and cravings is recommended. If cravings and use of nicotine and methamphetamine have been reduced to a level manageable with behavioral interventions, continue the patient's current dosage of medications. If cravings and use continue to be significant, consider increasing the dosage. The following examples are based on the author's experience:

- Bupropion + naltrexone 380 mg IM + NRT: the combination of bupropion and naltrexone injection with NRT (gum, lozenge, patch) is suggested for use as needed for breakthrough nicotine cravings.
- Methylphenidate, lisdexamfetamine, or atomoxetine ± NRT ± varenicline: Individuals with comorbid ADHD may experience greater benefit from this combination for the management of both ADHD and MUD. Those with a higher severity of TUD may need a combination of NRT and varenicline.
- Topiramate ± NRT ± varenicline: This combination should be considered for individuals with comorbid AUD or CUD. Note that topiramate may exacerbate ADHD and other cognitive symptoms.
- Cariprazine or risperidone ± NRT ± varenicline: This combination should be considered for individuals with psychotic and bipolar disorders (either primary or substance induced).

## Methamphetamine and Cannabis

Cannabis is one of the most-used substances in the world and the most-used illicit substance in the United States. In the United States and other countries, use rates have increased in the past decade because of legalization, greater access, permissive attitudes, and lower perceived risk (Manthey et al. 2021; Palamar et al. 2021). Cannabis products are used for the treatment of various physical and mental conditions, including pain, anxiety, and insomnia. $\Delta$-9-Tetrahydrocannabinol ($\Delta$-9 THC) and cannabidiol (CBD) are the two most common cannabinoids in the marijuana plant. THC acts as a partial agonist at the cannabinoid receptors $CB_1$ and $CB_2$ and is responsible for the major behavioral and subjective effects of cannabis, including euphoria, reward, withdrawal, and the development of cannabis use disorder (CaUD). In contrast,

**Table 6–3.** Medications for methamphetamine use disorder

| Medication | Dosage | Notes |
|---|---|---|
| **Stimulants** | | |
| Methylphenidate ER | Up to 180 mg/day | ER formulations may have lower risk of misuse. Strongly consider for patients with comorbid ADHD and MUD. May initiate at higher dosages rather than a slow titration from low dosages. Some patients may need dosing higher than that approved by the FDA, but going too far beyond FDA-approved dosages is not recommended because of limited evidence for safety and efficacy (i.e., 250 mg/day of lisdexamfetamine is not recommended). Adverse side effects may include irritability and hypomania or mania at higher dosages. |
| Lisdexamfetamine | 30 mg to >70 mg/day | |
| Atomoxetine | 80–100 mg | Nonstimulant option with low risk of misuse. May be effective for ADHD. |
| Bupropion + naltrexone | Bupropion XL 450 mg + IM naltrexone ER 380 mg q 3 weeks | Reduces methamphetamine use and cravings and depression. Consider for patients with comorbid AUD who would benefit from naltrexone. |
| Topiramate | 25–150 mg bid | Reduces amount of use and recurrence rates. Consider for patients with comorbid AUD, CUD, or migraines. May have cognitive side effects even at 50 mg/day and worsen ADHD. Twice-daily dosing may limit adherence. |
| Mirtazapine | 30–60 mg/day | At 30 mg/day, reduces methamphetamine use and sexual risk behaviors in cisgender men and transgender women who have sex with men. Consider for patients with depression and insomnia severity. Risk of weight gain may not be acceptable to some patients with MUD. |

**Table 6–3. Medications for methamphetamine use disorder** (*continued*)

| Medication | Dosage | Notes |
|---|---|---|
| Cariprazine | 1.5–6 mg/day | Reduced methamphetamine cravings and use in a small case series with two patients with severe MUD and multiple co-occurring disorders who did not respond to other treatments. Consider for patients with co-occurring psychosis or bipolar disorder. |
| **Antipsychotics** | | Consider for patients experiencing chronic psychotic symptoms (whether methamphetamine induced or primary psychotic disorder). Low evidence for reducing methamphetamine use and cravings but may improve treatment retention. Higher risk of extrapyramidal symptoms and neuroleptic malignant syndrome in stimulant users. Long-acting injectable equivalents preferred to improve adherence. |
| Risperidone | 0.5–6 mg/day | |
| Paliperidone | 3–12 mg/day | |

*Note.* AUD=alcohol use disorder; CUD=cocaine use disorder; ER=extended release; MUD=methamphetamine use disorder; TUD=tobacco use disorder; XL=extended release.

CBD acts as an antagonist at $CB_1$ receptors and a partial agonist at $CB_2$ receptors and has antireward effects. THC, CBD, and other cannabinoids are available in pure, isolated forms and can be consumed as edibles, smoked, or vaped. Cannabis potency, measured by the THC concentration in herbal cannabis products, has increased in the past decade in the United States and Europe. Higher THC concentration is associated with progression to the first symptom of CaUD, greater severity of CaUD, and increased risk of psychosis (Di Forti et al. 2019; ElSohly et al. 2021; Hines et al. 2020).

Concurrent use of cannabis is common among amphetamine users, particularly among those who inject amphetamines. One study found that amphetamine users were seven times more likely to use cannabis compared with nonusers (Massaro et al. 2017). Despite the high prevalence of cannabis and amphetamine co-use, few studies have examined the interaction between the two drugs. In our clinic, methamphetamine users report using cannabis to relieve agitation, anxiety, and insomnia associated with methamphetamine intoxication. Others use the combination to prolong and intensify the euphoric effects of methamphetamine. Many people continue using cannabis even when they have stopped using amphetamines or methamphetamine, which they see as carrying a higher risk. However, concurrent use of methamphetamine and cannabis is associated with a greater risk of psychosis, cognitive impairment, and neurotoxicity than either substance alone (Cuzen et al. 2015).

We did not find any studies examining pharmacotherapy for comorbid amphetamine use disorder and CaUD. There is a paucity of data to determine whether one treatment that reduces methamphetamine cravings would also reduce cannabis cravings, even if it may be effective for each substance alone. In our patient population, we choose medications that have individual data for use in MUD and CaUD and combine medications when appropriate. Taking a harm reduction approach may include using products with a lower THC concentration, using edibles, or transitioning to pure CBD. For patients using cannabis to treat various symptoms such as anxiety or insomnia, we recommend medications in place of cannabis.

## Naltrexone

A placebo-controlled trial of maintenance naltrexone 50 mg/day found it to reduce the reinforcing effects of cannabis and cannabis self-administration in daily users (Haney et al. 2015). An open-label pilot trial with naltrexone injection reduced frequency but not quantity of use. Only 3 of 12 participants reported abstinence (Notzon et al. 2018). As discussed earlier, naltrexone injection combined with bupropion may reduce methamphetamine use. There are currently no data on the effectiveness of naltrexone for the comorbidity of methamphetamine use and cannabis use, but these trials suggest it has potential for reducing both methamphetamine and cannabis cravings and use.

## N-Acetylcysteine

Studies of N-acetylcysteine (NAC) for CaUD have been mixed for promoting abstinence and reducing cravings. NAC may be more likely to be effective in adolescents (younger than 21 years) and at higher dosages (2,400 mg/day) (Sharma et al. 2022). We use NAC in our clinic for adolescents with CaUD in addition to medications used to treat MUD. However, prognosis depends on patient motivation and engagement in other aspects of treatment.

## Gabapentin

Gabapentin (1,200 mg/day in divided doses) reduced cannabis withdrawal, cravings, and use in a small RCT (Brezing and Levin 2018). A challenge when using gabapentin to treat CaUD in the context of MUD is the limited literature on the effects of gabapentin when combined with other commonly used medications for MUD. Gabapentin combined with topiramate, for example, may carry greater risks of cognitive impairment than either medication alone. However, gabapentin combined with naltrexone has been shown to be effective and well tolerated for AUD. We extrapolate from these studies on alcohol that this combination may be tolerable. Data on the combination of gabapentin and stimulants are limited. One case study examined gabapentin and methylphenidate use in a patient with comorbid ADHD and bipolar disorder (Hamrin and Bailey 2001). In summary, gabapentin may be a reasonable option for patients who experience significant cannabis withdrawal and cravings, but if other medications are used, drug-drug interactions should be carefully monitored.

## Cannabidiol

There is emerging evidence for CBD to reduce cannabis cravings and use, but the research is new, and its effectiveness in larger populations has yet to be seen. One study found that CBD in 400-mg and 800-mg doses was efficacious at reducing cannabis use, withdrawal, and craving (Freeman et al. 2020). Preclinical studies suggest the potential of CBD in reducing stimulant use and recurrence (Razavi et al. 2021).

# ADHD and Stimulant Use

ADHD has a high prevalence among stimulant users. One Australian study found that the rate of ADHD among methamphetamine and cocaine users was 45% (Kaye et al. 2013). Other studies identified ADHD in more than 50% of participants with methamphetamine use (Miovský et al. 2021). Thus, it is important that clinicians screen and provide treatment for ADHD in all patients with SUD. Concerns about misuse and diversion may make some clinicians reluctant to treat ADHD using stimulants in this population. However, treatment of ADHD has been shown to reduce substance use and to improve psychiatric comorbidities and quality of life. Furthermore, individuals with stimulant use disorder and ADHD may need higher dosages of stimulants to improve ADHD symptoms and psychosocial functioning, but the dosage may stabilize after 2 years. These improvements may be more gradual than in patients with ADHD alone (Chamakalayil et al. 2021; Skoglund et al. 2017). The benefits of treating ADHD with stimulants may outweigh the risks of misuse and diversion in many patients. Practical strategies to reduce these risks include using extended-release preparations with lower misuse potential (i.e., methylphenidate ER or lisdexamfetamine), urine drug testing, and frequent follow-up. Before initiating treatment, we inform patients of clinic guidelines for drug testing and follow-up. We also follow up with them monthly for at least the initial 12 months of treatment until they have demonstrated stability for a sustained period. If there is a recurrence of use or suspicion of misuse, we increase the frequency of appointments and urine drug testing (e.g., from monthly to biweekly).

# Clinical Practice

We have presented several medication options for stimulant use disorder, but these have yet to demonstrate consistent effectiveness in clinical trials or real-world settings for treatment outcomes such as retention, reduced use, and abstinence. In the clinic, we have found that basic principles of care such as the therapeutic alliance significantly affect patient outcomes. Several patients attribute their improvement to our doctor-patient relationship, which motivates them to attend their appointments and follow recommendations. Other principles include stabilizing acute medical or psychiatric conditions first. For example, a patient's psychosis must be stabilized with an antipsychotic before a deeper SUD evaluation and treatment can begin. As with any management of chronic conditions, a relapsing-remitting course should be expected. Recurrences are approached as added information to help the clinician and the patient understand what works and what needs to be changed. It is also necessary to regroup when patient and clinician goals do not align. Ambivalence toward change is expected and celebrated as part of an important rational decision-making process. The clinician helps the patient verbalize their ambivalence, which helps to reduce impulsive reactions.

# Case Example

A 25-year-old veteran with MUD and TUD has been admitted four times for methamphetamine-induced psychosis. With each hospitalization, her psychosis improves with risperidone and she is discharged after a few days, only to return 1–2 weeks later with the same symptoms. She reports auditory hallucinations and mild paranoia even when not acutely intoxicated and does not continue her medications as an outpatient for fear of being harmed while sleeping. She takes methamphetamine to stay on watch. These behaviors have significantly interfered with her life and have made her unable to attend follow-up appointments.

This veteran has struggled to engage in her recovery meaningfully and should be assessed for barriers to care, including housing, financial stability, and transportation needs. She would benefit from a residential treatment program and case management to promote treatment retention. Psychotherapeutically, motivational interviewing should be incorporated into every encounter to guide her in making healthy decisions and build rapport. Pharmacologically, a long-acting injectable such as paliperidone palmitate should be considered for her persistent methamphetamine psychosis. During this patient's hospitalization, a nicotine patch and as-needed gum or lozenge should be available for nicotine cravings and withdrawal. When her psychotic symptoms have stabilized, the clinician should assess for other psychiatric comorbidities such as depression, anxiety, and ADHD. Although stimulants can be helpful for MUD, they carry a risk of worsening her psychosis in the acute period. Therefore, if she continues to have significant methamphetamine cravings, the clinician should consider adding atomoxetine, topiramate, or oral naltrexone, with later transition to intramuscular formulation if well tolerated. The choice of medications may depend on the possibility of comorbid ADHD and the likelihood of adherence to daily to twice-daily dosing.

# Conclusion

Treating stimulant use disorders continues to be challenging for patients and clinicians. Although we have discussed potentially helpful medications, we must emphasize that none of these has shown consistent and robust efficacy. Therefore, pharmacotherapy must be combined with psychotherapy and psychosocial interventions. We support our patients in their journey to create a meaningful life outside substance use, including attaining employment, building a sober support network, and engaging or reengaging with their families.

# References

Anthenelli RM, Benowitz NL, West R, et al: Neuropsychiatric safety and efficacy of varenicline, bupropion, and nicotine patch in smokers with and without psychiatric disorders (EAGLES): a double-blind, randomised, placebo-controlled clinical trial. Lancet 387(10037):2507–2520, 2016 27116918

Aryan N, Banafshe HR, Farnia V, et al: The therapeutic effects of methylphenidate and matrix-methylphenidate on addiction severity, craving, relapse and mental health in the methamphetamine use disorder. Subst Abuse Treat Prev Policy 15(1):72, 2020 32977820

Blevins D, Seneviratne C, Wang X-Q, et al: A randomized, double-blind, placebo-controlled trial of ondansetron for the treatment of cocaine use disorder with post hoc pharmacogenetic analysis. Drug Alcohol Depend 228(Nov):109074, 2021 34600264

Blondal T, Gudmundsson LJ, Olafsdottir I, et al: Nicotine nasal spray with nicotine patch for smoking cessation: randomised trial with six year follow up. BMJ 318(7179):285–288, 1999 9924052

Bohadana A, Nilsson F, Rasmussen T, et al: Nicotine inhaler and nicotine patch as a combination therapy for smoking cessation: a randomized, double-blind, placebo-controlled trial. Arch Intern Med 160(20):3128–3134, 2000 11074742

Brezing CA, Levin FR: The current state of pharmacological treatments for cannabis use disorder and withdrawal. Neuropsychopharmacology 43(1):173–194, 2018 28875989

Brose LS, Hitchman SC, Brown J, et al: Is the use of electronic cigarettes while smoking associated with smoking cessation attempts, cessation and reduced cigarette consumption? A survey with a 1-year follow-up. Addiction 110(7):1160–1168, 2015 25900312

Cahill K, Stevens S, Perera R, et al: Pharmacological interventions for smoking cessation: an overview and network meta-analysis. Cochrane Database Syst Rev 2013(5):CD009329, 2013 23728690

Castells X, Cunill R, Pérez-Mañá C, et al: Psychostimulant drugs for cocaine dependence. Cochrane Database Syst Rev 9(9):CD007380, 2016 27670244

Chaiton M, Diemert L, Cohen JE, et al: Estimating the number of quit attempts it takes to quit smoking successfully in a longitudinal cohort of smokers. BMJ Open 6(6):e011045, 2016 27288378

Chamakalayil S, Strasser J, Vogel M, et al: Methylphenidate for attention-deficit and hyperactivity disorder in adult patients with substance use disorders: good clinical practice. Front Psychiatry 11:540837, 2021 33574770

Chan B, Freeman M, Kondo K, et al: Pharmacotherapy for methamphetamine/amphetamine use disorder: a systematic review and meta-analysis. Addiction 114(12):2122–2136, 2019a 31328345

Chan B, Kondo K, Freeman M, et al: Pharmacotherapy for cocaine use disorder: a systematic review and meta-analysis. J Gen Intern Med 34(12):2858–2873, 2019b 31183685

Cuzen NL, Koopowitz S-M, Ferrett HL, et al: Methamphetamine and cannabis abuse in adolescence: a quasi-experimental study on specific and long-term neurocognitive effects. BMJ Open 5(1):e005833, 2015 25636791

Dale LC, Hurt RD, Offord KP, et al: High-dose nicotine patch therapy: percentage of replacement and smoking cessation. JAMA 274(17):1353–1358, 1995 7563559

Di Forti M, Quattrone D, Freeman TP, et al: The contribution of cannabis use to variation in the incidence of psychotic disorder across Europe (EU-GEI): a multicentre case-control study. Lancet Psychiatry 6(5):427–436, 2019 30902669

ElSohly MA, Chandra S, Radwan M, et al: A comprehensive review of cannabis potency in the United States in the last decade. Biol Psychiatry Cogn Neurosci Neuroimaging 6(6):603–606, 2021 33508497

Ezard N, Clifford B, Dunlop A, et al: Safety and tolerability of oral lisdexamfetamine in adults with methamphetamine dependence: a phase-2 dose-escalation study. BMJ Open 11(5):e044696, 2021 34006547

Epstein DH, Marrone GF, Heishman SJ, et al: Tobacco, cocaine, and heroin: craving and use during daily life. Addict Behav 35(4):318–324, 2010 19939575

Freeman TP, Hindocha C, Baio G, et al: Cannabidiol for the treatment of cannabis use disorder: a phase 2a, double-blind, placebo-controlled, randomised, adaptive Bayesian trial. Lancet Psychiatry 7(10):865–874, 2020 32735782

Gatch MB, Flores E, Forster MJ: Nicotine and methamphetamine share discriminative stimulus effects. Drug Alcohol Depend 93(1–2):63–71, 2008 17961933

Gonzales D, Rennard SI, Nides M, et al: Varenicline, an alpha4beta2 nicotinic acetylcholine receptor partial agonist, vs sustained-release bupropion and placebo for smoking cessation: a randomized controlled trial. JAMA 296(1):47–55, 2006 16820546

Gray KM, Carpenter MJ, Lewis AL, et al: Varenicline versus bupropion XL for smoking cessation in older adolescents: a randomized, double-blind pilot trial. Nicotine Tob Res 14(2):234–239, 2012 21778151

Guglielmo R, Martinotti G, Quatrale M, et al: Topiramate in alcohol use disorders: review and update. CNS Drugs 29(5):383–395, 2015 25899459

Hamrin V, Bailey K: Gabapentin and methylphenidate treatment of a preadolescent with attention deficit hyperactivity disorder and bipolar disorder. J Child Adolesc Psychopharmacol 11(3):301–309, 2001 11642481

Han B, Compton WM, Jones CM, et al: Methamphetamine use, methamphetamine use disorder, and associated overdose deaths among US adults. JAMA Psychiatry 78(12):1329–1342, 2021 34550301

Haney M, Rubin E, Foltin RW: Aripiprazole maintenance increases smoked cocaine self-administration in humans. Psychopharmacology (Berl) 216(3):379–387, 2011 21373790

Haney M, Ramesh D, Glass A, et al: Naltrexone maintenance decreases cannabis self-administration and subjective effects in daily cannabis smokers. Neuropsychopharmacology 40(11):2489–2498, 2015 25881117

Harrell PT, Montoya ID, Preston KL, et al: Cigarette smoking and short-term addiction treatment outcome. Drug Alcohol Depend 115(3):161–166, 2011 21163592

Hartmann-Boyce J, McRobbie H, Butler AR, et al: Electronic cigarettes for smoking cessation. Cochrane Database Syst Rev 4(4):CD010216, 2021 33913154

Heikkinen M, Taipale H, Tanskanen A, et al: Association of pharmacological treatments and hospitalization and death in individuals with amphetamine use disorders in a Swedish nationwide cohort of 13,965 patients. JAMA Psychiatry 80(1):31–39, 2022 36383348

Hines LA, Freeman TP, Gage SH, et al: Association of high-potency cannabis use with mental health and substance use in adolescence. JAMA Psychiatry 77(10):1044–1051, 2020 32459328

Howes S, Hartmann-Boyce J, Livingstone-Banks J, et al: Antidepressants for smoking cessation. Cochrane Database Syst Rev 4(4):CD000031, 2020 32319681

Johnson BA, Roache JD, Ait-Daoud N, et al: A preliminary randomized, double-blind, placebo-controlled study of the safety and efficacy of ondansetron in the treatment of cocaine dependence. Drug Alcohol Depend 84(3):256–263, 2006 16631323

Kampangkaew JP, Spellicy CJ, Nielsen EM, et al: Pharmacogenetic role of dopamine transporter (SLC6A3) variation on response to disulfiram treatment for cocaine addiction. Am J Addict 28(4):311–317, 2019 31087723

Kampman KM, Pettinati HM, Lynch KG, et al: A double-blind, placebo-controlled trial of topiramate for the treatment of comorbid cocaine and alcohol dependence. Drug Alcohol Depend 133(1):94–99, 2013 23810644

Kaye S, McKetin R, Duflou J, et al: Methamphetamine and cardiovascular pathology: a review of the evidence. Addiction 102(8):1204–1211, 2007 17565561

Kaye S, Darke S, Torok M: Attention deficit hyperactivity disorder (ADHD) among illicit psychostimulant users: a hidden disorder? Addiction 108(5):923–931, 2013 23227816

Koegelenberg CFN, Noor F, Bateman ED, et al: Efficacy of varenicline combined with nicotine replacement therapy vs varenicline alone for smoking cessation: a randomized clinical trial. JAMA 312(2):155–161, 2014 25005652

Konstenius M, Jayaram-Lindström N, Guterstam J, et al: Methylphenidate for attention deficit hyperactivity disorder and drug relapse in criminal offenders with substance dependence: a 24-week randomized placebo-controlled trial. Addiction 109(3):440–449, 2014 24118269

Kosmider L, Cox S, Zaciera M, et al: Daily exposure to formaldehyde and acetaldehyde and potential health risk associated with use of high and low nicotine e-liquid concentrations. Sci Rep 10(1):6546, 2020 32300142

Levin FR, Mariani JJ, Specker S, et al: Extended-release mixed amphetamine salts vs placebo for comorbid adult attention-deficit/hyperactivity disorder and cocaine use disorder: a randomized clinical trial. JAMA Psychiatry 72(6):593–602, 2015 25887096

Lynch KG, Plebani J, Spratt K, et al: Varenicline for the treatment of cocaine dependence. J Addict Med 16(2):157–163, 2022 33840773

Magee JC, Lewis DF, Winhusen T: Evaluating nicotine craving, withdrawal, and substance use as mediators of smoking cessation in cocaine- and methamphetamine-dependent patients. Nicotine Tob Res 18(5):1196–1201, 2016 26048168

Manthey J, Freeman TP, Kilian C, et al: Public health monitoring of cannabis use in Europe: prevalence of use, cannabis potency, and treatment rates. Lancet Reg Health Eur 10(Nov):100227, 2021 34806072

Massaro LTS, Abdalla RR, Laranjeira R, et al: Amphetamine-type stimulant use and conditional paths of consumption: data from the Second Brazilian National Alcohol and Drugs Survey. Br J Psychiatry 39(3):201–207, 2017 28700012

Meredith CW, Jaffe C, Yanasak E, et al: An open-label pilot study of risperidone in the treatment of methamphetamine dependence. J Psychoactive Drugs 39(2):167–172, 2007 17703711

Meredith CW, Jaffe C, Cherrier M, et al: Open trial of injectable risperidone for methamphetamine dependence. J Addict Med 3(2):55–65, 2009 21769001

Miller SC, Fiellin DA, Rosenthal RN, et al (eds): The ASAM Principles of Addiction Medicine, 6th Edition. Philadelphia, PA, Wolters Kluwer, 2019

Minozzi S, Cinquini M, Amato L, et al: Anticonvulsants for cocaine dependence. Cochrane Database Syst Rev 2015(4):CD006754, 2015 25882271

Miovský M, Lukavská K, Rubášová E, et al: Attention deficit hyperactivity disorder among clients diagnosed with a substance use disorder in the therapeutic communities: prevalence and psychiatric comorbidity. Eur Addict Res 27(2):87–96, 2021 32781442

Morisano D, Bacher I, Audrain-McGovern J, et al: Mechanisms underlying the co-morbidity of tobacco use in mental health and addictive disorders. Can J Psychiatry 54(6):356–367, 2009 19527556

National Institute on Drug Abuse: Drug Overdose Death Rates. Bethesda, MD, National Institute on Drug Abuse, 2021. Available at: https://www.drugabuse.gov/drug-topics/trends-statistics/overdose-death-rates. Accessed January 29, 2021.

Newton TF, Reid MS, De La Garza R, et al: Evaluation of subjective effects of aripiprazole and methamphetamine in methamphetamine-dependent volunteers. Int J Neuropsychopharmacol 11(8):1037–1045, 2008 18664303

Notzon DP, Kelly MA, Choi CJ, et al: Open-label pilot study of injectable naltrexone for cannabis dependence. Am J Drug Alcohol Abuse 44(6):619–627, 2018 29420073

Oslin DW, Pettinati HM, Volpicelli JR, et al: The effects of naltrexone on alcohol and cocaine use in dually addicted patients. J Subst Abuse Treat 16(2):163–167, 1999 10023615

Palamar JJ, Le A, Han BH: Quarterly trends in past-month cannabis use in the United States, 2015–2019. Drug Alcohol Depend 219(February):108494, 2021 33434791

Pani PP, Trogu E, Vacca R, et al: Disulfiram for the treatment of cocaine dependence. Cochrane Database Syst Rev (1):CD007024, 2010 20091613

Pennings EJM, Leccese AP, Wolff FA: Effects of concurrent use of alcohol and cocaine. Addiction 97(7):773–783, 2002 12133112

Pettinati HM, Kampman KM, Lynch KG, et al: A double blind, placebo-controlled trial that combines disulfiram and naltrexone for treating co-occurring cocaine and alcohol dependence. Addict Behav 33(5):651–667, 2008 18079068

Pettinati HM, Kampman KM, Lynch KG, et al: A pilot trial of injectable, extended-release naltrexone for the treatment of co-occurring cocaine and alcohol dependence. Am J Addict 23(6):591–597, 2014 25251201

Poling J, Oliveto A, Petry N, et al: Six-month trial of bupropion with contingency management for cocaine dependence in a methadone-maintained population. Arch Gen Psychiatry 63(2):219–228, 2006 16461866

Razavi Y, Keyhanfar F, Shabani R, et al: Therapeutic effects of cannabidiol on methamphetamine abuse: a review of preclinical study. Iran J Pharm Res 20(4):152–164, 2021 35194436

Ricci V, Di Salvo G, Maina G: Remission of persistent methamphetamine-induced psychosis after cariprazine therapy: presentation of a case report. J Addict Dis 40(1):145–148, 2022 34180372

Rodriguez Cruz J, Sahlsten Schölin J, Hjorth S: Case report: cariprazine in a patient with schizophrenia, substance abuse, and cognitive dysfunction. Front Psychiatry 12:727666, 2021 34489766

Roll JM, Higgins ST, Budney AJ, et al: A comparison of cocaine-dependent cigarette smokers and non-smokers on demographic, drug use and other characteristics. Drug Alcohol Depend 40(3):195–201, 1996 8861397

Sachs DPL: Effectiveness of the 4-mg dose of nicotine polacrilex for the initial treatment of high-dependent smokers. Arch Intern Med 155(18):1973–1980, 1995 7575051

Schmitz JM, Lindsay JA, Green CE, et al: High-dose naltrexone therapy for cocaine-alcohol dependence. Am J Addict 18(5):356–362, 2009 19874153

Schottenfeld RS, Chawarski MC, Sofuoglu M, et al: Atomoxetine for amphetamine-type stimulant dependence during buprenorphine treatment: a randomized controlled trial. Drug Alcohol Depend 186(May):130–137, 2018 29573648

Sharma R, Tikka SK, Bhute AR, et al: N-acetyl cysteine in the treatment of cannabis use disorder: a systematic review of clinical trials. Addict Behav 129(June):107283, 2022 35189496

Shorter D, Lindsay JA, Kosten TR: The alpha-1 adrenergic antagonist doxazosin for treatment of cocaine dependence: a pilot study. Drug Alcohol Depend 131(1–2):66–70, 2013 23306096

Skoglund C, Brandt L, D'Onofrio B, et al: Methylphenidate doses in attention deficit/hyperactivity disorder and comorbid substance use disorders. Eur Neuropsychopharmacol 27(11):1144–1152, 2017 28935267

Substance Abuse and Mental Health Services Administration: The DAWN Report: Emergency department visits involving methamphetamine: 2007 to 2011. June 19, 2014. Available at: https://www.samhsa.gov/data/sites/default/files/DAWN_SR167_EDVisitsMeth_06-12-14/DAWN-SR167-EDVisitsMeth-2014.htm. Accessed February 27, 2022.

Substance Abuse and Mental Health Services Administration: Highlights for the National Survey on Drug Use and Health. Rockville, MD, Substance Abuse and Mental Health Services Administration, 2022. Available at: https://www.samhsa.gov/data/sites/default/files/2021-10/2020_NSDUH_Highlights.pdf. Accessed January 11, 2022.

Tashkin D, Kanner R, Bailey W, et al: Smoking cessation in patients with chronic obstructive pulmonary disease: a double-blind, placebo-controlled, randomised trial. Lancet 357(9268):1571–1575, 2001 11377644

Tonstad S, Farsang C, Klaene G, et al: Bupropion SR for smoking cessation in smokers with cardiovascular disease: a multicentre, randomised study. Eur Heart J 24(10):946–955, 2003 12714026

Tran AX, Ho TT, Varghese Gupta S: Role of CYP2B6 pharmacogenomics in bupropion-mediated smoking cessation. J Clin Pharm Ther 44(2):174–179, 2019 30578565

Triantafyllou GA, Tiberio PJ, Zou RH, et al: Long-term outcomes of EVALI: a 1-year retrospective study. Lancet Respir Med 9(12):e112–e113, 2021 34710356

Trivedi MH, Walker R, Ling W, et al: Bupropion and naltrexone in methamphetamine use disorder. N Engl J Med 384(2):140–153, 2021 33497547

Truong TT, Li B: Case series: cariprazine for treatment of methamphetamine use disorder. Am J Addict 31(1):85–88, 2022 34713943

Tsai H, Lee J, Hedlin H, et al: Methamphetamine use association with pulmonary diseases: a retrospective investigation of hospital discharges in California from 2005 to 2011. ERJ Open Res 5(4):00017–02019, 2019 31637253

U.S. Food and Drug Administration: FDA Drug Safety Communication: FDA revises description of mental health side effects of the stop-smoking medicines Chantix (varenicline) and Zyban (bupropion) to reflect clinical trial findings. February 2019. Available at: https://www.fda.gov/drugs/drug-safety-and-availability/fda-drug-safety-communication-fda-revises-description-mental-health-side-effects-stop-smoking. Accessed December 31, 2022.

Vogeler T, McClain C, Evoy KE: Combination bupropion SR and varenicline for smoking cessation: a systematic review. Am J Drug Alcohol Abuse 42(2):129–139, 2016 26809272

Wagena EJ, Knipschild PG, Huibers MJH, et al: Efficacy of bupropion and nortriptyline for smoking cessation among people at risk for or with chronic obstructive pulmonary disease. Arch Intern Med 165(19):2286–2292, 2005 16246996

Wang G, Ma L, Liu X, et al: Paliperidone extended-release tablets for the treatment of methamphetamine use disorder in Chinese patients after acute treatment: a randomized, double-blind, placebo-controlled exploratory study. Front Psychiatry 10:656, 2019 31607961

Winhusen TM, Kropp F, Theobald J, et al: Achieving smoking abstinence is associated with decreased cocaine use in cocaine-dependent patients receiving smoking-cessation treatment. Drug Alcohol Depend 134(January):391–395, 2014 24128381

Winhusen T, Theobald J, Kaelber DC, et al: The association between regular cocaine use, with and without tobacco co-use, and adverse cardiovascular and respiratory outcomes. Drug Alcohol Depend 214(Sept):108136, 2020 32623147

# 7

# Opioids and Co-occurring Substance Use

Thanh Thuy Truong, M.D.
M. Asif Khan, M.D., M.R.O.
Nidal Moukaddam, M.D., Ph.D.

*The current* opioid epidemic began in the 1990s with the introduction of OxyContin (oxycodone hydrochloride) and extensive marketing by Purdue Pharma that led to the integration of pain as the fifth vital sign. The three waves of overdose deaths began with prescription opioids in the late 1990s, transitioning to heroin overdoses in 2010 and then to synthetic opioid overdoses with drugs such as fentanyl and fentanyl analogs in 2013. We are now in the fourth wave of overdose deaths secondary to combined synthetic opioids and stimulants. Nearly 73% of opioid-related overdose deaths involved synthetic opioids in 2019, which further accelerated during the 2020 coronavirus SARS-CoV-2 disease (COVID-19) pandemic, with a 38.4% increase (Centers for Disease Control and Prevention 2020). A significant number of deaths were linked to methamphetamine co-use (Mattson et al. 2021). Although medications for opioid use disorder (OUD) are effective, clinicians and patients continue to be challenged by co-occurring substance use disorders (SUDs). The treatment of OUD is extensively covered in other texts and resources (Miller et al. 2019); thus, in this chapter we focus on the pharmacological management of co-occurring SUDs. An overview of medications for OUD is presented in Table 7–1.

**Table 7–1.    Medications for opioid use disorder**

| Medication | Dosing | Considerations |
|---|---|---|
| **Opioid agonist treatment** | | |
| Methadone[a] | Inpatient withdrawal management: Initiate treatment with 10–30 mg (2.5–10 mg in patients with low opioid tolerance), reassess q 2–4 hours and increase dosage by 5–10 mg as needed to a maximum dosage of 30–40 mg in first 24 hours. Order naloxone prn (0.1 mg IV/IM q 1–2 minutes prn) for signs of overdose.<br><br>Maintenance: Titrate by 10 mg every ~ 5 days based on patient sedation, withdrawal symptoms, and craving. Usual daily dosage ranges from 60 mg to 120 mg. | Inpatient: contact patient's OTP to obtain previous dosage of methadone, then continue current dosage. If cannot confirm dosage, then treat as though patient is opioid naive. |
| Buprenorphine[b] | Induction: COWS score must be ≥6 prior to induction (at ≥14 for fentanyl users). If lower, then reschedule. | Partial agonism creates a ceiling effect on respiratory depression and euphoria. Naloxone added to buprenorphine deters misuse and diversion. |

**Table 7–1.** Medications for opioid use disorder (*continued*)

| Medication | Dosing | Considerations |
|---|---|---|
| Buprenorphine[b] (*continued*) | Buprenorphine/naloxone film or sublingual tablet:<br><br>Day 1: Start with 2–4 mg, reassess after 1–2 hours. If COWS score ≥6, then give another 2–4 mg. If withdrawal is relieved, patient may be released with one dose. Maximum dosage is 8 mg, although this may be higher for fentanyl users.<br><br>Day 2: Give total dosage of day 1, then monitor for 1–2 hours. If COWS score ≥6, give another 4 mg. Repeat depending on COWS score for a maximum dosage of 16 mg. Prescribe 1-week supply and reassess. Most patients are maintained on 8–16 mg/day, although higher dosages up to 32 mg/day may be needed for some, e.g., fentanyl users).<br><br>Extended-release injection: Establish tolerability with oral buprenorphine, then start with 300-mg injection. Follow ≥26 days later with 100-mg second dose; may consider 300 mg for second injection in patients still experiencing craving or withdrawal symptoms.<br><br>Maintenance: 100 mg monthly | Microdosing protocols reduce withdrawal by gradually replacing full agonist with low doses of buprenorphine. A variety of protocols have been reported in the case literature for transitioning from short-acting opioids and methadone to buprenorphine. These are less well studied and require significant clinical monitoring and follow-up during the titration process (Soyka 2021). |

**Table 7–1.    Medications for opioid use disorder** (*continued*)

| Medication | Dosing | Considerations |
|---|---|---|
| **Opioid antagonist** | | |
| Naltrexone | Oral naltrexone not recommended unless dosing is supervised. If used, start at 25 mg/day for 2–3 days, then increase to 50 mg/day. Some patients may benefit from 100 mg/day.<br><br>Extended-release injection: 380 mg q 4 weeks. Consider q 3 weeks in those with breakthrough cravings. | Naltrexone has shown effectiveness comparable with buprenorphine for craving and relapse (Lee et al. 2018). It should be used only after completion of a medically managed withdrawal from opioids, which makes the transition to naltrexone challenging (see "Switching Therapies" rows below). May use naloxone challenge (0.1 mg IV or SC) to ensure completed withdrawal prior to administration. |
| **α₂-Adrenergic agonists for withdrawal management** | | |
| Clonidine | For COWS score of 8–12, give 0.1 mg.<br><br>For COWS score > 12, give 0.2 mg q 4–6 hours prn up to a maximum dosage of 1.2 mg/day. On day 5, start tapering by 0.1–0.2 mg/day. | Clonidine and lofexidine have equivalent efficacy, but lofexidine may be better tolerated with less hypotension. Use of lofexidine is limited by cost. Both are used as adjuncts to maintenance treatment with buprenorphine, methadone, or naltrexone. Treatment with α₂-adrenergic agonists alone for OUD is not recommended. |

**Table 7–1.** Medications for opioid use disorder (*continued*)

| Medication | Dosing | Considerations |
|---|---|---|
| Lofexidine | Initial: 0.18 mg q 5–6 hours during peak withdrawal symptoms (first 5–7 days after last opioid use). Adjust according to symptoms up to a maximum 0.72 mg per dose, or 2.88 mg/day; may continue up to 14 days if needed. | Side effects include hypotension, bradycardia, syncope, and QT prolongation. Do not give if BP >90/60, HR <60, and/or orthostatic hypotension is present. Monitor ECG if lofexidine is combined with methadone, due to higher risk of QT prolongation. |
| **Switching therapies** | | |
| Buprenorphine to methadone | No delay needed. Titrate methadone according to withdrawal symptoms, craving, and sedation. | |
| Methadone to buprenorphine (Soyka 2021) | Reduce methadone to 30–40 mg/day or less. Patient remains on dosage for ≥7 days. Discontinue methadone at least 24 hours before buprenorphine induction. Use COWS score to guide induction per above. | May need adjunct medications (e.g., clonidine, NSAIDs) for opioid withdrawal. Various protocols have been developed to transition patients without methadone taper and withdrawal, including microdosing and bridging with other opioids. However, these are limited to case reports. We recommend medical supervision if using one of these protocols for high-risk patients. |
| Naltrexone to buprenorphine or methadone | Begin buprenorphine or methadone ~1 day after last oral dose of naltrexone and ~28 days after last IM dose of naltrexone. | |

**Table 7–1.   Medications for opioid use disorder** *(continued)*

| Medication | Dosing | Considerations |
|---|---|---|
| Buprenorphine or methadone to extended-release naltrexone | Taper buprenorphine or methadone gradually and discontinue. Wait 7–14 days before initiating treatment with naltrexone. | Transition may be difficult because of withdrawal symptoms and increased risk of relapse (Lee et al. 2018). We recommend medically supervised withdrawal (residential or inpatient) to reduce risk of relapse and overdose. Protocols have been developed using escalating low-dose naltrexone to transition patients on buprenorphine to naltrexone. An RCT comparing a low-dose naltrexone protocol with standard treatment found no significant differences. Both groups benefited from ancillary medications for opioid withdrawal (Comer et al. 2020). Low-dose naltrexone is unavailable at accessible pharmacies. |

*Note.*   COWS is recommended for assessing opioid withdrawal.

BP = blood pressure; COWS = Clinical Opiate Withdrawal Scale; ECG = electrocardiogram; HR = heart rate; NSAIDs = nonsteroidal anti-inflammatory drugs; OTP = opiate treatment program; OUD = opioid use disorder; RCT = randomized controlled trial; SC = subcutaneous; SL = sublingual.

[a]Can be given inpatient, but maintenance treatment must be through a certified OTP.

[b]Office-based buprenorphine 8 mg SL tablet = buprenorphine/naloxone 8 mg/2 mg SL film = buprenorphine/naloxone 5.7 mg/1.4 mg SL tablet.

# Opioids and Tobacco or Nicotine

The prevalence of tobacco smoking among individuals with OUD is high, ranging from 92% to 95% in those with OUD not receiving treatment and from 85%–98% for those receiving methadone. Even patients without OUD who receive opioid prescriptions for chronic pain are nearly twice as likely to smoke. This high prevalence is also seen in international samples, with an estimated 85% of people receiving OUD medications also smoking cigarettes (Elkader et al. 2009; Guydish et al. 2016). The likelihood of smoking among individuals with OUD was equivalent for males and females, but the predictors of smoking severity were significantly different; opioid craving was positively correlated with the number of cigarettes smoked among males, whereas anxiety was correlated with the number of cigarettes smoked among females (McHugh et al. 2020). Electronic (e-)cigarette use has also increased among smokers with OUD with the intent of harm reduction or quitting smoking. However, pilot studies on e-cigarettes have not shown efficacy in promoting smoking cessation. Most individuals using e-cigarettes continue to smoke cigarettes (Baldassarri et al. 2019; Felicione et al. 2019).

Several studies examined the relationship between opioids and smoking, with some showing a positive relationship between methadone and buprenorphine dose and the number of cigarettes. Richter et al. (2007) found that patients taking methadone increase their smoking within the first 2 hours following the methadone dose. Patients attribute their increased smoking in the context of opioid agonist treatment (OAT) and other drug use to increased enjoyment of both substances, habit, a ritual of pairing both, or relief from withdrawal. Some patients also smoke to manage their dislike of methadone taste, whereas others find that methadone aids smoking by reducing throat discomfort and cough (McCool and Paschall Richter 2003). Patients with chronic pain may use nicotine to relieve pain or to potentiate the analgesic effects of opioids. Although acute nicotine use has short-term analgesic effects through endogenous opioid release, ongoing use exacerbates pain by sensitizing pain receptors, decreasing pain tolerance, and increasing pain awareness (Ditre et al. 2011). Neurobiological mechanisms may also explain why opioids and nicotine prime one another. Opioids interact with nicotinic acetylcholine receptors, whereas nicotine stimulates the release of endogenous opioids that bind to μ opioid receptors (Lichenstein et al. 2019). Regardless of the underlying reasons, it is critical to address co-occurring tobacco use in all patients recovering from an SUD because those who continue or initiate smoking are more likely to relapse than nonsmokers. Patients who achieve smoking abstinence appear to have better substance and psychiatric treatment outcomes in addition to numerous health benefits (Weinberger et al. 2017). Clinicians should be aware that because of these interactions between opioids and nicotine, quitting may be more challenging for people with OUD even though most patients in OUD treatment desire smoking cessation. Low-intensity behavioral interventions such as Screening, Brief Intervention, and Referral to Treatment (SBIRT) and quitlines are insufficient for this population compared with the general population. Studies have found negligible, or 0%, cessation rates among people with OUD who also smoke. Motivational interviewing also shows disappointing results in this population (Vlad et al. 2020). Therefore, patients with co-occurring tobacco use disorder (TUD) and OUD need pharmacotherapy as a first-line intervention.

## Medications for Tobacco Use Disorder in Patients With Opioid Use Disorder

A summary of medications for TUD is provided in Chapter 6, "Stimulants and Co-occurring Substance Use." FDA-approved pharmacological interventions include nicotine replacement therapy (NRT), bupropion, and varenicline. The response to these medications is generally lower among people with OUD compared with those without OUD:

- *NRT:* Although NRT only modestly increases rates of abstinence, patients with OUD are more likely to quit with high-dose NRT (21-mg or higher-dose patch), combination NRT (patch plus gum), and extended NRT (24 weeks) (Vlad et al. 2020).
- *Bupropion:* Bupropion has much less evidence to support smoking cessation in patients with OUD than in other populations. One small study in patients receiving bupropion found that it had a significantly negative effect on treatment retention (58% in bupropion group vs. 90% in placebo group) despite contingency management. Rates of smoking cessation did not differ between groups (Mooney et al. 2008). Although the reasons for the high attrition rate in the bupropion group are unclear, this potential negative outcome should be considered when selecting treatment. Other trials combining contingency management with bupropion also found no significant difference in abstinence rates, although adherence to bupropion was low. Only one small, uncontrolled trial combining motivational interviewing for TUD with bupropion had higher abstinence rates (14%) (Vlad et al. 2020).

- *Varenicline:* Several trials have investigated varenicline for smoking cessation in patients with OUD. Contrary to the drug's success in patients without OUD, it has not shown consistent efficacy in this population. In a study with 315 patients receiving methadone, varenicline did not increase abstinence rates compared with NRT or placebo. Similar to bupropion, varenicline had low adherence (Stein et al. 2013). A trial comparing varenicline with placebo found that it increased abstinence rates (10.5% vs. 0%), but these effects were not maintained after treatment stopped (Nahvi et al. 2014). Other trials have found similar results, either that varenicline was poorly adhered to and failed to produce a statistically significant effect or that the effects were modest and not sustained (Vlad et al. 2020).

## Clinical Practice

Several of our patients have reported increased tobacco use and craving after initiating OAT. For example, one female patient increased from one pack per day to three packs per day. We have seen these effects with varying intensity in each patient. We ask our patients to monitor changes in tobacco use as they stabilize on OAT. Given the negligible rates of smoking cessation with behavioral intervention, we recommend initiating pharmacotherapy with combination NRT, adjusting the dosage for the number of cigarettes smoked (see Chapter 6), as soon as a patient enters OUD treatment. If combination NRT is insufficient, consider switching to varenicline with short-acting NRT for breakthrough cravings (e.g., gum, lozenges). Although the combination of varenicline and nicotine patch has not been studied in this population, it has shown improved efficacy in other groups with co-occurring alcohol use disorder (AUD), who also historically have a poorer response to standard treatment approaches (King et al. 2022). With informed consent, we have tried combining bupropion with combination NRT or varenicline plus short- and long-acting NRT, depending on tolerability. Our patients have had an improved response with these combinations compared with each intervention alone, but the rates of nicotine cessation are still low. We have also attempted to time medications to accommodate increased cravings at certain times of the day (i.e., taking varenicline 1–2 hours before buprenorphine or methadone dose or an anticipated high craving time, such as dinner). Admittedly, this strategy has worked in very few patients. We employ motivational interviewing for tobacco use at each appointment and encourage harm reduction methods. Some patients have reported improved respiratory function after switching to e-cigarettes and tapering nicotine over years rather than months.

# Opioids and Cannabis

The opioid epidemic has spurred novel ideas and research into potentially useful substances to help patients reduce opioid use and relieve pain. Cannabis has been investigated for its potential role in analgesia and OUD treatment. Cannabinoid and opioid receptors are both active in brain regions involved in analgesia, including the periaqueductal gray, raphe nuclei, central medial thalamic nuclei, and spinal cord. Cannabinoid $CB_2$ receptors indirectly stimulate opioid receptors, suggesting that cannabinoids may enhance opioid analgesia. Preclinical studies support the opioid-sparing effects of cannabis, such that lower doses of opioids were required to produce the same analgesia when coadministered with Δ-9-tetrahydrocannabinol (Δ-9 THC). There is no well-substantiated evidence for this opioid-sparing effect in humans because of a lack of high-quality randomized controlled trials (RCTs) (Nielsen et al. 2017). However, despite the mixed and low-quality evidence of this potential benefit, several states have moved ahead in approving medical cannabis as an indication for OUD. Expectedly, cannabis dispensaries became more aggressive in marketing cannabis as a treatment for OUD and cannabidiol (CBD) to prevent opioid withdrawal, without rigorous supporting evidence (Shover et al. 2020; Voelker 2018).

## Epidemiology

Our understanding of the societal impact of cannabis legalization on OUD continues to evolve. Thus far, legalization seems to correlate with lower odds of any opioid use, chronic opioid use, and high-risk opioid use (Shah et al. 2019). Among people with OUD, cannabis use is widespread. Rosic et al. (2017) found that the prevalence of cannabis use disorder (CaUD) in patients with OUD who were receiving methadone was 28% ($n=935$). A subsequent evaluation showed that of 2,315 patients receiving buprenorphine/naloxone or methadone for OUD, 51% reported past month cannabis use, of which 68% reported daily use. In this sample, 75% reported that cannabis use did not affect OAT. A small proportion of patients reported improved opioid cravings (6.9%) and opioid withdrawal symptoms (8.3%). An even smaller percentage (2.4%) reported a negative impact of cannabis use on OAT. Daily cannabis users had lower odds of opioid use. However, nearly 50% reported adverse side effects from cannabis, including impairments in cognition, motivation, and school and work performance (Rosic et al. 2021). Cannabis is also used in the community for opioid withdrawal. In a survey of 200 community opioid users, 62.5% had used cannabis to treat withdrawal, and most found it helpful for anxiety, tremors, and insomnia. Only 6% reported cannabis worsened opioid withdrawal. Interestingly, females reported greater relief from withdrawal than males (Bergeria et al. 2020).

## Treatment Outcomes With Co-use of Cannabis and Opioids

A reduction in opioid use is only one outcome, and multiple studies have examined whether this relationship leads to a higher quality of life. In a cohort of 450 patients with chronic pain, cannabis and opioid co-use was not associated with differences in pain intensity and disability versus opioid use alone but was associated with elevated anxiety and depression symptoms, opioid misuse, and other substance use. However, these results do not establish cannabis as a cause but suggest a different vulnerability in the co-using population (Rogers et al. 2019). A systematic review in 2020 did not find consistent evidence to support the benefits or detriment of cannabis co-use because most studies did not detect a statistically significant association between cannabis use and treatment outcomes (Lake and St Pierre 2020). A Cochrane review concluded that the benefits of cannabis use for chronic neuropathic pain might outweigh the harms. However, the evidence of cannabis for pain relief outcomes may reflect the exclusion of participants with a history of SUDs and other comorbidities (Mücke et al. 2018). Thus, from these results, it is not clear that cannabis improves treatment outcomes in patients prescribed opioids for chronic pain.

Although several other studies have examined cannabis co-use, they did not specify whether the participants met criteria for CaUD. Having multiple SUDs generally leads to greater impairment than having one SUD alone. In a study comparing patients with co-occurring CaUD and OUD with those with either disorder alone, patients with the co-occurring conditions were more likely to be homeless, have a history of psychiatric hospitalizations, use other substances, and have serious mental illness and personality disorders. The group with co-occurring conditions was not, however, associated with a higher frequency of any pain diagnoses. Although the number of opioid prescriptions was actually lower in the group with co-occurring conditions, patients in this group experienced more adverse events (De Aquino et al. 2019). These results indicate a need to treat both disorders when the patient is engaged in OUD treatment. For patients receiving OAT, cannabis inhibits cytochrome P450 (CYP) 3A4 buprenorphine levels (Vierke et al. 2021).

## Medications for Cannabis Use Disorder and Opioid Use Disorder

We did not find any studies of pharmacotherapy for treatment of combined CaUD and OUD. We do not have evidence to inform whether off-label medications demonstrating modest efficacy for CaUD would be effective when co-occurring OUD exists. Among medications detailed in Chapter 6, our patients have tolerated the combination of N-acetylcysteine with medications for OUD. However, its effectiveness in reducing cannabis use and craving is highly inconsistent, and adherence is generally poor unless the patient has supervised dosing by family. We have also combined gabapentin with OAT, although with caution, because of an elevated risk of overdose and gabapentin misuse. Patients have responded better to this combination, partly because of relief of cannabis withdrawal and pain. More recently, many patients have reported preferential use of only CBD or low THC formulations instead of prescribed medications. CBD has been investigated for various SUDs because of its low-reinforcing properties. CBD treatment for CaUD has one positive RCT (Freeman et al. 2020). For OUD, one study reported that coadministration of CBD 400 mg/day and 800 mg/day and fentanyl was well tolerated without significant adverse events (Manini et al. 2015). A subsequent double-blind, placebo-controlled RCT found that CBD 400 mg/day and 800 mg/day for 3 days effectively reduced cue-induced opioid craving and cue-induced anxiety compared with placebo in patients who were abstinent from opioids and not receiving medications for OUD ($n=42$). The effect was seen 1 week after the final administration of CBD, suggesting a prolonged impact. Notably, most participants also smoked tobacco and had undiagnosed CaUD (Hurd et al. 2015, 2019).

## Clinical Practice

No medications have demonstrated consistent effectiveness for CaUD alone, and there is an even greater dearth of information about individuals with co-occurring use disorders. Although CBD shows promise, we need larger trials showing safety and effectiveness to confidently recommend it as a treatment. In our experience, as with tobacco use, it is not uncommon for cannabis use to receive less focus during OUD treatment, especially in the early recovery stages when the patient is achieving stability, likely because of the high lethality of OUD. However, many patients increase cannabis use because they perceive it to carry lower risks, which may lead to other impairments. Not all patients develop CaUD, but the long-term impact of low-level cannabis use remains unclear. When we raise the issue of cannabis and tobacco use, many patients request to curb the discussion, preferring "to quit one drug at a time." This dynamic poses significant challenges in treatment outcomes because immediately challenging the patient may disrupt rapport. Some of our patients have shared that they have a knee-jerk defensive attitude for fear of criticism about their cannabis use, despite recognizing its harms. In the spirit of motivational interviewing, we recommend assessing readiness, asking the patient what they already know about cannabis, asking for permission to share information that might be relevant to them, then asking them what they think of the information. For patients who have already self-transitioned to CBD, we discuss harm reduction measures, such as obtaining CBD from a reputable dispensary that ensures its purity. For patients who decline to address cannabis or other substance use, we recommend collaborating with the patient to continually assess their overall function and quality of life and troubleshoot different relevant aspects. Quite often, the substance eventually comes up as a topic of conversation.

# Opioids and Alcohol

Opioids and alcohol or sedatives are intertwined in neurotransmitter systems and in epidemiological findings. Heavy drinking, opioid misuse, and chronic pain are a nexus to be examined when treating patients with comorbid use disorders. AUD is a major societal concern that equates to and even exceeds the costs of OUD, with alcohol use estimated to contribute to 5% of worldwide global disease burden according to the World Health Organization (2014).

## Epidemiology

Among individuals with OUD, more than half of those surveyed also used alcohol, with 30% exceeding recommended levels (Soyka 2015). Globally, research trends show that alcohol outcomes are worse in those with OUD, and AUD outcomes are worse in those who use opioids or have chronic pain. Sustained alcohol use is linked to poorer OUD outcomes, with more than 20% of deaths in opioid-dependent individuals being related to use of other drugs or alcohol (Frank et al. 2015). The 2015 National Survey on Drug Use and Health (NSDUH) revealed that people who have misused alcohol were also more likely to have misused prescription drugs (Hughes et al. 2017). The 2012–2013 National Epidemiologic Survey on Alcohol and Related Conditions–III (NESARC-III) conducted interviews based on DSM-5 criteria using the National Institute on Alcohol Abuse and Alcoholism's Alcohol Use Disorder and Associated Disabilities Interview Schedule–5 (AUDADIS-5), and the results highlighted increased prevalence of AUD and other addictive disorders in individuals with OUD (American Psychiatric Association 2013; Saha et al. 2016). Specific research targeting populations who have both AUD or sedative use disorder and OUD is lacking. Examining Medicare records from 2007 to 2014, Acevedo et al. (2022) found that hospitalizations for AUD or OUD increased among adults age 65 or older and that a subpopulation with comorbid OUD and AUD were found to have higher rates of mental illness and circulatory and endocrine issues during hospitalizations. Emergency department visits involving both AUD and OUD cost more than visits for either disease alone (Xierali et al. 2021). The presence of dual disorders (AUD, OUD) in treatment programs may also negatively influence the odds of getting medication-assisted treatment for OUD (Mintz et al. 2021).

A cross-sectional examination of the National Ambulatory Medical Care Survey from 2014 to 2016 revealed 17.1 million and 21.7 million visits involving patients with an OUD or AUD diagnosis, respectively, but a decrease in visits for AUD treatment and an increase in visits for OUD treatments (Evoy et al. 2020). The publicity and increased education surrounding the opioid epidemic may have helped popularize OUD treatments, whereas medications for AUD remain woefully underused.

## Clinical Practice

The most important step clinicians can take in patients with concomitant alcohol or sedative and opioid use is to investigate and assess the extent of use and then the extent of problematic use. Trajectories of concomitant use can include alcohol or sedatives before opioids, simultaneous use, or use of sedatives and alcohol after opioids. Users may report alcohol use as part of an entirely different routine (i.e., nighttime drinking) that is unrelated to social or peer-pressure-driven opioid use. The ubiquitous presence of alcohol in everyday life makes its use challenging to assess and avoid.

Screening for substance use can be done with structured questionnaires, such as the Alcohol Use Disorders Identification Test (AUDIT), or with unstructured questions. Optimal interview-style questions can begin with open-ended inquiries (e.g., "Have you used substances this past week?") but should also include follow-up questions on specific substances. Patients with OUD who consider opioids their drug of choice may not report other substances if they do not see them as problematic. Inquiring about pain is another crucial aspect of the interview. Patients frequently return to using alcohol when their pain is poorly controlled or exacerbated, even when they are no longer taking opioids (Jakubczyk et al. 2016). Similar issues arise with sedative use, whereas individuals with chronic pain report more benzodiazepine use when pain is ill controlled or interferes more with their life (Nielsen et al. 2015).

Assessments for social issues, trauma, mood, and other psychiatric disorders are crucial when dual SUDs are suspected. Patients who report alcohol and sedative use tend to present with more complex OUD clinical treatment pictures (Hartzler et al. 2010) and are more likely to drop out of OUD treatment with methadone or buprenorphine sooner (Tsui et al. 2016). Suicide risk is also increased in individuals with both OUD and sedative use or AUD (Rizk et al. 2021). There are no specific treatment guidelines for comorbid OUD and alcohol or sedative use. In considering treatment for this population, the following principles may be helpful:

- AUD tends to be undertreated compared with OUD. Buprenorphine and methadone treatments enhance treatment retention. AUD may then be targeted independently once OUD is managed.
- Avoidance of polypharmacy and reduction in risk of respiratory depression are major goals of treatment design and psychoeducation.
- Behavioral therapies, including cognitive-behavioral therapy, coping skills, mindfulness-based cognitive-behavioral therapy, and contingency management, are helpful for both alcohol or sedative and opioid use. However, individuals with dual SUDs do best in comprehensive treatments that include psychotropic agents and psychotherapy.
- Clinicians should have a low threshold for referral to a higher level of care (i.e., residential or inpatient treatment) if they have concerns about alcohol withdrawal with abstinence or risk of overdose.

## Pharmacotherapy for Comorbid Alcohol Use Disorder and Opioid Use Disorder

The literature has not examined any specific medications for comorbid AUD and OUD; therefore, these recommendations are based on our clinical experience. Specific medications that target both AUD and OUD are helpful (see Chapter 5, "Alcohol and Co-occurring Substance Use," for specific dosing of medications for AUD) (Soyka 2015). Although extended-release naltrexone is highly recommended, many patients with OUD will be receiving OAT and thus cannot use naltrexone. Acamprosate and disulfiram would not interfere with buprenorphine or methadone. Although we have combined topiramate with buprenorphine and methadone, it has been shown to worsen cognition in patients taking methadone. Therefore, we recommend titrating topiramate slowly and monitoring closely for these side effects (Rass et al. 2015). Active alcohol use also impairs cognition, which must be considered by clinicians weighing risks and benefits. We also add gabapentin to the treatment, especially if the patient has neuropathic pain. However, gabapentin may enhance the reinforcing effects of opioids and alcohol in patients with dual disorders (AUD, OUD), so use should be carefully monitored (Castillo et al. 2022). Baclofen may also be added to OAT and is especially helpful for patients with liver disorders.

# Opioids and Stimulants

Colloquially known as a "speedball" or "goofball," use of an opioid and a stimulant concurrently is common in the community and among individuals receiving OAT. The NSDUH documented significant increases in the use of methamphetamine and methamphetamine combined with other substances over the past decade (Hughes et al. 2017). Between 2015 and 2018, 40.4% of methamphetamine users reported prescription opioid misuse, and 16.9% reported heroin use. A number of studies have investigated this trend across the United States. In one cross-sectional multistate study of rural communities ($N=3,048$), 79% of people using drugs reported methamphetamine use in the past 30 days. Most participants who reported using any opioid or methamphetamine used them concurrently (63%) (Ellis et al. 2018; Jones 2020; Korthuis et al. 2022). This surge has been seen globally, with European and Asian countries also seeing an increase in multi-substance use involving opioids and stimulants (Hazani et al. 2022; United Nations 2020).

## Morbidity and Mortality

A survey of goofball users in the Seattle area found that concomitant use of methamphetamine and opioids is associated with increased injection drug use in high-risk areas of the body, such as the jugular vein, and fentanyl use, contributing to greater psychiatric and medical comorbidity. People who are co-using are more likely to have infections secondary to drug use, including abscesses, infected blood clots or blood infection, and endocarditis. Notably, the authors found that goofball users were more likely to be female, unstably housed or homeless, and recently incarcerated (Glick et al. 2021). Another study in Dayton, Ohio, found that methamphetamine and opioid co-use was associated with homelessness and injection heroin and fentanyl use (Daniula-ityte et al. 2020). Nonfatal overdose was greatest in people using both meth-amphetamine and opioids (22%) compared with those using opioids alone (14%) or methamphetamine alone (6%) (Korthuis et al. 2022). Opioids are frequently involved in fatal drug overdoses involving methamphetamine and cocaine. In 2018, the overdose death rate for illicit psychostimulants sur-passed the rate for prescription opioids.

Individuals using both opioids and methamphetamine were more likely to have a severe mental illness compared with those using opioids alone. Anxiety, depression, and psychosis are more prevalent and severe. One study found that the severity of negative symptoms in stimulant-induced psychosis is sec-ondary to opioids rather than the stimulant (Hazani et al. 2022; Shearer et al. 2020). The mechanisms behind these observations are unclear, but animal studies show higher neurotoxicity of co-use compared with use of either drug alone (Tian et al. 2017). Among patients in treatment for OUD, both cocaine use and methamphetamine use have been associated with poor treatment re-tention and lower opioid abstinence (Proctor et al. 2015; Tsui et al. 2020).

## Motivations for Co-use

Co-use of methamphetamine and opioids appears to yield greater rewarding effects than use of either drug alone, possibly from a greater elevation of do-pamine in the nucleus accumbens (Hazani et al. 2022). Qualitative interviews of users echoed this finding because individuals reported that small amounts of methamphetamine prolonged heroin intoxication, delaying heroin with-drawal. Stimulants are also used to prevent oversedation with opioids and to mitigate opioid withdrawal. In turn, individuals use opioids to reduce agita-tion and overexcitability with severe stimulant intoxication, making the "come down" less unpleasant. Among patients in OUD treatment, stimulants relieve the psychological urge to be "high." Some individuals transition to methamphetamine use from opioid use as a harm reduction strategy because they perceive methamphetamine to have less risk of overdose (Lopez et al. 2021; Palmer et al. 2020). These findings reflect the motivations we have heard from our patients through the years.

## Treatment

Stimulant use disorders and OUD are challenging to treat individually, and the complexity is greatly increased when they occur together. The clinician must combine psychosocial, psychotherapeutic, and pharmacological interventions to treat both conditions. Off-label medications for stimulant use disorders are covered in Chapter 6. Several studies have investigated adjunctive medications for co-occurring stimulant use disorders and OUD, with inconsistent efficacy. Most of the studies were conducted in patient populations receiving OAT. Many opioid treatment clinics discharge patients who continue to use illicit stimulants. However, we recommend continuing to treat the patient despite confirmed use. If available, contingency management may have synergistic effects with pharmacotherapy to produce better outcomes. For co-occurring disorders, we combine the medications in Table 6–1 (for cocaine use disorder [CUD]) and in Table 6–3 (for methamphetamine use disorder [MUD]) with medications for OUD (Table 7–1). In a large cohort study ($N=22,946$) of individuals with OUD receiving buprenorphine, stimulant treatment days were associated with 19% increased odds of drug-related poisoning but 36% decreased odds of attrition from buprenorphine treatment. Although this study did not specify whether stimulants were prescribed for stimulant use disorders or ADHD, this finding suggests that there may be a net gain with stimulants added to medications for OUD when appropriate (Mintz et al. 2022). However, the higher odds of drug poisoning warrant cautious prescribing, which may include practices such as frequent follow-up, limited prescriptions, and using the lowest effective dose.

## Strategies for Cocaine Use Disorder in Patients Receiving Opioid Agonist Treatment

Specific considerations to treat patients with CUD who are receiving OAT include the following:

- **Increased buprenorphine dose:** A double-blind, placebo-controlled RCT found that higher doses of buprenorphine (8–16 mg/day sublingual liquid, equivalent to 16–32 mg/day sublingual tablet) were associated with reduced cocaine and opioid use in patients with co-occurring disorders (Montoya et al. 2004).
- **Methadone versus buprenorphine:** A meta-analysis found that OAT with methadone is associated with higher rates of abstinence from both heroin and cocaine than buprenorphine (Castells et al. 2009).
- **Nonstimulant and stimulant medications:**
  - *Disulfiram 125–500 mg/day:* We combine disulfiram with buprenorphine or methadone. Any patient taking disulfiram should be educated on disulfiram's reaction with alcohol.

- *Sustained- or extended-release bupropion:* As discussed in Chapter 6, bupropion combined with contingency management reduced cocaine use in a 6-month trial with patients treated with methadone (Poling et al. 2006).

- *Stimulants:* The literature shows mixed results for methylphenidate, dextroamphetamine, and lisdexamfetamine combined with OAT, but some patients experience reduced cocaine craving and use (Castells et al. 2009; Palis et al. 2021). We have found stimulants to be useful in our patient population with regular monitoring. Stimulants should be considered for patients with comorbid ADHD.

- *Modafinil:* Although modafinil demonstrated efficacy in patients with CUD, it did not outperform placebo in a 2022 RCT for patients with CUD receiving methadone (DeVito et al. 2022).

- *Other medications:* Although topiramate has been found to be effective for CUD, an RCT did not find it to be effective for retention or cocaine abstinence in patients treated with methadone (Umbricht et al. 2014). Doxazosin has not been studied in a population with co-use, but we have used it in our patients taking buprenorphine and had success in reducing cocaine cravings and use. If the patient has PTSD or nightmares, consider adding doxazosin first if nightmares are frequent and severe.

## Strategies for Methamphetamine Use Disorder in Patients Receiving Opioid Agonist Treatment

Table 6–3 details various treatments found effective for MUD. Specific considerations include the following:

- *Atomoxetine 80 mg:* An RCT that added atomoxetine to buprenorphine/naloxone for OUD demonstrated reduced methamphetamine cravings and a higher proportion of negative urine drug screens results than placebo (Schottenfeld et al. 2018).

- *Stimulants:* The combination of methylphenidate and Matrix Model treatment resulted in significant reductions in methamphetamine use, cravings, addiction severity, and relapse rates, while also improving mental health (Aryan et al. 2020). We have combined other stimulants such as lisdexamfetamine and extended-release mixed amphetamine salts with OAT with higher rates of success among patients with more severe MUD. We recommend strongly considering stimulants for patients with comorbid ADHD.

- *Mirtazapine:* No studies have examined mirtazapine in a co-using population. However, we have used mirtazapine to treat symptoms such as anxiety, depression, insomnia, and low appetite in this patient population.
- *Antipsychotics:* Cariprazine showed efficacy in our case series and in other case reports for both methamphetamine and opioid craving in patients with co-occurring disorders. It is especially beneficial for patients with bipolar disorder or psychotic disorder (Truong and Li 2022). We have used long-acting injectable paliperidone and risperidone to treat methamphetamine-induced psychosis and to increase treatment retention.

# Clinical Practice and Case Presentation

The management of stimulant use disorders in patients with OUD has unique challenges. The following case provides an example of how to approach evaluation and treatment of such patients. We discuss different modalities of medication management, psychiatric comorbidity, and the reasons and rationale for a patient's SUD.

## Case Example

C.S. is a 36-year-old white male who presents to the Veteran Affairs clinic to treat his OUD. His psychiatric history is significant for PTSD due to military combat from several deployments to the Middle East. During his last deployment, he was involved in a Humvee accident in which his vehicle flipped over, resulting in severe physical trauma. Since the accident, C.S. has had chronic back pain, which was treated with opioids. Pain management with opioids led to development of OUD, which progressed to intravenous heroin use. Aside from chronic back pain, C.S. has no other medical comorbidities. He is currently living with his very supportive parents. After many years of using various illicit drugs, including heroin, and several failed stints in residential treatment, C.S. finally wants to get "clean." His urine drug screen (UDS) is positive for opioids, cocaine, methamphetamines, and THC.

During his intake, C.S. states, "I have a lot of pain, so I take heroin, oxy, and whatever opioids I can get my hands on. I took buprenorphine in rehab; however, when I got out of rehab, I went back to using heroin. I use coke and meth because I like the way it makes me feel, and it numbs my PTSD. I do smoke a lot of weed because it helps control my anxiety and helps with my PTSD. I want to get off these drugs and have a better life because I can't live like this anymore." In the past, C.S. has been prescribed buprenorphine with some success. However, his adherence and motivation to use the medication were suboptimal.

C.S. provided a considerable amount of information and showed insight into the drugs he was using. He uses several illicit drugs as surrogates for psychiatric medications to help with his PTSD and anxiety. In this case, the clinician must prioritize the conditions to stabilize. First and foremost, they must address his OUD because C.S. is in danger of overdosing. Therefore, the clinician needs to help C.S. stop his pattern of cravings, withdrawals, and use of opioids. Because C.S. has chronic pain requiring opioids, the clinician cannot use naltrexone as a treatment option to address both the patient's OUD and his stimulant use disorder. Buprenorphine can be used to address both his opioid use and pain.

Treatment was initiated with one sublingual tablet of buprenorphine/naloxone 8 mg/2 mg combined medication. C.S. was also started on mirtazapine 15 mg to address his anxiety, sleep, and PTSD-associated nightmares and began attending therapy sessions with an addiction therapist. He was seen for a follow-up appointment after 1 week on the medications and stated that he slept slightly better, with less anxiety at night. He had some pain relief but was still craving opioids. His UDS was positive for cocaine, methamphetamine, and THC but was negative for opioids. His buprenorphine/naloxone was increased to 16 mg/4 mg to address pain and opioid craving. Mirtazapine was maintained at 15 mg, and he was started on venlafaxine to address anxiety, PTSD, and pain.

C.S. was again seen in 1 week (2 weeks after starting buprenorphine/naloxone, 16 mg/4 mg). He stated that he was doing much better and felt his pain was better controlled with the increased dose of buprenorphine/naloxone. C.S. stated that his anxiety and PTSD symptoms have improved, but his sleep remains poor. C.S.'s UDS was positive for THC and methamphetamine. He reported no longer using any opioids and THC, and he also stopped using cocaine. However, he is still using methamphetamine because he likes how it makes him feel. C.S. was seen for several more weeks to titrate and optimize his medications. His mood and affect all improved, and his PTSD symptoms were much more manageable. His therapy sessions were going well, and his pain was significantly better. C.S.'s medications were buprenorphine/naloxone 16 mg/4 mg daily, mirtazapine 15 mg at bedtime, and venlafaxine 112.5 mg/day. His UDS was positive for only methamphetamines and negative for all other illicit drugs and alcohol.

When asked about his reasons for continued methamphetamine use, C.S. stated that he had cut down significantly on using methamphetamine but still used it every other day. Although his PTSD had improved and he was in much less pain, he could not stop using methamphetamine. C.S. stated, "I feel like myself, and I feel normal when I take meth." When asked about sleep, C.S. reported that despite taking 15 mg of mirtazapine, he was still not sleeping well. He was noted to be drinking energy drinks during his office visits. Further inquiry revealed frequent use of beverages with high caffeine content. C.S. admitted that he is easily distracted and has poor concentration, which are improved by caffeine. A thorough review of his childhood history revealed academic struggles and other symptoms indicative of ADHD. The clinician posited that C.S. might have been self-medicating with methamphetamine and high-dose caffeine drinks. C.S. was started on lisdexamfetamine 20 mg/day to help with his concentration and, although counterintuitive, anxiety and sleep.

After 1 week taking lisdexamfetamine, C.S. stated that he felt better than he had in his entire life. He could function and not feel anxious and distracted. His sleep had improved, and he was able to stop using methamphetamines. His UDS was negative for all substances. C.S.'s medications, along with therapy, were effective for OUD, MUD, THC use, chronic pain, PTSD, and ADHD. C.S.'s final medications were buprenorphine/naloxone 16 mg/4 mg daily for OUD and pain; mirtazapine 15 mg at bedtime for mood, anxiety, and sleep; venlafaxine 112.5 mg/day for mood, PTSD, and chronic pain; and lisdexamfetamine 40 mg/day for ADHD.

# Conclusion

The opioid crisis has taken countless lives and continues to ravage families and communities. Managing OUD and co-occurring disorders necessitates a multidisciplinary team with medical management, psychiatry and addiction care, peer recovery, psychotherapy, contingency management, psychosocial interventions, and case management. Essentially, individuals struggling with these conditions must rebuild their lives toward recovery. Both clinician and patient may feel that the path to change is never quite fast or easy enough and is filled with dangerous obstacles. Most clinicians treating patients with OUD have had some patients die from overdose or from other drug-related causes. Patients have often witnessed the deaths of their friends. Although these experiences may drive the initial motivation to enter treatment, they also compound trauma, increasing the risk for multi-substance use and overdose. It is not uncommon for clinicians and patients to feel frustrated, burned out, and hopeless. We recommend that clinicians prioritize their self-care. Strategies such as mindfulness, reflection, and peer consultation are essential for providers during long-term patient care.

# References

Acevedo A, Rodriguez Borja I, Alarcon Falconi TM, et al: Hospitalizations for alcohol and opioid use disorders in older adults: trends, comorbidities, and differences by gender, race, and ethnicity. Subst Abuse 16(Aug):11782218221116733, 2022 35966614

American Psychiatric Association: Diagnostic and Statistical Manual of Mental Disorders, 5th Edition. Arlington, VA, American Psychiatric Association, 2013

Aryan N, Banafshe HR, Farnia V, et al: The therapeutic effects of methylphenidate and matrix-methylphenidate on addiction severity, craving, relapse and mental health in the methamphetamine use disorder. Subst Abuse Treat Prev Policy 15(1):72, 2020 32977820

Baldassarri SR, Fiellin DA, Savage ME, et al: Electronic cigarette and tobacco use in individuals entering methadone or buprenorphine treatment. Drug Alcohol Depend 197(Apr):37–41, 2019 30769264

Bergeria CL, Huhn AS, Dunn KE: The impact of naturalistic cannabis use on self-reported opioid withdrawal. J Subst Abuse Treat 113(June):108005, 2020 32359667

Castells X, Kosten TR, Capella D, et al: Efficacy of opiate maintenance therapy and adjunctive interventions for opioid dependence with comorbid cocaine use disorders: a systematic review and meta-analysis of controlled clinical trials, in Database of Abstracts of Reviews of Effects (DARE): Quality-Assessed Reviews. York, UK, Centre for Reviews and Dissemination, 2009. Available at: https://www.ncbi.nlm.nih.gov/books/NBK78542. Accessed December 15, 2022.

Castillo F, Jones JD, Luba RR, et al: Gabapentin increases the abuse liability of alcohol alone and in combination with oxycodone in participants with co-occurring opioid and alcohol use disorder. Pharmacol Biochem Behav 221(Nov):173482, 2022 36244527

Centers for Disease Control and Prevention: Overdose deaths accelerating during COVID-19: expanded prevention efforts needed. CDC Newsroom Releases, December 17, 2020. Available at: https://www.cdc.gov/media/releases/2020/p1218-overdose-deaths-covid-19.html. Accessed December 30, 2022.

Comer SD, Mannelli P, Alam D, et al: Transition of patients with opioid use disorder from buprenorphine to extended-release naltrexone: a randomized clinical trial assessing two transition regimens. Am J Addict 29(4):313–322, 2020 32246728

Daniulaityte R, Silverstein SM, Crawford TN, et al: Methamphetamine use and its correlates among individuals with opioid use disorder in a midwestern U.S. city. Subst Use Misuse 55(11):1781–1789, 2020 32441178

De Aquino JP, Sofuoglu M, Stefanovics E, et al: Adverse consequences of co-occurring opioid use disorder and cannabis use disorder compared to opioid use disorder only. Am J Drug Alcohol Abuse 45(5):527–537, 2019 31112429

DeVito EE, Poling J, Babuscio T, et al: Modafinil does not reduce cocaine use in methadone-maintained individuals. Drug Alcohol Depend Rep 2(Mar):100032, 2022 36310662

Ditre JW, Brandon TH, Zale EL, et al: Pain, nicotine, and smoking: research findings and mechanistic considerations. Psychol Bull 137(6):1065–1093, 2011 21967450

Elkader AK, Brands B, Selby P, et al: Methadone-nicotine interactions in methadone maintenance treatment patients. J Clin Psychopharmacol 29(3):231–238, 2009 19440076

Ellis MS, Kasper ZA, Cicero TJ: Twin epidemics: the surging rise of methamphetamine use in chronic opioid users. Drug Alcohol Depend 193(Dec):14–20, 2018 30326396

Evoy KE, Roccograndi L, Le S, et al: National outpatient medication utilization for opioid and alcohol use disorders from 2014 to 2016. J Subst Abuse Treat 119(Dec):108141, 2020 33138926

Felicione NJ, Enlow P, Elswick D, et al: A pilot investigation of the effect of electronic cigarettes on smoking behavior among opioid-dependent smokers. Addict Behav 91(Apr):45–50, 2019 30006020

Frank D, Mateu-Gelabert P, Guarino H, et al: High risk and little knowledge: overdose experiences and knowledge among young adult nonmedical prescription opioid users. Int J Drug Policy 26(1):84–91, 2015 25151334

Freeman TP, Hindocha C, Baio G, et al: Cannabidiol for the treatment of cannabis use disorder: a phase 2a, double-blind, placebo-controlled, randomised, adaptive Bayesian trial. Lancet Psychiatry 7(10):865–874, 2020 32735782

Glick SN, Klein KS, Tinsley J, et al: Increasing heroin-methamphetamine (goofball) use and related morbidity among Seattle area people who inject drugs. Am J Addict 30(2):183–191, 2021 33301230

Guydish J, Passalacqua E, Pagano A, et al: An international systematic review of smoking prevalence in addiction treatment. Addiction 111(2):220–230, 2016 26392127

Hartzler B, Donovan DM, Huang Z: Comparison of opiate-primary treatment seekers with and without alcohol use disorder. J Subst Abuse Treat 39(2):114–123, 2010 20598831

Hazani HM, Naina Mohamed I, Muzaimi M, et al: Goofballing of opioid and methamphetamine: the science behind the deadly cocktail. Front Pharmacol 13:859563, 2022 35462918

Hughes A, Williams MR, Lipari RN, et al: Prescription drug use and misuse in the United States: results from the 2015 National Survey on Drug Use and Health. Ann Intern Med 167(5):293–301, 2017 28761945

Hurd YL, Yoon M, Manini AF, et al: Early phase in the development of cannabidiol as a treatment for addiction: opioid relapse takes initial center stage. Neurotherapeutics 12(4):807–815, 2015 26269227

Hurd YL, Spriggs S, Alishayev J, et al: Cannabidiol for the reduction of cue-induced craving and anxiety in drug-abstinent individuals with heroin use disorder: a double-blind randomized placebo-controlled trial. Am J Psychiatry 176(11):911–922, 2019 31109198

Jakubczyk A, Ilgen MA, Kopera M, et al: Reductions in physical pain predict lower risk of relapse following alcohol treatment. Drug Alcohol Depend 158(Jan):167–171, 2016 26653340

Jones CM: Patterns and characteristics of methamphetamine use among adults—United States, 2015–2018. MMWR Morb Mortal Wkly Rep 69(12):317–323, 2020 32214077

King A, Vena A, de Wit H, et al: Effect of combination treatment with varenicline and nicotine patch on smoking cessation among smokers who drink heavily: a randomized clinical trial. JAMA Netw Open 5(3):e220951, 2022 35244704

Korthuis PT, Cook RR, Foot CA, et al: Association of methamphetamine and opioid use with nonfatal overdose in rural communities. JAMA Netw Open 5(8):e2226544, 2022 35969400

Lake S, St Pierre M: The relationship between cannabis use and patient outcomes in medication-based treatment of opioid use disorder: a systematic review. Clin Psychol Rev 82(Dec):101939, 2020 33130527

Lee JD, Nunes EV Jr, Novo P, et al: Comparative effectiveness of extended-release naltrexone versus buprenorphine-naloxone for opioid relapse prevention (X:BOT): a multicentre, open-label, randomised controlled trial. Lancet 391(10118):309–318, 2018 29150198

Lichenstein SD, Zakiniaeiz Y, Yip SW, et al: Mechanisms and clinical features of co-occurring opioid and nicotine use. Curr Addict Rep 6(2):114–125, 2019 32864292

Lopez AM, Dhatt Z, Howe M, et al: Co-use of methamphetamine and opioids among people in treatment in Oregon: a qualitative examination of interrelated structural, community, and individual-level factors. Int J Drug Policy 91(May):103098, 2021 33476863

Manini AF, Yiannoulos G, Bergamaschi MM, et al: Safety and pharmacokinetics of oral cannabidiol when administered concomitantly with intravenous fentanyl in humans. J Addict Med 9(3):204–210, 2015 25748562

Mattson CL, Tanz LJ, Quinn K, et al: Trends and geographic patterns in drug and synthetic opioid overdose deaths—United States, 2013–2019. MMWR Morb Mortal Wkly Rep 70(6):202–207, 2021 33571180

McCool RM, Paschall Richter K: Why do so many drug users smoke? J Subst Abuse Treat 25(1):43–49, 2003 14512107

McHugh RK, Janes AC, Griffin ML, et al: Clinical correlates of smoking status in men and women with opioid use disorder. Subst Use Misuse 55(7):1054–1058, 2020 32037945

Miller SC, Fiellin DA, Rosenthal RN, et al (eds): The ASAM Principles of Addiction Medicine, 6th Edition. Philadelphia, PA, Wolters Kluwer, 2019

Mintz CM, Presnall NJ, Xu KY, et al: An examination between treatment type and treatment retention in persons with opioid and co-occurring alcohol use disorders. Drug Alcohol Depend 226(Sept):108886, 2021 34245997

Mintz CM, Xu KY, Presnall NJ, et al: Analysis of stimulant prescriptions and drug-related poisoning risk among persons receiving buprenorphine treatment for opioid use disorder. JAMA Netw Open 5(5):e2211634, 2022 35544135

Montoya ID, Gorelick DA, Preston KL, et al: Randomized trial of buprenorphine for treatment of concurrent opiate and cocaine dependence. Clin Pharmacol Ther 75(1):34–48, 2004 14749690

Mooney ME, Poling J, Gonzalez G, et al: Preliminary study of buprenorphine and bupropion for opioid dependent smokers. Am J Addict 17(4):287–292, 2008 18612883

Mücke M, Phillips T, Radbruch L, et al: Cannabis-based medicines for chronic neuropathic pain in adults. Cochrane Database Syst Rev 3(3):CD012182, 2018 29513392

Nahvi S, Ning Y, Segal KS, et al: Varenicline efficacy and safety among methadone maintained smokers: a randomized placebo-controlled trial. Addiction 109(9):1554–1563, 2014 24862167

Nielsen S, Lintzeris N, Bruno R, et al: Benzodiazepine use among chronic pain patients prescribed opioids: associations with pain, physical and mental health, and health service utilization. Pain Med 16(2):356–366, 2015 25279706

Nielsen S, Sabioni P, Trigo JM, et al: Opioid-sparing effect of cannabinoids: a systematic review and meta-analysis. Neuropsychopharmacology 42(9):1752–1765, 2017 28327548

Palis H, Marchand K, Peachey GS, et al: Exploring the effectiveness of dextroamphetamine for the treatment of stimulant use disorder: a qualitative study with patients receiving injectable opioid agonist treatment. Subst Abuse Treat Prev Policy 16(1):68, 2021 34530878

Palmer A, Scott N, Dietze P, et al: Motivations for crystal methamphetamine-opioid co-injection/co-use amongst community-recruited people who inject drugs: a qualitative study. Harm Reduct J 17(1):14, 2020 32106854

Poling J, Oliveto A, Petry N, et al: Six-month trial of bupropion with contingency management for cocaine dependence in a methadone-maintained population. Arch Gen Psychiatry 63(2):219–228, 2006 16461866

Proctor SL, Copeland AL, Kopak AM, et al: Predictors of patient retention in methadone maintenance treatment. Psychol Addict Behav 29(4):906–917, 2015 26098127

Rass O, Umbricht A, Bigelow GE, et al: Topiramate impairs cognitive function in methadone-maintained individuals with concurrent cocaine dependence. Psychol Addict Behav 29(1):237–246, 2015 25365653

Richter KP, Hamilton AK, Hall S, et al: Patterns of smoking and methadone dose in drug treatment patients. Exp Clin Psychopharmacol 15(2):144–153, 2007 17469938

Rizk MM, Herzog S, Dugad S, et al: Suicide risk and addiction: the impact of alcohol and opioid use disorders. Curr Addict Rep 8(2):194–207, 2021 33747710

Rogers AH, Bakhshaie J, Buckner JD, et al: Opioid and cannabis co-use among adults with chronic pain: relations to substance misuse, mental health, and pain experience. J Addict Med 13(4):287–294, 2019 30557213

Rosic T, Naji L, Bawor M, et al: The impact of comorbid psychiatric disorders on methadone maintenance treatment in opioid use disorder: a prospective cohort study. Neuropsychiatr Dis Treat 13(May):1399–1408, 2017 28579787

Rosic T, Kapoor R, Panesar B, et al: The association between cannabis use and outcome in pharmacological treatment for opioid use disorder. Harm Reduct J 18(1):24, 2021 33622351

Saha TD, Kerridge BT, Goldstein RB, et al: Nonmedical prescription opioid use and DSM-5 nonmedical prescription opioid use disorder in the United States. J Clin Psychiatry 77(6):772–780, 2016 27337416

Schottenfeld RS, Chawarski MC, Sofuoglu M, et al: Atomoxetine for amphetamine-type stimulant dependence during buprenorphine treatment: a randomized controlled trial. Drug Alcohol Depend 186:130–137, 2018 29573648

Shah A, Hayes CJ, Lakkad M, et al: Impact of medical marijuana legalization on opioid use, chronic opioid use, and high-risk opioid use. J Gen Intern Med 34(8):1419–1426, 2019 30684198

Shearer RD, Howell BA, Bart G, et al: Substance use patterns and health profiles among US adults who use opioids, methamphetamine, or both, 2015–2018. Drug Alcohol Depend 214(Sept):108162, 2020 32652380

Shover CL, Vest NA, Chen D, et al: Association of state policies allowing medical cannabis for opioid use disorder with dispensary marketing for this indication. JAMA Netw Open 3(7):e2010001, 2020 32662844

Soyka M: Alcohol use disorders in opioid maintenance therapy: prevalence, clinical correlates and treatment. Eur Addict Res 21(2):78–87, 2015 25413371

Soyka M: Transition from full mu opioid agonists to buprenorphine in opioid dependent patients: a critical review. Front Pharmacol 12(Nov):718811, 2021 34887748

Stein MD, Caviness CM, Kurth ME, et al: Varenicline for smoking cessation among methadone-maintained smokers: a randomized clinical trial. Drug Alcohol Depend 133(2):486–493, 2013 23953658

Tian X, Ru Q, Xiong Q, et al: Neurotoxicity induced by methamphetamine-heroin combination in PC12 cells. Neurosci Lett 647(Apr):1–7, 2017 28274858

Truong TT, Li B: Case series: cariprazine for treatment of methamphetamine use disorder. Am J Addict 31(1):85–88, 2022 34713943

Tsui JI, Lira MC, Cheng DM, et al: Chronic pain, craving, and illicit opioid use among patients receiving opioid agonist therapy. Drug Alcohol Depend 166(Sept):26–31, 2016 27422763

Tsui JI, Mayfield J, Speaker EC, et al: Association between methamphetamine use and retention among patients with opioid use disorders treated with buprenorphine. J Subst Abuse Treat 109(Feb):80–85, 2020 31810594

Umbricht A, DeFulio A, Winstanley EL, et al: Topiramate for cocaine dependence during methadone maintenance treatment: a randomized controlled trial. Drug Alcohol Depend 140(July):92–100, 2014 24814607

United Nations: UNODC Report on East and Southeast Asia: Continued Growth in the Supply of Methamphetamine While Synthetic Opioids Spread. New York, United Nations Office on Drugs and Crime, May 2020. Available at: http://www.unodc.org/unodc/en/frontpage/2020/May/unodc-report-on-east-and-southeast-asia_-continued-growth-in-the-supply-of-methamphetamine-while-synthetic-opioids-spread.html. Accessed November 30, 2022.

Vierke C, Marxen B, Boettcher M, et al: Buprenorphine-cannabis interaction in patients undergoing opioid maintenance therapy. Eur Arch Psychiatry Clin Neurosci 271(5):847–856, 2021 31907614

Vlad C, Arnsten JH, Nahvi S: Achieving smoking cessation among persons with opioid use disorder. CNS Drugs 34(4):367–387, 2020 32107731

Voelker R: States move to substitute opioids with medical marijuana to quell epidemic. JAMA 320(23):2408–2410, 2018 30484825

Weinberger AH, Platt J, Esan H, et al: Cigarette smoking is associated with increased risk of substance use disorder relapse: a nationally representative, prospective longitudinal investigation. J Clin Psychiatry 78(2):e152–e160, 2017 28234432

World Health Organization: Global Status Report on Alcohol and Health: 2014. Geneva, World Health Organization, 2014

Xierali IM, Day PG, Kleinschmidt KC, et al: Emergency department presentation of opioid use disorder and alcohol use disorder. J Subst Abuse Treat 127(Aug):108343, 2021 34134862

# 8

# Trinity Combinations

## Daryl Shorter, M.D.

*Patients* with multi-substance use disorder (MSUD), which is sometimes interchangeably referred to as polysubstance use disorder, can be particularly challenging when a clinical approach is being crafted. Both patient and clinician satisfaction can be substantially complicated and reduced in cases in which multiple substances are involved, creating further challenges for building rapport, developing shared goals, and decision-making in clinical care.

Polysubstance use represents a particular challenge for patients, given that treatment retention and completion are less likely among persons who use three or more substances. Studies have found that individuals with MSUD experience greater negative consequences from use and worsened treatment outcomes. In a 2017 study of veterans with substance use disorders (SUDs) ($N$=472,624), subjects with higher levels of MSUD (24% with two or three SUDs, 2.7% with more than three SUDs) were more likely to be unhoused and have medical illness, such as hepatic disease (Bhalla et al. 2017). Veterans with higher levels of MSUD were also more likely to have psychiatric illnesses, including schizophrenia, bipolar disorder, personality disorders, and major depressive disorder, and to have multiple psychotropic medication prescription fills. Additionally, higher levels of MSUD were associated with greater service utilization, including psychiatric inpatient care and residential and rehabilitative treatment. Of note, this study also found that veterans identifying as African American were more likely to experience higher levels of MSUD; however, the contribution of social determinants of mental health, such as race/ethnicity, has yet to be fully elucidated and remains an active focus of research.

There has been a substantial focus in the literature on the characteristics of persons with MSUD as well as the trajectories of their use. Perhaps unsurprisingly, rates of long-term persistence of SUD (e.g., 3-year follow-up) have been found to be highest among persons with MSUD (Evans et al. 2017). In one analysis of stimulant users, for example, those who used a combination of powder cocaine, alcohol, and cannabis and those using a combination of non-prescribed opioids, alcohol, cannabis, crack cocaine, and powder cocaine had poorer physical and mental health status, greater severity of substance use, and higher treatment service utilization (Timko et al. 2018).

Given the substantial mental health and psychosocial challenges associated with polysubstance use, it is even more critical that these conditions be aggressively managed in the clinical setting—a treatment approach that can, and should, include use of pharmacotherapy. In this chapter, we discuss the management of patients who have three significant SUDs.

# General Approach to Treatment

Although crafting a comprehensive and evidence-supported treatment of poly-substance use disorders can be challenging, developing a clinical strategy that allows for psychiatric triage and considers the patient's short- and long-term goals can enhance shared decision-making between the clinician and patient and clarify the role of pharmacotherapy in management. Using the following five-step approach can help with determining how to proceed with care:

1. Thoroughly evaluate all substances used.
2. Triage the patient and provide treatment for any substances associated with life-threatening withdrawal or acute psychiatric symptoms in the context of substance intoxication or withdrawal.
3. Once the patient is through acute withdrawal or their psychiatric symptoms stabilize, develop an understanding of their goals for treatment.
4. Offer evidence-supported pharmacotherapy aimed at either establishing abstinence or reducing harms.
5. Check in frequently with the patient and be open to revising the plan as necessary.

## Step 1: Thoroughly Evaluate Substances Used

Individuals engage in polysubstance use for many reasons. Some use multiple substances concurrently to create a synergistic effect, enhancing euphoria or other drug-related experiences. They may combine substances with opposing effects, which adds to the complexity of determining which substance(s) to address first in treatment and in what order. For example, some patients may use one substance for its primary effect, then use other substances to diminish symptoms associated with drug withdrawal or to reduce drug craving. Still others may use various substances primarily on the basis of the desired effect at the time of use, drug availability, or other factors such as cost.

In addition to specific drug effects, patients may also experience psychiatric symptoms that are similar to symptoms of substance intoxication or withdrawal. It is crucial to determine whether psychiatric symptoms are present that require immediate intervention or the patient's symptoms will resolve with the end of acute drug effects and require post-acute withdrawal monitoring. Mood changes, such as elevation or dysphoria, are especially common at the time of presentation to treatment. Mood elevation reflects the euphoria typically seen during intoxication, and dysphoria is often observed during withdrawal. Symptoms of psychosis, including paranoid ideation and perceptual distortions such as auditory or visual hallucinations, can complicate evaluation in the acute setting and make it difficult to determine which substances were ingested. Altered sensorium, decreased alertness, and sedation also may be acute drug effects that affect the clinician's ability to collect a patient's history. In such cases, collateral information from others can provide vital clues, particularly when employed alongside drug testing (see Chapter 4, "Laboratory Testing").

The traditional substance use history focuses on details regarding the patient's use patterns (i.e., first use, last use), the frequency, and the amount used (see Chapter 2, "General Approach to Patients With Multi-substance Use Disorders"). It is also essential to scrutinize the pattern and relationship of substances to each other within the patient's use constellation. When assessing patients with multi-substance use, it is necessary to determine not only those substances currently being used but the temporal relationship between them (Table 8–1). Clinicians should inquire about the substances last used in order to determine which symptoms of substance withdrawal to monitor. By understanding the relationship between substances and their desired effects, clinicians can provide optimal guidance to patients about which substances to discontinue immediately, which to taper gradually, and the order in which to taper them.

## Step 2: Triage Patient and Treat Emergent Cases

Once a complete history is obtained, a psychiatric triage should be performed to determine the presence of any substances associated with life-threatening withdrawal (e.g., alcohol, benzodiazepines, barbiturates). If acute withdrawal

Table 8–1.    Sample questions for collecting history of multi-substance use

In a typical episode of substance use, which substance(s) do you use first or in combination?

What effect(s) are you seeking when using? For how long do you generally experience these effects?

Which substance(s) might you use to reduce withdrawal?

Are there substances that you use to reduce cravings for another type or category of substance?

Which substance(s) did you most recently use prior to your presentation?

management for one or more substances is necessary, admission for inpatient medical or psychiatric services may be warranted. Clinical practice guidelines for managing acute alcohol or sedative-hypnotic withdrawal should be followed, along with routine monitoring of vital signs and administering medications such as benzodiazepines to stabilize or prevent autonomic instability, seizures, or delirium.

If the acute withdrawal is not life-threatening but the symptoms can be reduced or alleviated, the clinician should consider providing pharmacotherapeutic support. Assessment begins with an inquiry about past episodes of the withdrawal syndrome and includes determining the severity level at presentation. Scales such as the Clinical Institute Withdrawal Assessment for Alcohol–Revised (CIWA-Ar) and Brief Alcohol Withdrawal Scale (BAWS) allow for an objective assessment to help guide clinical decision-making regarding the need for medications. In cases in which opioid withdrawal syndrome is anticipated, clinicians may consider using opioid agonist medications such as buprenorphine/naloxone and methadone and nonopioid medications such as the $\alpha_2$-adrenergic agonists clonidine and lofexidine. It is no longer clinically appropriate to recommend or endorse a process of abrupt cessation, or "quitting cold turkey," because it forces patients to go through unnecessary discomfort, reduces their likelihood of completing withdrawal, and worsens treatment retention and clinical outcomes. Concurrent treatment of acute psychiatric symptoms, such as substance-induced mania or psychosis, may also be required following initial evaluation (see Chapter 2).

## Step 3: Understand the Patient's Goals for Treatment

Patients and clinicians may not always agree on a treatment approach. When regularly using multiple substances, patients may consider one substance particularly problematic due to factors such as negative family or social consequences, individual drug cost, and availability. The clinician's priorities may deviate from these patient concerns, particularly when substances are present that complicate or become life-threatening during withdrawal (e.g., alcohol, benzodiazepines) or cause or exacerbate psychiatric symptoms (e.g., psychostimulant worsening of psychosis). Therefore, while creating a plan of action, clinicians must clearly understand the patient's treatment goals. They should first ask whether abstinence is a treatment goal. If so, does the patient seek abstinence from all substances or do they intend to change the pattern of use for only one of several substances used? By gathering this information, the clinician can gain a more comprehensive understanding of the patient's relationship with abstinence.

In cases in which abstinence is not the goal, clinicians must meet their patients where they are in terms of their motivation and readiness to change. Although providing psychoeducation on the dangers of withdrawal is important, trying to scare or push patients into total abstinence without first exploring deeper can generate distance and conflict between clinician and patient, causing patients to feel unheard and perhaps making it less likely that they will engage in care. If harm reduction is the patient's stated treatment goal, the clinician should inquire what harm reduction means to them. Operating from this framework, the clinician can help patients establish ideal substance use in terms of an amount and frequency that lower their harm risks. The clinician should also discuss and review other behaviors related to substance use that the patient would like to reduce (i.e., driving while under the influence, engaging in unsafe sex). Another important part of this patient conversation focuses on helping them decide how they will know their harm reduction plan is not working or requires modification or when they should consider incorporating a trial of abstinence or a higher level of treatment services.

## Step 4: Offer Pharmacotherapy to Establish Abstinence or Reduce Harms

Despite the substantial dangers posed to patients with multiple drug use, information in the clinical trial literature is scant regarding the pharmacotherapeutic management of these complex conditions. However, the principles and strategies discussed in previous chapters can help create a standardized approach to the patient's clinical management. In addition to considering medications, particularly in cases in which harm reduction is the patient's goal, additional services such as referral for primary care or specialty medical services (e.g., infectious disease treatment for HIV, hepatitis B and C) are likely appropriate.

## Step 5: Check in With Patient and Revise Plan as Necessary

Because a one-size-fits-all approach is extremely challenging to employ when working with patients with SUDs, flexibility and willingness to continuously revise the plan are critical. Reframing difficulties and challenges that patients face as opportunities for improving the overall treatment strategy can go a long way in reducing patients' guilt and shame over experiencing craving or a recurrence of use. Often, the constraints of clinical schedules that do not allow frequent follow-up (i.e., weekly or more) mean that, unfortunately, many patients do not receive clinical reinforcement of tools and strategies to promote harm reduction or abstinence. When patients are struggling, the clinician should consider increasing the number of patient encounters per week. Consultation with nursing and peer recovery specialists can be a valuable part of crafting a team-based approach to SUD management in which between-visit contact can be incorporated to support the patient and promote retention in care.

# Trinity Combinations

When patients present requesting treatment for SUD and have multiple substances in their recent use history, one challenge for clinicians is determining how to structure the management of multi-substance withdrawal. However, prior to prescribing medications, clinicians should first determine whether inpatient hospitalization or withdrawal management ("detox") services are necessary. Using the American Society of Addiction Medicine (ASAM) Patient Placement Criteria (American Society of Addiction Medicine 2022) or another standardized evaluation is clinically appropriate and helpful in removing much of the subjectivity from the evaluation and in making decisions based on objective findings and data. A free interview guide based on the ASAM criteria can be downloaded at www.asam.org/asam-criteria.

For patients admitted to an inpatient or residential facility, it is possible to utilize either a fixed-dose or symptom-triggered strategy for managing withdrawal from substances such as alcohol, sedative/hypnotics, and opioids. A fixed-dose strategy is characterized by a standard, preset amount of medication tapered over several days. This strategy may be considered for withdrawal management when monitoring is limited for various reasons (e.g., staff shortages, clinical or nursing staff unfamiliar with managing withdrawal). However, whenever possible, we prefer using a symptom-triggered approach in which objective signs of withdrawal are measured via standardized scales, and medication is administered on the basis of the patient's demonstrated need for pharmacological assistance. This strategy is helpful in cases in which it is not possible to confirm the amount of substance ingested prior to admission. It also ensures that patients are not undertreated for withdrawal because of concern that they are seeking medications, a highly stigmatizing concern that is, unfortunately, all too prevalent in our treatment settings. Creating a standardized approach to medication management of multi-substance withdrawal syndrome (Table 8–2) can help ensure that patients receive the appropriate dosages of medications, reduce patient and clinician anxiety and frustration, and increase the likelihood of retaining patients in care throughout the withdrawal management phase.

# Management of Opioid-Involved Multi-substance Withdrawal

When opioids are one of the drug categories in the patient's constellation of substances, clinicians must first choose between using opioid agonist therapy (OAT) and symptom management with clonidine. This decision should be made in collaboration with the patient, who must understand both the risks and benefits of both approaches. Opioid withdrawal symptom control with buprenorphine/naloxone induction or methadone is likely to be superior to that achieved with clonidine or other ancillary medications for bone pain or myalgia (e.g., nonsteroidal anti-inflammatory drugs, acetaminophen), anxiety (e.g., benzodiazepines), or insomnia (e.g., trazodone). However, patients may express concern or reticence regarding the long-term implications of OAT, particularly because they may worry about the need to be prescribed these medications for some time. It is important to review with patients the evidence supporting stabilization and maintenance with buprenorphine/naloxone and its superiority to taper in terms of treatment retention and reduced

Table 8–2.    Multi-substance withdrawal management
              strategies

| Substances involved | Medication strategy |
|---|---|
| Opioids, alcohol, and tobacco or nicotine | Use symptom-triggered COWS protocol for buprenorphine induction and stabilization. |
| | Use symptom-triggered CIWA-Ar or BAWS protocol for management of alcohol withdrawal syndrome using benzodiazepine. |
| | Offer combination NRT (long-acting, i.e., patch, plus short-acting, i.e., gum, lozenge), bupropion, or varenicline. |
| Opioids, alcohol, and psychostimulant | Use symptom-triggered COWS protocol for buprenorphine/naloxone induction and stabilization. |
| | Use symptom-triggered CIWA-Ar or BAWS protocol for alcohol withdrawal syndrome management. |
| | Once alcohol withdrawal syndrome has resolved, initiate treatment of co-occurring alcohol and psychostimulant use disorders with topiramate, naltrexone , or disulfiram. Note that initiation of topiramate during withdrawal may be helpful. |
| Opioids, benzodiazepines, and psychostimulant | Use symptom-triggered COWS protocol for buprenorphine/naloxone induction and stabilization. |
| | Convert reported benzodiazepine dosage to equivalent dosage in long-acting formulation (e.g., clonazepam) and initiate gradual, flexible taper. |
| | Incorporate evidence-supported medication for treatment of stimulant use disorder (see Tables 8–3 and 8–4). |
| Alcohol or sedative, psychostimulant, and cannabis | Use symptom-triggered CIWA-Ar or BAWS protocol for alcohol withdrawal syndrome management. |
| | If sedative-hypnotic withdrawal syndrome is a concern, use CIWA-B to assess withdrawal severity; convert reported benzodiazepine dosage to equivalent dosage in long-acting formulation (e.g., clonazepam) and initiate gradual, flexible taper. |

**Table 8–2.** **Multi-substance withdrawal management strategies** *(continued)*

| Substances involved | Medication strategy |
|---|---|
| Alcohol or sedative, psychostimulant, and cannabis *(continued)* | Incorporate evidence-supported medication for treatment of stimulant use disorder.<br><br>Although evidence is weaker, consider addition of medications to reduce cannabis withdrawal and craving such as gabapentin and *N*-acetylcysteine. |

*Note.* BAWS = Brief Alcohol Withdrawal Scale; CIWA-Ar = Clinical Institute Withdrawal Assessment for Alcohol–Revised; CIWA-B = Clinical Institute Withdrawal Assessment for Benzodiazepines; COWS = Clinical Opiate Withdrawal Scale; NRT = nicotine replacement therapy.

opioid use (Wakeman et al. 2020). Furthermore, in light of the potential risks associated with increased exposure to fentanyl and accidental opioid overdose, simply managing opioid withdrawal symptoms or tapering/discontinuing agonist therapy places the patient at risk for negative or fatal consequences that far exceed the risks posed by maintenance therapy.

If the patient selects management of OUD with agonist therapy, either buprenorphine/naloxone or methadone, then pharmacotherapy for the comorbid SUDs can be initiated concurrently or immediately following stabilization of the opioid withdrawal syndrome. If alcohol has been a prominent part of the patient's use constellation, then monitoring and assessing the severity of alcohol withdrawal syndrome are appropriate. Using a symptom-triggered protocol, the clinician should prescribe an intermediate-acting benzodiazepine (e.g., lorazepam) or long-acting benzodiazepine (e.g., chlordiazepoxide or diazepam) for patients with either a CIWA score greater than 10 or a BAWS score greater than 4. We recommend checking the patient's liver enzymes prior to selecting a benzodiazepine, when possible, to confirm that hepatic function has not been compromised (alanine transaminase, aspartate transaminase less than 3 times upper limit of normal). If the liver enzymes are significantly elevated or the patient is older than 65 years, then lorazepam is recommended because of its metabolism via glucuronidation, which is less affected by hepatic disease. Unlike chlordiazepoxide and diazepam, lorazepam also lacks active metabolites that can accumulate and lead to excess sedation.

In some cases, patients may achieve only partial relief from opioid withdrawal and craving while pharmacotherapy is being used to treat another SUD. Using the COWS and CIWA-Ar scales concurrently can guide which medication(s), if any, should be adjusted or if encouragement and psychological support are needed instead to reassure the patient that their symptoms are being adequately monitored and will gradually resolve with time. Clinicians may worry about concurrently using an opioid, even a partial agonist, alongside a benzodiazepine. However, in cases of severe alcohol withdrawal and concomitant opioid withdrawal, this may be necessary. Although there are risks to combining OAT with a benzodiazepine, the potential risk of severe and untreated alcohol withdrawal may be even greater.

# Management of Benzodiazepine-Involved Multi-substance Withdrawal

In cases in which patients present with both OUD and sedative-hypnotic (benzodiazepine) use disorder, once opioid withdrawal syndrome has been stabilized, addressing the benzodiazepine is appropriate, particularly given the potential synergistic effect with the opioid. At the time of admission (or shortly thereafter), the clinician should transition the patient to a long-acting benzodiazepine such as clonazepam at relatively equivalent dosages and institute a gradual taper (Medscape 2021).

One complication with using an equivalent-dosage strategy is that it is often not possible to verify or confirm the amount of benzodiazepine being taken at the time of presentation. Furthermore, if patients have been obtaining benzodiazepines from street-based sources, sometimes referred to as "street benzos," these pressed pills may not have the amount of benzodiazepine advertised. Therefore, admitting the patient to an inpatient unit or withdrawal management program allows them to be monitored continuously for withdrawal symptoms using a scale such as the Clinical Institute Withdrawal Assessment for Benzodiazepines (CIWA-B). Benzodiazepine dosing can be symptom-triggered on the first day. On the second day, the total amount of benzodiazepines needed on the first day can be dosed on a fixed schedule, then gradually tapered. If the patient has not been admitted to a facility and outpatient treatment is being attempted, then calculating an equivalent dosage of the short-acting benzodiazepine and converting it to a long-acting benzodiazepine is appropriate.

There is no established protocol for a benzodiazepine taper, but evidence supports a gradual taper over a period of weeks. Generally, although clinicians may try to reduce the amount of benzodiazepine by 10% per week (Soyka 2017), in practice, many patients need prescribers to "hang in" with them, providing substantial support, establishing rapport and trust, and incrementally decreasing the dosage at intervals when the patient feels the most comfortable with and prepared for dosage reduction. For example, if a patient reports a recent or current stressor, it is clinically inappropriate to rigidly adhere to a taper schedule and reduce the dosage of a benzodiazepine while the patient is experiencing psychological strain. Instead, clinicians should hold at the current dosage until the patient reports readiness or agreement with dosage reduction. This approach may require frequent check-ins and patient visits; thus, using clinical extenders and nursing staff to check in with patients is ideal (and can be helpful).

# Management of Stimulant-Involved Multi-substance Withdrawal

Because psychostimulant withdrawal is not associated with the likelihood of mortality, inpatient admission or withdrawal management is not always warranted. However, in cases in which concurrent psychiatric symptoms of depression and suicidal ideation, mania, or psychosis are present, admission may be necessary. Thus, acute withdrawal management is required in addition to stabilizing the patient psychiatrically. Even in cases in which patients are not experiencing acute psychiatric crises, some patients are admitted on the basis of other factors that place them at increased risk of recurrence (e.g., poor social support, unsafe living conditions). Ultimately, regardless of whether they are admitted to an inpatient or residential treatment program, frank discussions with patients about the management of stimulant withdrawal in the context of other substance withdrawal syndromes are warranted.

Patients may wonder whether there are medications that can be used to reduce their craving or other abstinence-related symptoms of discomfort. Although currently no medications have been FDA-approved for treatment of stimulant use disorder, several have shown a positive signal in clinical trials. These may be potential interventional options (Tables 8–3 and 8–4). Consider use of these medications as a component of the overall pharmacotherapeutic treatment offering. Patients with MSUD are incredibly challenging to engage and retain in treatment. As such, the untreated discomfort of stimulant withdrawal, particularly in the context of other types of abstinence syndromes, may be one of the primary factors contributing to adverse treatment outcomes, behavioral challenges such as irritability, and increased risk of early treatment termination or discharge. Withholding potentially helpful medica-

**Table 8–3.** Methamphetamine pharmacotherapy

| Medication | Proposed mechanism of action | Target effects |
|---|---|---|
| Bupropion (Anderson et al. 2015; Elkashef et al. 2008; Heinzerling et al. 2014; Shoptaw et al. 2008) | Dopamine and norepinephrine reuptake inhibition | Reduce methamphetamine use in users with low severity |
| Mirtazapine (Coffin et al. 2020; Colfax et al. 2011) | Enhance dopamine and norepinephrine by blocking presynaptic $\alpha_2$-adrenergic and/or 5-HT$_{2C}$ receptors | Reduce methamphetamine use and HIV risk behaviors |
| Methylphenidate (Ling et al. 2014; Tiihonen et al. 2012) | Enhance dopamine and norepinephrine by reuptake inhibition at DAT/NET | Reduce craving (may be better in heavy users) |
| Naltrexone (Jayaram-Lindström et al. 2008) | Opioid antagonist | Reduce methamphetamine use, reduce craving |
| Intramuscular naltrexone plus bupropion (Trivedi et al. 2021) | Combination therapy | Reduce methamphetamine use, decrease treatment attrition |

*Note.* DAT=dopamine transporter; 5-HT$_{2C}$=serotonin type 2 receptor; NET=norepinephrine transporter.

Table 8–4.    Cocaine pharmacotherapy

| Medication | Proposed mechanism of action | Target effects |
|---|---|---|
| Bupropion 300 mg/day | Dopamine and norepinephrine reuptake inhibition | Combined with contingency management, reduce cocaine use |
| Topiramate (Johnson et al. 2013; Kampman et al. 2004, 2013) | GABA and glutamate modulation | Reduce cocaine use |
| Mixed amphetamine salts plus topiramate (Levin et al. 2020) | Enhance dopamine and norepinephrine by reuptake inhibition at DAT/NET; glutamate modulation | Reduce cocaine use, reduce craving (better in heavy users) |
| Modafinil 200–400 mg/day (Dackis et al. 2012) | Enhance dopamine and norepinephrine by blocking presynaptic $\alpha_2$-adrenergic and/or $5\text{-HT}_{2C}$ receptors | Reduce cocaine use in males |

*Note.*    $5\text{-HT}_{2C}$ = serotonin type 2 receptor.

tions from patients in an effort to adhere to archaic notions of "getting clean" and "going cold turkey" is no longer appropriate because the punishment and suffering are potentially avoidable.

Based on the psychiatric symptoms present at the time of assessment, the patient's history of experiences with psychiatric medications, the potential for drug-drug interactions, and the patient's medical and psychosocial history, clinicians should select a medication that might help reduce stimulant craving. For example, in patients with a long-standing history of chronic depression who use methamphetamine and engage in high-risk sexual behaviors, clinicians should consider adding mirtazapine because it has been shown to reduce methamphetamine use and to lower HIV risk behaviors. It has the additional benefit of helping reduce insomnia, which can be a complicating treatment factor. Furthermore, from a harm reduction standpoint, the risk associated with prescribing mirtazapine is far outweighed by the risk of continuing methamphetamine use and/or HIV risk behaviors. Thus, medication can and should be a cornerstone component of the clinician's pharmacotherapeutic strategy despite the lack of FDA approval.

# Management of Cannabis-Involved Multi-substance Withdrawal

Given the vastly higher potency of cannabinoid (Δ-9-tetrahydrocannabinol [Δ-9 THC]) products used by patients more recently, we recommend medication to assist with managing cannabis withdrawal, particularly when cannabis is used in combination with other substances. Again, if retaining the patient in treatment remains the central goal, then it is important to convey a sense of hope and to express willingness to work with them, validating and addressing their concerns, which includes managing cannabis withdrawal.

Although the evidence supporting medications such as gabapentin and N-acetylcysteine (NAC) is weak, they still represent our current best options for managing cannabis withdrawal. Managing withdrawal becomes especially important when we consider that—just as high-potency THC presents a risk from a mental health standpoint during its use and intoxication—withdrawal from high-potency THC, particularly in the absence of pharmacotherapeutic support or taper, poses a risk to continued treatment engagement.

# Guiding Principles

Admittedly, patients with MSUD can be challenging to treat. However, keeping in mind certain guiding principles can help to make this work more rewarding for both patients and clinicians:

- Abstinence syndrome, regardless of substance, is difficult for patients to get through. It is critical to recognize that even if the withdrawal is not life-threatening, it still warrants attention and is important to treat.
- Providing pharmacotherapy to reduce withdrawal-related discomfort represents an important strategy for early engagement and retention of patients in treatment.
- The use of pharmacotherapy during this early period can be a bridge to the ongoing use of medications for both SUD and symptoms related to mental health.
- Medication management may be one of the primary reasons that patients remain engaged in care, which then affords an opportunity to use psychotherapeutic strategies such as motivational interviewing, contingency man-

agement, and cognitive-behavioral therapy to further bolster a desire to uphold change.

- Clinicians should adjust expectations and ideas regarding what constitutes treatment success. Going from using four substances regularly to total abstinence overnight is incredibly challenging for the vast majority of persons with MSUD. By meeting patients where they are and ensuring their continued engagement in care, the likelihood of achieving positive change over time increases, leading to greater satisfaction for both patients and clinicians, as well as improved potential for positive outcomes.

# References

American Society of Addiction Medicine: ASAM Criteria Intake Assessment Guide. Rockville, MD, American Society of Addiction Medicine, 2022. Available at: https://www.asam.org/asam-criteria/criteria-intake-assessment-form. Accessed December 4, 2022.

Anderson AL, Li S-H, Markova D, et al: Bupropion for the treatment of methamphetamine dependence in non-daily users: a randomized, double-blind, placebo-controlled trial. Drug Alcohol Depend 150(May):170–174, 2015 25818061

Bhalla IP, Stefanovics EA, Rosenheck RA: Clinical epidemiology of single versus multiple substance use disorders: polysubstance use disorder. Med Care 55(Sept):S24–S32, 2017 28806363

Coffin PO, Santos G-M, Hern J, et al: Effects of mirtazapine for methamphetamine use disorder among cisgender men and transgender women who have sex with men: a placebo-controlled randomized clinical trial. JAMA Psychiatry 77(3):246–255, 2020 31825466

Colfax GN, Santos GM, Das M, et al: Mirtazapine to reduce methamphetamine use: a randomized controlled trial. Arch Gen Psychiatry 68(11):1168–1175, 2011 22065532

Dackis CA, Kampman KM, Lynch KG, et al: A double-blind, placebo-controlled trial of modafinil for cocaine dependence. J Subst Abuse Treat 43(3):303–312, 2012 22377391

Elkashef AM, Rawson RA, Anderson AL, et al: Bupropion for the treatment of methamphetamine dependence. Neuropsychopharmacology 33(5):1162–1170, 2008 17581531

Evans EA, Grella CE, Washington DL, et al: Gender and race/ethnic differences in the persistence of alcohol, drug, and poly-substance use disorders. Drug Alcohol Depend 174(May):128–136, 2017 28324815

Heinzerling KG, Swanson A-N, Hall TM, et al: Randomized, placebo-controlled trial of bupropion in methamphetamine-dependent participants with less than daily methamphetamine use. Addiction 109(11):1878–1886, 2014 24894963

Jayaram-Lindström N, Hammarberg A, Beck O, et al: Naltrexone for the treatment of amphetamine dependence: a randomized, placebo-controlled trial. Am J Psychiatry 165(11):1442–1448, 2008 18765480

Johnson BA, Ait-Daoud N, Wang X-Q, et al: Topiramate for the treatment of cocaine addiction: a randomized clinical trial. JAMA Psychiatry 70(12):1338–1346, 2013 24132249

Kampman KM, Pettinati H, Lynch KG, et al: A pilot trial of topiramate for the treatment of cocaine dependence. Drug Alcohol Depend 75(3):233–240, 2004 15283944

Kampman KM, Pettinati HM, Lynch KG, et al: A double-blind, placebo-controlled trial of topiramate for the treatment of comorbid cocaine and alcohol dependence. Drug Alcohol Depend 133(1):94–99, 2013 23810644

Levin FR, Mariani JJ, Pavlicova M, et al: Extended release mixed amphetamine salts and topiramate for cocaine dependence: a randomized clinical replication trial with frequent users. Drug Alcohol Depend 206(Jan):107700, 2020 31753736

Ling W, Chang L, Hillhouse M, et al: Sustained-release methylphenidate in a randomized trial of treatment of methamphetamine use disorder. Addiction 109(9):1489–1500, 2014 24825486

Medscape: Benzodiazepine equivalency chart: benzodiazepine equivalency. Medscape, September 20, 2021. Available at: https://emedicine.medscape.com/article/2172250-overview. Accessed January 14, 2023.

Shoptaw S, Heinzerling KG, Rotheram-Fuller E, et al: Randomized, placebo-controlled trial of bupropion for the treatment of methamphetamine dependence. Drug Alcohol Depend 96(3):222–232, 2008 18468815

Soyka M: Treatment of benzodiazepine dependence. N Engl J Med 376(12):1147–1157, 2017 28328330

Tiihonen J, Krupitsky E, Verbitskaya E, et al: Naltrexone implant for the treatment of polydrug dependence: a randomized controlled trial. Am J Psychiatry 169(5):531–536, 2012 22764364

Timko C, Han X, Woodhead E, et al: Polysubstance use by stimulant users: health outcomes over three years. J Stud Alcohol Drugs 79(5):799–807, 2018 30422794

Trivedi MH, Walker R, Ling W, et al: Bupropion and naltrexone in methamphetamine use disorder. N Engl J Med 384(2):140–153, 2021 33497547

Wakeman SE, Larochelle MR, Ameli O, et al: Comparative effectiveness of different treatment pathways for opioid use disorder. JAMA Netw Open 3(2):e1920622, 2020 32022884

# 9

# Novel Psychoactive Substances

Thanh Thuy Truong, M.D.

*Novel* psychoactive substances (NPSs) refer to emerging psychoactive substances, most of which are synthetic and have effects similar to common substances. The NPSs include synthetic cannabis, synthetic cathinones, synthetic opioids, hallucinogens, and other plant-derived substances such as kratom. These substances emerged as legal alternatives to standard substances and are easily accessible in convenience stores and on the internet. Some substances (i.e., kratom and delta-8) are marketed as having milder effects than common drugs and carrying health benefits. The Synthetic Drug Abuse Prevention Act of 2012 banned synthetic cathinones and synthetic cannabis, but newer similar compounds continue to be produced (Office of National Drug Control Policy 2014). The literature has limited information on the pharmacological management of these substance use disorders. In this chapter we provide a broad overview of each NPS, with a summary in Table 9–1.

## Note on Urine Toxicology Screening

Standard urine toxicology screens do not detect NPSs. Separate screening is required for each synthetic substance category. However, many of these substances likely evade detection. Therefore, all patients using substances should be screened for NPSs during the clinical encounter and given psychoeducation about their potential dangers, especially patients using potentially counterfeit substances.

**Table 9–1.** Summary of novel psychoactive substances

| Category | Street names | Mechanism | Clinical effects | Management |
|---|---|---|---|---|
| **Opioid-like substances** | | | | |
| Fentanyl and analogs | China White, Dance Fever, Great Bear, Poison | μ opioid receptor agonist | Euphoria, analgesia, sedation, severe respiratory depression, overdose | Intoxication or overdose: treat similarly to opioid overdose with naloxone and supportive care. Use disorder: treat with medications for opioid use disorder with buprenorphine and methadone. Naltrexone has not been examined. |
| Kratom | Thang, kakuam, thom, ketum, biak | Postsynaptic $\alpha_2$-adrenergic receptor agonist, μ opioid receptor partial agonist | Stimulant effects at low doses, opioid effects at high doses; risk of sedation, respiratory depression, overdose | |
| Tianeptine | ZaZa, Tianna Red | μ opioid receptor agonist | Euphoria, analgesia, sedation, severe respiratory depression, overdose | |

**Table 9–1.** Summary of novel psychoactive substances (*continued*)

| Category | Street names | Mechanism | Clinical effects | Management |
|---|---|---|---|---|
| **Stimulant-like substances** | | | | |
| Synthetic cathinones | Bath salts, Blue Silk, Purple Wave, Vanilla Sky | Increases levels of norepinephrine, serotonin, and dopamine by inhibiting reuptake and promoting release | Increased alertness, hypertension, tachycardia, agitation, aggression, psychosis, seizures, acute kidney injury, cardiac arrest | Intoxication: prescribe benzodiazepines for agitation, hypertension, and seizures. For severe hypertension, give phentolamine and avoid β-blockers. Prescribe antipsychotics for psychosis and agitation. Monitor for QTc prolongation, especially if antipsychotics are used. Provide supportive management for other physiological symptoms. |
| **Cannabinoid-like substances** | | | | |
| Synthetic cannabis | Spice, K2, Kush | Potent full agonists at the $CB_1$ and $CB_2$ receptors | Agitation, psychosis, hypertension, tachycardia, acute kidney injury | Intoxication: prescribe benzodiazepines for agitation, hypertension, and seizures. For severe hypertension, give phentolamine and avoid β-blockers. Provide supportive management for other physiological symptoms. Prescribe antipsychotics for psychosis and agitation. |

**Table 9–1.    Summary of novel psychoactive substances (*continued*)**

| Category | Street names | Mechanism | Clinical effects | Management |
|---|---|---|---|---|
| **Cannabinoid-like substances (*continued*)** | | | | |
| Δ8 THC | Delta-8, D8 | Partial agonist at $CB_1$ and $CB_2$ receptors | Euphoria, drowsiness, analgesia, altered time perception, tremor, anxiety, psychosis | Intoxication: provide reassurance and supportive treatment and benzodiazepines and antipsychotics for agitation and psychosis. Use disorder: literature is limited. Consider using medications for cannabis use disorder such as NAC and gabapentin. |
| Sedatives and hypnotics | Legal benzodiazepine, research chemicals, fake Xanax, liquid Xanax | Positive allosteric modulators of GABA receptors | Euphoria, drowsiness, loss of coordination, amnesia, respiratory depression | Intoxication and overdose: provide supportive management; consider naloxone for possible comorbid opioid overdose. Flumazenil may reverse overdose but carries a risk of seizures. Use disorder: consider transitioning to clonazepam and taper over weeks to months. |

**Table 9–1.** Summary of novel psychoactive substances *(continued)*

| Category | Street names | Mechanism | Clinical effects | Management |
|---|---|---|---|---|
| **Synthetic hallucinogens** | | | | |
| 2C-I, 2C-C, 2C-B | 2C-B, Nexus, 2's, Toonies, Bromo, Spectrum, Venus | Partial agonist of $5\text{-HT}_{2A}$, $5\text{-HT}_{2B}$, and $5\text{-HT}_{2C}$ receptors; inhibits serotonin, norepinephrine, and dopamine transporter | Stimulant and hallucinogen effects: altered perception, nausea, vomiting, tachycardia, hypertension, seizures | Intoxication: Provide reassurance and symptom-specific supportive management. Prescribe benzodiazepines for severe agitation. |
| NBOMe (N-methoxybenzyl) | N-bomb, Smiles, 25I, 25C, 25B | $5\text{HT}_{2A}$ receptor agonist, $\alpha_1$-adrenergic agonist | Agitation, tachycardia, hypertension, delirium, hallucinations, seizures, hyperthermia | |

*Note.* 5-HT=serotonin; CB=cannabinoid receptor; Δ8 THC=Δ-8-tetrahydrocannabinol; NAC=N-acetylcysteine.

# Opioid-Like Substances

## Fentanyl

Fentanyl and fentanyl analogs have been widely distributed as counterfeit prescription opioids or mixed in multiple substances, including other opiates and stimulants. Fentanyl is 50–100 times more potent than morphine, and its analogs can be 10,000 times more potent than morphine (Suzuki and El-Haddad 2017). Synthetic opioids were responsible for 73% of all opioid-related deaths in 2019 (Mattson et al. 2021). Pharmacotherapy for synthetic opioid use disorder (OUD) is clinically similar to that for other OUDs, with opioid agonist (methadone or buprenorphine) or opioid antagonist (naltrexone) treatment. However, no high-quality data are currently available on the efficacy of these standard treatments for fentanyl use disorder. Opioid withdrawal with a Clinical Opiate Withdrawal Scale (COWS) score of 14 is recommended before proceeding with buprenorphine induction in fentanyl users. The injectable extended-release formulation, buprenorphine XR, has several advantages, including ensured compliance, more stable and higher serum levels than other formulations, and reduced risk of diversion. It may be preferred in synthetic opioid users because the likelihood of blocking fentanyl is higher. A 2020 case series examined rapid induction with buprenorphine XR injection in five heroin users who also used synthetic opioids. Participants who received ≥16 mg of sublingual buprenorphine on two consecutive days tolerated the buprenorphine XR 300 mg injection. Within 24 hours after administration, withdrawal symptoms were controlled (Mariani et al. 2020). Every patient should receive a naloxone spray kit for overdose rescue. Clinicians should consider these kits for individuals using stimulants, given the frequent adulteration of illicit stimulants with fentanyl. Patients and their families should be provided training on using naloxone and informed that multiple doses may be needed. Some patients have required continuous intravenous naloxone while hospitalized.

## Kratom

Kratom is derived from the plant *Mitragyna speciosa*. Commonly brewed in tea or chewed, it has been used in Asia for euphoria and analgesia and to prevent opium withdrawal. As an unscheduled substance, it has become significantly more popular in the United States and is easily bought in stores and on the internet. Individuals who use kratom perceive the drug as being low risk and having health benefits. The psychoactive compounds in kratom mitragynine and 7-hydroxymitragynine (7-OH-MG) are partial agonists at the μ opioid receptor. Mitragynine is the more prevalent alkaloid, and it has a weaker affinity to the μ opioid receptor than morphine. However, 7-OH-MG is 13 times more potent than morphine. Kratom has stimulant effects when used at low doses (<5 g) and opioid-like effects at high doses (>5 g) (Eastlack et al. 2020). As a result, it is used nonmedically for opioid withdrawal and as a harm reduction approach for OUD. However, heavy users also experience kratom withdrawal and cravings that are as severe as those for other opioids. Kratom overdose resembles an opioid toxidrome and may be reversed with naloxone. For patients with kratom use disorder, buprenorphine/naloxone has demonstrated efficacy in some case reports and in this author's experience (Weiss and Douglas 2021).

### Tianeptine

Tianeptine is a tricyclic antidepressant approved in Europe, Asia, and Latin America that emerged in the United States as a misused drug. It acts as a full agonist at the μ opioid receptor and has euphoric properties similar to those of other opioid agonists (Zahran 2018). Although a prescription dose ranges from 25 mg/day to 50 mg/day, recreational doses have been reported to be up to 3,000 mg. Fatal and nonfatal tianeptine toxicities have been reported in case literature (Bakota et al. 2018). Tianeptine withdrawal and overdose resemble those with opioids. Tianeptine overdose was successfully reversed with naloxone in a case report (Ari et al. 2010). Another case report documented successful treatment using buprenorphine/naloxone in a patient with tianeptine withdrawal and use disorder (Trowbridge and Walley 2019).

# Synthetic Stimulants and Cannabinoids

### Synthetic Cathinones

Cathinones are compounds with stimulant properties that are found in the *Catha edulis* plant, or khat. Synthetic cathinones, also commonly known as bath salts, are cathinone derivatives with more potent stimulant effects. 3,4-Methylenedioxypyrovalerone (MDPV) is one of many synthetic cathinones and is 10 times more potent and reinforcing than cocaine (McClenahan et al. 2020). Synthetic cathinone intoxication is associated with extreme aggression, agitation, psychosis, seizures, and cardiac arrest. Agitation associated with intoxication is treated with benzodiazepines and antipsychotics. Medical interventions are similar to those for other types of stimulant overdose, such as cooling for hyperthermia, benzodiazepines and nitrates for myocardial infarction, phentolamine for hypertension, and intravenous fluids for rhabdomyolysis. Clinicians should avoid $\beta$-blockers for hypertension because they can lead to unopposed $\alpha_1$ receptor agonism, resulting in worsened vasoconstriction and hypertension. There is no known treatment for synthetic cathinone use disorder, and it is unknown whether treatments for other stimulant use disorders would extrapolate to treatment for synthetic cathinones. MDPV vaccines are currently being developed and show promise in animal models (Nguyen et al. 2017).

## Synthetic Cannabinoids

Synthetic cannabinoids are a diverse group of chemicals that became widespread as "legal" cannabis. They are sold in colorful wrapping under names such as K2, Spice, and Kush. Synthetic cannabinoids are full agonists at the cannabinoid $CB_1$ and $CB_2$ receptors, binding with much higher potency than $\Delta$-9-tetrahydrocannabinol ($\Delta$-9 THC) found in the cannabis plant. Products also often contain other unknown chemicals that add to their toxicity. Intoxication is associated with agitation, psychosis, and medical sequelae such as hypertension, tachycardia, acute kidney injury, and death. Agitation is managed with benzodiazepines and antipsychotics. Like for synthetic cathinones, there is no known treatment for synthetic cannabis use disorder (CaUD), and it is unknown whether treatments for CaUD would be effective. Vaccines against synthetic cannabinoids are currently being developed and tested in animal models (Lin et al. 2020).

## Δ-8-Tetrahydrocannabinol

$\Delta$-8 THC emerged as another form of "legal" cannabis. It is a naturally occurring alkaloid found in smaller amounts in the cannabis plant. However, the $\Delta$-8 THC products on the market are synthesized from cannabidiol, which is found in large amounts in hemp. $\Delta$-8 THC is advertised as having milder effects than $\Delta$-9 THC and a range of health benefits such as improving sleep and anxiety. Similar to $\Delta$-9 THC, it is consumed via edibles or vaping. Poorly regulated $\Delta$-8 THC products may contain other unknown chemicals generated during the synthetic process. $\Delta$-8 THC intoxication and toxicity may manifest with psychosis, agitation, vomiting, anxiety, and confusion (Livne et al. 2022). Psychosis and agitation are responsive to antipsychotics and benzodiazepines. Chronic users may experience persistent psychosis even after a period of abstinence and may need continued treatment with antipsychotics. No clinical studies examining treatments for $\Delta$-8 THC addiction are yet available. Our clinical experience suggests that medications for CaUD, such as N-acetylcysteine and gabapentin, may be effective in reducing cravings and cannabis withdrawal.

# Novel Sedatives and Hypnotics

In recent years, NPSs with benzodiazepine-like properties have propagated as legal or counterfeit versions of prescribed benzodiazepines. Some of these have properties similar to their pharmaceutical counterparts, whereas others have unpredictable effects. Although some benzodiazepines are authorized medications in some countries (e.g., etizolam in Japan), others are synthesized via the chemical modification of known benzodiazepines and then sold on the internet. Among these are phenazepam, etizolam, and flualprazolam, which were placed under the international drug control system in 2020. As of February 2021, the European Union's Early Warning System was monitoring 30 new benzodiazepines, such as flubromazolam, meclonazepam, and diclazepam (European Monitoring Centre for Drugs and Drug Addiction 2021). Most of the novel benzodiazepines are sold as tablets, powders, capsules, blotters, or sprays at an affordable price; patients have claimed to have bought hundreds of counterfeit alprazolam tablets for less than $100. The pharmacodynamic effects of new benzodiazepines mirror those of their authorized versions, described as having euphoric, anxiolytic, sedative, muscle relaxant, and amnestic properties. Their potency greatly varies, and they have been associated with toxicity and overdose fatalities, especially when mixed with opioids and alcohol (Orsolini et al. 2020).

Recognizing intoxication and overdose is challenging because these substances lead to symptoms similar to those of opiates (e.g., respiratory depression, sedation), and they are not often detected in urine toxicology screens. Clinicians should be on high alert for these presentations, especially if the patient is not responsive to standard treatments such as naloxone for opioid overdose. Management of new benzodiazepine overdose reported in the case literature has included supportive care and flumazenil. In one case report of flubromazolam intoxication, the patient was comatose and required recurrent flumazenil injections. However, flumazenil should be used with caution in mixed benzodiazepine overdose because it can induce seizures. Supportive care is the preferred treatment approach. Information on the management of withdrawal and addiction to novel benzodiazepines is limited to case reports (Edinoff et al. 2022). We have managed these patients similarly to those with sedative-hypnotic use disorders, using long-acting benzodiazepines such as clonazepam and tapering over several months. Motivational enhancement therapy, cognitive-behavioral therapy, and psychoeducation are essential aspects of treatment

# Novel Hallucinogens

Serotonergic hallucinogens (psychedelics), such as lysergic acid diethylamide (LSD), psilocybin, and 3,4-methylenedioxymethamphetamine (MDMA), have reemerged as having potential benefit for depression and PTSD. Although these substances are presently restricted to clinical research, the decriminalization of psychedelic drugs in certain states has made them more readily available for nonmedical use. N,N-Dimethyltryptamine (DMT) is another hallucinogen found in plants and animal venoms. Ayahuasca is the common name for various plant extracts containing DMT consumed in a brew. Mescaline is found in the peyote cactus and used in traditional Native American ceremonies (Tullis 2021). Psychedelics share a primary mechanism via activation of the serotonin type 2A ($5\text{-HT}_{2A}$) receptor. Repeated administration of classic hallucinogens such as LSD and psilocybin leads to very rapid development of tolerance from downregulation of $5\text{-HT}_{2A}$ receptors, which limits their addiction liability. Generally, hallucinogens have common physiological and subjective effects, including nausea, vomiting, visual distortions and illusions, altered perception of time, depersonalization and/or derealization, and sense of connectedness and meaning. Many users report a profound spiritual experience and clarity about various life decisions. Some individuals use psychedelics in lower doses (microdosing) as self-medication for anxiety, depression, or emotional well-being.

A number of designer synthetic hallucinogens have become popular and accessible on the internet. These novel hallucinogens have higher potency and toxicity than classic psychedelics and include NBOMe (N-methoxybenzyl, also known as 25I-NBOMe, 25C-NBOMe, and 25B-NBOMe) and the 2C family (2C-I, 2C-C, 2C-B), which have a phenethylamine structure common to MDMA and the amphetamines. In addition to hallucinogenic effects from $5\text{-HT}_{2A}$ agonism, they cause sympathomimetic symptoms such as tachycardia, hypertension, hyperthermia, seizures, and excited delirium. NBOMe and 2C fatalities secondary to cardiopulmonary arrest have been reported. Management of hallucinogen intoxication usually involves supportive care. Mild symptoms may be relieved with gentle reassurance and placement in a calm and quiet environment. Agitation and excited delirium are managed with benzodiazepines. Antipsychotic medications may be used with caution because they may cause QT prolongation and increase the risk of sudden cardiac death (Dean et al. 2013; Minns 2015). Other supportive measures, such as fluids and cooling, are used for dehydration and hyperthermia. Pharmacotherapy for hallucinogen use disorder has not been established, and treatment centers on behavioral interventions. One small study showed that citalopram attenuates the effects of MDMA, but no literature has been published on whether these results would extend to the designer phenethylamine hallucinogens (Liechti et al. 2000).

# Conclusion

Experimentation has been essential for discovering new ideas and medications throughout human history. "Psychonauts" seek to understand altered states of consciousness, usually through experimenting with psychedelics. Their efforts may have partially contributed to the resurgence of psychedelic research for psychiatric ailments. However, NPSs have inundated the drug scene and are becoming increasingly obscure in their short- and long-term pharmacological effects. While some have potential therapeutic implications (i.e., mitragynine for opiate use disorder), the indulgent marketing around these substances' legality and health benefits is of concern. We must provide psychoeducation to guide our patients through balancing perceived benefits, safety, and curiosity with the potential dangers of using NPSs.

# References

Ari M, Oktar S, Duru M: Amitriptyline and tianeptine poisoning treated by naloxone. Hum Exp Toxicol 29(9):793–795, 2010 20498036

Bakota EL, Samms WC, Gray TR, et al: Case reports of fatalities involving tianeptine in the United States. J Anal Toxicol 42(7):503–509, 2018 29566235

Dean BV, Stellpflug SJ, Burnett AM, et al: 2C or not 2C: phenethylamine designer drug review. J Med Toxicol 9(2):172–178, 2013 23494844

Eastlack SC, Cornett EM, Kaye AD: Kratom-pharmacology, clinical implications, and outlook: a comprehensive review. Pain Ther 9(1):55–69, 2020 31994019

Edinoff AN, Nix CA, Odisho AS, et al: Novel designer benzodiazepines: comprehensive review of evolving clinical and adverse effects. Neurol Int 14(3):648–663, 2022 35997362

European Monitoring Centre for Drugs and Drug Addiction: New Benzodiazepines in Europe: A Review. Luxembourg, Publications Office of the European Union, 2021

Liechti ME, Baumann C, Gamma A, et al: Acute psychological effects of 3,4-methylenedioxymethamphetamine (MDMA, "Ecstasy") are attenuated by the serotonin uptake inhibitor citalopram. Neuropsychopharmacology 22(5):513–521, 2000 10731626

Lin M, Lee JC, Blake S, et al: Broadly neutralizing synthetic cannabinoid vaccines. JACS Au 1(1):31–40, 2020 34467269

Livne O, Budney A, Borodovsky J, et al: Delta-8 THC use in US adults: sociodemographic characteristics and correlates. Addict Behav 133(Oct):107374, 2022 35644057

Mariani JJ, Mahony A, Iqbal MN, et al: Case series: rapid induction onto long acting buprenorphine injection for high potency synthetic opioid users. Am J Addict 29(4):345–348, 2020 32167629

Mattson CL, Tanz LJ, Quinn K, et al: Trends and geographic patterns in drug and synthetic opioid overdose deaths—United States, 2013–2019. MMWR Morb Mortal Wkly Rep 70(6):202–207, 2021 33571180

McClenahan SJ, Gunnell MG, Owens SM, et al: Active vaccination reduces reinforcing effects of MDPV in male Sprague-Dawley rats trained to self-administer cocaine. Psychopharmacology (Berl) 237(9):2613–2620, 2020 32500210

Minns A: NBOMe drugs. California Poison Control System, August 12, 2015. Available at: https://calpoison.org/news/nbome-drugs. Accessed November 5, 2022.

Nguyen JD, Bremer PT, Ducime A, et al: Active vaccination attenuates the psychostimulant effects of α-PVP and MDPV in rats. Neuropharmacology 116(Apr):1–8, 2017 27956054

Office of National Drug Control Policy: Synthetic drugs (a.k.a. K2, Spice, bath salts, etc.). Washington, DC, The White House, 2014. Available at: https://obamawhitehouse.archives.gov/ondcp/ondcp-fact-sheets/synthetic-drugs-k2-spice-bath-salts. Accessed September 26, 2021.

Orsolini L, Corkery JM, Chiappini S, et al: "New/designer benzodiazepines": an analysis of the literature and psychonauts' trip reports. Curr Neuropharmacol 18(9):809–837, 2020 31933443

Suzuki J, El-Haddad S: A review: fentanyl and non-pharmaceutical fentanyls. Drug Alcohol Depend 171(Feb):107–116, 2017 28068563

Trowbridge P, Walley AY: Use of buprenorphine-naloxone in the treatment of tianeptine use disorder. J Addict Med 13(4):331–333, 2019 30550394

Tullis P: How ecstasy and psilocybin are shaking up psychiatry. Nature 589(7843):506–509, 2021 33505033

Weiss ST, Douglas HE: Treatment of kratom withdrawal and dependence with buprenorphine/naloxone: a case series and systematic literature review. J Addict Med 15(2):167–172, 2021 32858563

Zahran TE: Characteristics of tianeptine exposures reported to the national poison data system—United States, 2000–2017. MMWR Morb Mortal Wkly Rep 67(30):815–818, 2018 30070980

# 10

# Co-occurring Psychiatric and Substance Use Disorders

Nancy C. Shenoi, M.D.
Mark Yurewicz, M.D.

*Currently,* the body of knowledge regarding the interplay of substance use disorders (SUDs) and mental health disease pales in comparison to the understanding of SUDs and mental health conditions independent of each other. There are both clear indicators of strong correlations between these conditions and a growing understanding of bidirectional effects between them in relation to biological factors and psychosocial (environmental) events.

In this chapter, we broadly focus on pharmacological interventions for dual, or co-occurring, diagnoses of psychiatric disorders and independent SUDs. We refer readers to other texts that extensively cover the management of psychiatric-induced symptoms of substance withdrawal and intoxication. The number of studies dedicated to specific interventions for co-occurring conditions is growing. Review articles and meta-analyses are starting to emerge. To offer further confidence for providers in managing this unique intersection of disease, we also offer evidence of relevant correlations to help predict disease course, treatment response, and other clinical hurdles. Long-standing evidence exists for the correlation between the prevalence of and worsened morbidity for psychiatric disorders and SUDs. As of 2020, 37.9 million adults in the United States, more than 15% of the population, met the criteria for an SUD. Of adults with an SUD, 17 million (44.9%) also had a psychiatric condition. Even before the start of the coronavirus SARS-CoV-2 disease (COVID-19) pandemic, the incidence of major depressive episodes grew from 2017 to 2020 for both sexes and in all age groups younger than 50 years. In general, co-occurring SUDs increase the risk for worse psychiatric outcomes, although not universally or uniformly. Suicidality is strikingly more prevalent and serious for American adults with SUDs, regardless of other psychiatric conditions. Past-year serious suicidal thoughts were experienced by 14.2% of adults with SUDs versus 3.2% of adults without SUDs (Nunes and Weiss 2019).

Heavy substance use is often linked with more frequent and more severe symptoms. For example, daily or near-daily cannabis use doubled the risk for a major depressive episode in American adults (from 7.1% to 16.9% prevalence). A co-occurring SUD also fairly consistently complicates mental health treatment access, treatment retention (both pharmacological and psychosocial), and treatment response. As of 2020, of the 17 million American adults with past-year SUD and a psychiatric condition, 49.5% received no care for either condition; 42% received care for only mental health; and only 5.7%, or 960,000, received care for both SUD and mental health—the standard of care (Substance Abuse and Mental Health Services Administration 2021).

# Alcohol

## Alcohol and Mood Disorders

A few topics in the management of alcohol use disorder (AUD) and comorbid mood disorders are considered here: epidemiology, appropriate diagnosis, triage, addressing suicidality, and tailoring treatment.

### *Epidemiology*

Alcohol use and AUD are highly prevalent among individuals with depressive disorders and bipolar disorders. Epidemiological studies give a broad overview of the correlation between AUD and depressive disorders. Core studies include the Epidemiologic Catchment Area (ECA), the National Comorbidity Survey (NCS), and the National Epidemiologic Survey on Alcohol and Related Conditions (NESARC), as well as the recurring National Survey on Drug Use and Health (NSDUH). In DSM-IV (American Psychiatric Association 1994), the odds ratio of alcohol dependence in patients with major depressive disorder (MDD) and dysthymia (persistent depressive disorder in

DSM-5; American Psychiatric Association 2022) ranged from 1.6 to 3.7, with the highest odds ratio in females with MDD reported at 4.1 in the NCS. Bipolar disorder has a stronger link with alcohol dependence (OR 4.6–5.7). The NCS demonstrated an exceptionally high connection in males for alcohol dependence and bipolar disorders, with an odds ratio of 12.0 versus 5.3 for females (Nunes and Weiss 2019).

Given that alcohol-induced depressive and manic episodes are frequent and their management differs from that of primary major depressive episodes and manic episodes, completing a thorough clinical evaluation, with a psychiatric history, collateral information, and examination, is essential. Alcohol-induced depressive disorders are common. *Diagnostic Issues in Substance Use Disorders: Refining the Research Agenda for the DSM-V* (Saunders et al. 2007) presented extensive data in support of prolonged mood and anxiety symptoms beyond just the intoxication and withdrawal phase. In a 12-month prospective study of 200 people with AUD, heavy drinking predicted depressive symptoms the following month. At 3 months and 12 months, only those still drinking reported ongoing depression. Also, in patients with active AUD, depressive symptoms often remit with 1 month of sobriety with no other medication. The incidence decreased from 42% to 6% in one study and from 67% to 13% in another study with sobriety. Furthermore, the worldwide incidence of MDD in those with AUD is 15%, nearly identical to that for MDD overall, suggesting that at least a significant portion of the increased incidence of depressive symptoms in individuals with AUD could be attributed in some way to the effects of alcohol itself (Schuckit 2006).

### Suicidality

Any lifetime alcohol use in adults correlates with a relative risk of 1.65 for suicidal ideation or behavior (Amiri and Behnezhad 2020). AUD is the second most common mental health condition worldwide among individuals who die from suicide. Furthermore, acute alcohol intoxication drastically increases the risk of suicidal behavior; between 2003 and 2009, 24% of men and 17% of women who died from suicide in the United States had a blood alcohol level (BAL) above 0.08 g/dL. There is a dose-dependent ratio for suicide risk and alcohol exposure: the odds ratio of suicide attempts increases from 2.71 at the lowest levels of BAL to 37.18 when BAL is above 0.10 g/dL (Conner and Bagge 2019). In our fiduciary role in caring for mental health beyond SUDs, keeping this point in mind and sharing it with patients and family are worthy tasks given the finality of suicide. Providing this information to patients and families, without pressure or expectation, may further inform their goals for either harm reduction or abstinence and may help shape their recovery maintenance plans.

### Tailoring Care for Major Depressive Disorder

Both medication and psychosocial interventions can be adjusted for patients who have co-occurring depressive disorders and AUD. Most studies have not found that selective serotonin reuptake inhibitors (SSRIs) reduce excessive drinking in patients with comorbid AUD and depressive disorders, although they reduce depressive symptoms. However, medications for AUD, such as naltrexone and disulfiram, have been shown to be effective and safe for use with co-occurring MDD (Petrakis et al. 2007). In one study of 254 outpatients at three Veterans Affairs (VA) clinics, participants with depression who were receiving disulfiram reported fewer cravings over time than those with depression who received naltrexone. Several trials have found that combining naltrexone and disulfiram may be more effective than either medication alone (Pettinati et al. 2010). Currently, no literature has shown topiramate or acamprosate to have efficacy for depressive symptoms in co-occurring depression and AUD.

### Tailoring Care for Bipolar Disorder

Bipolar disorder is highly comorbid with AUD, with rates more than 3 times higher among patients with bipolar disorder than in the general population (Hirschfeld et al. 2010). Alcohol use may also affect pharmacotherapies for bipolar disorder. For instance, alcohol-related dehydration may raise lithium concentration to toxic levels. Hepatic dysfunction from chronic alcohol use or hepatitis associated with intravenous substance use may alter the plasma levels of valproate, carbamazepine, and other psychotropics metabolized by the liver. Adjusted dosing and coordination with gastroenterology and internal medicine clinicians are critical in these circumstances. Mood stabilizers have been explored as potential therapeutic targets for comorbid bipolar disorder and AUD:

- *Lithium:* The two largest clinical trials evaluating the efficacy of lithium in treating comorbid depression and AUD found the effects of lithium to be no better than placebo when considering measures such as achieving abstinence and reducing number of drinking days, severity of depression, or severity of alcoholism (Frye and Salloum 2006).

- *Valproate/Divalproex:* An open randomized trial of divalproex found that it reduced alcohol withdrawal symptoms and was equally effective as standard chlordiazepoxide, with further improvements in abstinence persisting at 6-week follow-up (Longo et al. 2002).
- *Topiramate:* Topiramate, a mood stabilizer that facilitates GABA neurotransmission through an allosteric site on $GABA_A$ receptors, is thought to mediate the cravings and reinforcement associated with alcohol. However, it may serve better as an adjunct or in combination pharmacotherapy because multiple studies have suggested it is ineffective as monotherapy for bipolar disorder (Hirschfeld et al. 2010).

### Psychotherapy

A prevailing ideology used to be that AUD had to be addressed before the symptoms of bipolar disorder. However, noncompliance with treatment recommendations is a persistent challenge among patients with comorbid mood disorders and SUDs, which is why dual-diagnosis treatment with psychosocial support and behavioral interventions is essential. Currently, few psychotherapeutic interventions have been studied in a randomized study format. Cognitive-behavioral therapy (CBT) is considered the best-evidenced modality, with psychoeducation and family involvement being critical components of the patient experience (Grunze et al. 2021).

### Ketamine

Ketamine is an *N*-methyl-D-aspartate (NMDA) receptor antagonist known for its antidepressant effects in treating MDD or bipolar disorder. One clinical predictor of response to ketamine is a family history of AUD in a first-degree relative (Niciu et al. 2014). Efforts are under way to determine whether ketamine's antidepressant mechanism has more to do with opioid receptors than with NMDA receptor antagonism. One study reported that preadministered naltrexone blocks ketamine's antidepressant effects (Williams et al. 2018), although pilot data from another study indicated that these effects are not attenuated by naltrexone pretreatment (Yoon et al. 2019). As such, combining opiate receptor antagonism with ketamine treatment might reduce addiction risk when treating patients with comorbid AUD and MDD. Clinical ketamine therapies may prove to be a reliable treatment for patients with depression and other comorbid SUDs. In one systematic review of studies focused on treating AUD, cocaine use disorder (CUD), and opioid use disorder (OUD), ketamine treatment led to a decrease in cravings and decreased cocaine use rates.

Studies in AUD and OUD found improvements in abstinence rates among the ketamine groups, with durable effects for up to 2 years following infusions (Jones et al. 2018).

## Alcohol and Anxiety Disorders

Comorbid AUD and anxiety disorders are a common dual diagnosis, with epidemiological surveys revealing a global prevalence rate of AUD in 20%–40% of individuals with anxiety disorders. The most significant comorbid anxiety disorders are generalized anxiety disorder (GAD), social anxiety disorder, and panic disorder (Castillo-Carniglia et al. 2019). One theory is that acute alcohol consumption increases GABAergic activity to produce an anxiolytic effect, but that chronic alcohol use and alcohol withdrawal result in decreased GABA tone, which leads to increased anxiety. Overly active noradrenergic systems in the brain have been associated with anxiety, and alcohol withdrawal is associated with increased noradrenergic activity (Kushner et al. 2000). Interestingly, SSRIs, the gold standard of treatment for anxiety disorders, may make patients more vulnerable to the effects of pathological intoxication with alcohol. Case reports suggest that even moderate alcohol intoxication in people taking SSRIs can lead to disinhibition and, in some cases, even instances of violence and aggression (Menkes and Herxheimer 2014).

One clinical review determined that gabapentin effectively treats mild- to moderate-severity anxiety disorders such as GAD, social phobia, and performance anxiety (Ahmed et al. 2019). Gabapentin is effective in treating acute alcohol withdrawal, and for short-term recurrence prevention after medically managed alcohol withdrawal, by normalizing sleep. Because the liver does not metabolize it, gabapentin is a treatment option for patients with hepatic insufficiency and can even be considered in patients who are unable to tolerate acamprosate because of insufficient renal function (Anton et al. 2020). It is thus far unknown whether gabapentin can be used as a monotherapy and as a treatment for severe and recurrent anxiety.

## Social Anxiety and Alcohol Use Disorder

Individuals with social phobia fear the scrutiny of others, so using alcohol reduces their inhibition—a social lubricant, so to speak. However, consistently drinking alcohol during social encounters leads to AUD in up to 50% of affected individuals (Koyuncu et al. 2019). Because social anxiety disorder begins earlier than AUD, it is considered a risk factor for the development of AUD as per the self-medication hypothesis. In a randomized controlled trial

(RCT) examining the effectiveness of CBT for patients with AUD and social phobia compared with CBT for AUD alone, no significant benefits were observed when simultaneous adjunctive treatment targeting both social anxiety and AUD was administered. Surprisingly, the group that received combined treatment exhibited higher rates of alcohol use compared with the group that received alcohol treatment alone. This was attributed to the increased distress experienced during exposures in the social phobia treatment group. Despite both groups demonstrating improvement in social anxiety and alcohol use, no noticeable correlation between the improvement in social anxiety and the improvement in alcohol use was identified. These findings highlight the significance of considering the treatment order as an important factor (Randall et al. 2001).

## Alcohol and PTSD

PTSD and AUD frequently co-occur, but not many pharmacological options target both disorders successfully and simultaneously. After applying DSM-5 criteria (American Psychiatric Association 2013) to the U.S. veteran population, one study group found that 57% of individuals with PTSD in the past month also met criteria for current MDD, and among those with probable lifetime PTSD, 69% had a lifetime history of AUD (Department of Veterans Affairs and Department of Defense 2017).

## Treatment Considerations

When concurrently treating PTSD and AUD, it is imperative to avoid benzodiazepines, which are contraindicated because they may pose harm. They may exacerbate anxiety via discontinuation symptoms, a problem because patients with PTSD and AUDs are prone to elevated anxiety levels at baseline. Moreover, benzodiazepines may actually increase the risk of developing PTSD by 2 to 5 times among patients with a history of trauma and may complicate treatment because their side effects overlap with the core PTSD symptoms of avoidance, negative mood, inattention, amnesia, irritability, and impulsivity (Guina and Merrill 2018). Clinical evidence suggests that benzodiazepines interfere with fear conditioning, impeding recovery from trauma.

### Maintenance Pharmacotherapy

Generally, the standard of care for co-occurring PTSD and AUD involves simultaneous, ideally integrated, treatments spanning medical, psychiatric, psychotherapeutic, and social services. Other publications thoroughly review the diagnosis, assessment, and psychosocial management. Pharmacotherapy for AUD is detailed in Chapter 5, "Alcohol and Co-occurring Substance Use." Here we consider specific issues with AUD medications in individuals with PTSD:

- *Naltrexone and disulfiram:* Use of either naltrexone or disulfiram alone or both in combination is likely safe and effective for alcohol use, with sobriety demonstrating benefit for PTSD symptoms. In smaller studies and case reports, combining naltrexone with exposure psychotherapy for PTSD versus either separately did not cause worse treatment outcomes (Ralevski et al. 2014). Patients taking any combination of these medications who maintained sobriety had a significant improvement in PTSD symptoms.

- *Topiramate:* Despite side effects of transient cognitive slowing, one pharmacological agent with promise is topiramate (Varma et al. 2018). Topiramate has been studied in concurrent AUD and PTSD treatment and has been found to have benefit in AUD-related outcomes (potentially comparable, but not equal, to efficacy in AUD alone). Excitingly, patients had statistically significant improvement in hyperarousal symptoms, although not in regard to reexperiencing or avoidance symptoms. In a prospective 12-week randomized, double-blind study of topiramate treatment administered to veterans with comorbid PTSD and AUD, it reduced participants' frequency of alcohol use and alcohol craving more significantly than placebo. Topiramate also decreased PTSD symptom severity and reduced hyperarousal symptoms (Batki et al. 2014).

- *SSRIs:* SSRIs could help or hurt patients with comorbid AUD and PTSD and require some thought. At least sertraline appears to have different effects based on the duration and severity of either disease. SSRIs in patients with early-onset AUD may worsen alcohol outcomes, and sertraline may do the same in patients with early-onset AUD and late-onset PTSD. However, in the reverse setting, among individuals with early-onset PTSD and later-onset AUD, alcohol-related outcomes were significantly improved. In a double-blind RCT of 94 veterans given sertraline, the late-onset AUD and early-onset PTSD group drank less than one drink per day versus five drinks in the placebo group. Participants with early-onset AUD drank, on average, more than seven drinks per day while taking sertraline (Brady et al. 2005). In another study comparing desipramine and paroxetine, the authors reported that both equally helped with PTSD symptoms. However, only the tricyclic antidepressant (TCA) desipramine helped with alcohol-related outcomes (Na et al. 2022). With the arrival of newer antidepressants with fewer side effects, the TCAs have fallen out of favor as a first-line treatment. Nevertheless, they should remain in the clinician's arsenal for cases in which SSRIs are insufficient. Serotonin reuptake inhibitors such as sertraline and venlafaxine are the first-line treatment for PTSD.

- *Doxazosin:* An $\alpha_1$ antagonist similar to prazosin but with a longer half-life, doxazosin can help with both daytime and nighttime hyperarousal and with nighttime intrusive dreams. More than 10 clinical trials, several early reviews, and some meta-analyses show doxazosin helps reduce the number of drinking days and amounts consumed in patients with AUD (Burnette et al. 2022). Currently, there is preliminary work for an extensive RCT of doxazosin for co-occurring AUD and PTSD with extensive self-report, functional MRI, and other objective measures (Back et al. 2018).
- *β-Blockers:* Although frequently used off-label for various PTSD-related symptoms, β-blockers have no current evidence for treatment in AUD. They may mask alcohol withdrawal symptoms, which can be dangerous during acute withdrawal.

In summary, doxazosin may be preferred to prazosin for patients with AUD, nightmares, daytime arousal, or anxiety. Topiramate may be helpful for patients with AUD and PTSD-related hyperarousal along with any other potential target issue such as migraines, binge eating, nicotine or stimulant use, and weight loss. Finally, SSRIs may be more reliable in patients with long-standing PTSD that then contributes to AUD.

## Further Considerations: Tailoring Care

Choosing between multiple medications can be daunting. First, the clinician and the patient should remember that there will be no magic bullet, no perfectly correct answer to managing AUD and co-occurring conditions. We use evidence to guide our decision-making, but for any individual patient, this process is imprecise. Unreasonable expectations will hamper the collaborative decision-making process with the patient. With realistic expectations, the clinician may reasonably proceed by choosing medications that address multiple symptoms. An essential goal is to find a sustainable treatment option without intolerable side effects or other barriers so that the patient is more likely to take the medication regularly. Collaborative decision-making is essential to reducing treatment nonadherence.

# Opioids

## Opioids and Mood and Anxiety Disorders

Mood and anxiety disorders commonly occur comorbid with OUD. Fortunately, standard medications for each disorder often benefit one another, but they are not without potential pitfalls. Pharmacotherapy alone is insufficient to treat multiple comorbid conditions. Thus, psychosocial interventions are equally important. Positive research regarding use of CBT and motivational interviewing for AUD and MDD has not yet been robustly completed and replicated in dual OUD and mood disorders, although studies have shown promise for such treatments (Barry et al. 2019).

### Medication Considerations

Medications for OUD or for mood and anxiety disorders have demonstrated some effect on outcomes of the companion condition. In a meta-analysis including 1,948 patients, patients with OUD and depression had, on average, a 31% decrease in depressive symptoms with methadone treatment (Mohammadi et al. 2020). Although larger clinical trials of buprenorphine's effect on depressive symptoms often exclude OUD and other SUDs, smaller studies and retrospective analyses over the past 30 years have demonstrated an antidepressant effect from buprenorphine, which is thought to be due to its antagonism at κ opioid receptors (Kosten et al. 1990). Case studies also have reported success using buprenorphine as an augmenting agent for acute mania in patients with comorbid bipolar disorder and OUD stabilized on buprenorphine.

There is limited but growing evidence regarding the effects of antidepressants on comorbid depression and OUD on outcomes of either condition. Early data often included older medications such as TCAs and methadone and did not show consistent benefits (Torrens et al. 2005). The debate over dysphoria at the onset of naltrexone use persists, with studies both confirming and disproving its existence. Our personal experience suggests an uncommon, but potential, risk for naltrexone inducing either a dysregulated, dissociative, and activating dysphoria or anhedonic depressive symptoms. Some studies have demonstrated the opposite effect: in five clinical trials with 30–500 participants, naltrexone was often associated with mild, gradual improvement in anxiety and/or depressive symptoms comparable with or equal to that with buprenorphine (Latif et al. 2019).

### Drug-Drug Interactions

There are multiple concerns about interactions with the concurrent use of buprenorphine or methadone and common medications in mood disorders. The most likely of these are respiratory depression, overdose, and death. Despite the protective factors of buprenorphine's partial agonism, there remains an increased risk of overdose death when it is combined with centrally acting sedatives. With concurrent gabapentin use, this risk is doubled (Gomes et al. 2017). Concurrent pregabalin has a hazard ratio of 2.82, and Z-drugs carry a hazard ratio of 1.6 (Abrahamsson et al. 2017). An unlikely but possible lethal condition is serotonin syndrome when buprenorphine is combined with serotonergic antidepressants. A few case reports document buprenorphine precipitating serotonin syndrome in patients given a TCA (Isenberg et al. 2008). Similar interactions with concurrent use of bupropion have not been reported.

Methadone is more susceptible to pharmacokinetic interactions with medications metabolized by cytochrome P450 (CYP) 3A4, CYP2D6, or CYP2B6. Known interactions associated with these agents include 1) methadone leading to increased levels of duloxetine and imipramine, 2) decreased levels of methadone when it is administered with carbamazepine or topiramate, 3) increased levels of methadone when it is administered with fluvoxamine and quetiapine, and 4) a synergistic effect of methadone when it is administered with diphenhydramine (McCance-Katz et al. 2010). Naltrexone can be used with relatively little concern about pharmacokinetic medication interactions because it is metabolized through non-CYP pathways. However, a potential pharmacodynamic complication exists between naltrexone and ketamine. A prospective RCT with 30 patients reported that when treated with naltrexone first, participants received almost none of ketamine's antidepressant and antisuicidal properties, nor were its dissociative effects inhibited (Williams et al. 2018). These data have not been replicated in larger studies.

## Opioids and PTSD

Although there is relatively less research about the overlap between PTSD and OUD versus other SUDs, available data thus far indicate that OUD has the highest rate of comorbid PTSD compared with other SUDs. In one study, among persons with OUD, 44% had met criteria for PTSD in their lifetime, and 33% did so currently (Ecker and Hundt 2018). In a group of 113 patients seeking buprenorphine treatment, 80.5% reported some form of childhood trauma, 20% reported past sexual abuse, 39% reported physical abuse, 60%

reported emotional abuse, and 66% reported witnessing violence (Sansone et al. 2009).

There is interest in using the antidepressant effects of κ opioid receptor agents in the treatment of depression and PTSD. Early data indicate that buprenorphine treatment in comorbid PTSD and OUD can lead to improved PTSD outcomes. In one study, the response rates were 63% for patients receiving buprenorphine alone, equal to those of patients receiving methadone with an added TCA. A retrospective chart review through the VA system that included 165 patients over more than 2 years compared patients prescribed SSRIs, buprenorphine, or opioids. Those prescribed buprenorphine demonstrated a 24% decrease in PTSD symptoms compared with 1.16% in patients prescribed only SSRIs. However, the study included a narrow subset of patients with a higher incidence of chronic pain that may not be generalizable to the broader population (Madison and Eitan 2020).

As of 2022, only two antidepressants are FDA-approved for PTSD: sertraline and paroxetine. The VA system's extensive review of the evidence for psychoactive medications guided their recommendation for sertraline and venlafaxine and, potentially, prazosin for nightmares. A 2019 guideline for opioid use in patients with PTSD also acknowledged the lack of conclusive evidence that psychotherapy and medications effective for OUD and PTSD individually would be effective in patients with dual diagnoses (Bernardy and Montaño 2019). Still, the use of additional psychoactive medications, such as antipsychotics and mood stabilizers, has been common, but evidence regarding their efficacy is limited. Psychotropic medications (antidepressants, mood stabilizers, antipsychotics) are frequently involved in opioid-related deaths; the 2010 National Center for Health Statistics data on drug overdose deaths showed that antipsychotics were associated with 58% of all opioid overdose deaths in the United States and antidepressants were associated with 57.6% (Jones et al. 2013). The role of psychotropic medications in overdose deaths is unclear. However, people with comorbid mental health conditions and OUD generally have higher rates of negative outcomes, including overdose.

Among medications with evidence for use in PTSD treatment, prazosin is frequently used off-label for PTSD-associated nightmares and has minimal to no pharmacokinetic or pharmacodynamic interactions with the three FDA-approved medications for OUD when used properly. Clonidine is also effective for nightmares and may be used to reduce opioid withdrawal symptoms. In our experience, a few patients have also found clonidine to be helpful for opioid craving. On the other hand, benzodiazepines combined with opioid agonist treatment add a small but significant risk for respiratory depression. Notably, PTSD may predict a higher likelihood of OUD patients intentionally combining opioids and benzodiazepines (per one sample of 267 patients in the midwestern United States) (Ellis et al. 2022).

# Stimulants

Stimulants, including cocaine, methamphetamine, and prescription stimulants, have a close relationship with co-occurring psychiatric disorders. An earlier assumption was that people self-selected specific substances based on their psychological or physical symptoms; for example, they might choose cocaine to overcome fatigue and depletion states associated with depression or low self-esteem and self-assertiveness, whereas they might choose narcotics to reduce stress, rage, and dysphoria. Research now confirms that symptoms or diagnoses do not predict which substances people prefer. Instead, there is a complex interplay between substance use and psychiatric symptoms (Lembke 2012).

Thus far, no medications have been approved by the FDA for treatment of methamphetamine use disorder (MUD) or CUD. A number of medications have some degree of evidence for the management of stimulant use disorders (see Chapter 6, "Stimulants and Co-occurring Substance Use"); these include D-amphetamine, methylphenidate, modafinil, doxazosin, varenicline, antidepressants (i.e., serotonin-norepinephrine reuptake inhibitors [SNRIs], SSRIs, TCAs, bupropion, mirtazapine), antiepileptics (mainly topiramate), naltrexone, disulfiram, baclofen, ondansetron, and second-generation atypical antipsychotics. This section briefly discusses evidence for these medications in co-occurring psychiatric disorders.

## Stimulants and ADHD

Adults with ADHD have less educational attainment, more job dismissals, more traffic accidents and driver's license suspensions, and higher divorce rates because of their increased impulsivity and inattention (Mariani and Levin 2007). ADHD involves dysfunction in dopamine neurotransmission and can be treated using stimulant medications that increase dopamine levels. Methylphenidate compounds have been shown in uncontrolled trials to be effective in reducing ADHD symptoms and cocaine use. They have also been associated with decreased mortality risk when used to treat MUD. Lisdexamfetamine, another stimulant treatment for ADHD and binge-eating disorder, is associated with a 14% reduced risk of hospitalization and 57% reduced risk of death in patients with amphetamine use disorder during periods of medication compliance versus periods of medication noncompliance (Heikkinen et al. 2022). Stimulant treatment for ADHD lowers the risk of developing an SUD. ADHD without treatment is associated with earlier initiation of smoking tobacco and higher rates of regular tobacco use (Groenman et al. 2013).

The misuse potential for methylphenidate and amphetamine analogs is a concern. Using delayed-release formulations decreases the potential for misuse. Mechanisms to reduce diversion potential include urine toxicology testing and the careful documentation of all controlled substance prescriptions. Treating ADHD with nonstimulant pharmacotherapy minimizes the risk of diversion or drug misuse but comes at the expense of symptom control because stimulant medications are more effective in treating ADHD. It is important to review the patient's childhood history (preferably with collateral information) during an evaluation for ADHD. If collateral information or the childhood history is unavailable, the diagnosis of ADHD should be deferred until the patient has maintained a prolonged period of abstinence from substances.

## Stimulants and Mood Disorders

Generally, concurrent stimulant use and depressive disorders predict worse symptomatology. Patients experience dysphoria with stimulant withdrawal that can drive their prolonged use. A multisite study of 483 male patients with MUD revealed that 89.0% experienced comorbid depressive symptoms, with depression severity decreasing with increased abstinence time. Early-life exposure to methamphetamines was also connected with higher degrees of depression, suicidal ideation, and biological alterations to vasopressin and the hypothalamic-pituitary-adrenal axis. These neuroendocrine alterations were also correlated with worsening depression during withdrawal (Liu et al. 2021). Alternatively, anhedonia seems to be a core component of clinical depression in those with CUD. The pathophysiology of anhedonia in cocaine use is thought to be from chronic overstimulation of the CNS reward circuitry by cocaine, which leads to deficits in reward processing. This anhedonia may trigger a return to use after a period of abstinence or motivate ongoing cocaine use to feel pleasure (Crits-Christoph et al. 2018).

Various medications are used to treat comorbid stimulant and depressive disorders. Mirtazapine is an antidepressant that increases serotonin indirectly via antagonism of serotonin type 2 (5-HT$_2$) and type 3 (5-HT$_3$) receptors. It has demonstrated some utility in reducing methamphetamine use and high-risk sexual behaviors in men and transgender women who have sex with men independently of its effects on depression (Coffin et al. 2020). Bupropion, a dopamine and norepinephrine reuptake inhibitor, has been studied as a treatment for CUD and MUD. Although it has a very modest effect in reducing cocaine use, its efficacy is more substantial when combined with contingency management, a type of operant conditioning in which patients are rewarded for positive behavioral changes (Poling et al. 2006). A systematic review of contingency management for MUD revealed broader benefits with this intervention, including longer drug abstinence, higher utilization of medical services, and reductions in risky sexual behavior (Brown and DeFulio 2020). Desipramine and imipramine have also been associated with a reduction in depressive symptoms and cocaine use and cravings. CBT improves treatment retention among cocaine users with depression who are treated with desipramine (Carroll et al. 1995). Again, these results emphasize the synergistic effects of psychotherapeutic and psychosocial interventions with medications. Long-term aerobic exercise is another avenue for methamphetamine-dependent patients when combined with CBT and psychotherapy. Exercise reduces cravings, improves cognitive function, enhances inhibitory control, and lessens depressive and anxiety symptoms (Huang et al. 2020).

## Stimulants and Psychosis

Psychotic symptoms are commonly experienced by people who use stimulants. Symptoms include intense paranoid delusions and auditory or visual hallucinations. A systematic review in 2018 revealed that the frequency and quantity of methamphetamine use and the severity of MUD were the most consistent correlates of methamphetamine-related psychosis (Arunogiri et al. 2018). Psychotic symptoms usually resolve after stimulant use but may build up to a persistent psychotic disorder in chronic users. In fact, in a study based in Australia, the prevalence of psychosis among chronic methamphetamine users was 11 times that of the general public (McKetin et al. 2006). For individuals with stimulant use disorders, age at first use, duration of use, and severity of anxiety contribute to the severity of persistent psychotic symptoms. Stimulant use may also worsen psychotic episodes for individuals already diagnosed with schizophrenia. Because of sensitization, psychotic symptoms may also return for stimulant users even at reduced drug dosages.

The etiology of psychosis may not always be apparent for individuals who are using stimulants at the time their first-episode psychosis occurs. However, failing to treat psychotic symptoms could affect patient safety and quality of life. Antipsychotics are warranted for chronic psychotic symptoms that persist after stimulant cessation. An investigation of six RCTs found that aripiprazole, haloperidol, quetiapine, olanzapine, and risperidone were able to reduce or control a psychotic episode induced by amphetamine use without adverse effects, with no drug being superior to the others. However, an RCT comparing the second-generation antipsychotic olanzapine with haloperidol for methamphetamine-related psychosis found that olanzapine was better tolerated in terms of extrapyramidal symptoms (Shoptaw et al. 2009). As discussed in Chapter 6, aripiprazole may increase methamphetamine cravings. Benzodiazepines utilized in conjunction with antipsychotics can more effectively target agitated psychosis (Glasner-Edwards and Mooney 2014). Finally, a meta-analysis of treatment options showed that contingency management results in statistically significant reductions in stimulant use; incorporation of a community reinforcement approach or CBT in addition to contingency management makes the psychosocial treatment more effective (Farrell et al. 2019).

## Stimulants and Anxiety Disorders

Cocaine is used by some individuals as an anxiolytic, whereas others seek anxiolytics to alleviate anxiety symptoms associated with cocaine use and withdrawal. Among those with a lifetime use of cocaine among other substances, one-third have at least one lifetime anxiety disorder diagnosis. More specifically, cocaine use is associated with panic attacks, phobias, compulsions, and obsessions that can persist even after prolonged abstinence (Papatheofani et al. 2021). The degree of stimulant use also predicts anxiety risk. Among adolescents and young adults who report using cocaine, the risk of experiencing panic disorder and/or GAD is higher when individuals have CUD rather than only cocaine use.

The treatment of comorbid anxiety disorders and CUD requires a dual-diagnosis approach. In pharmacology studies, treatment with citalopram, fluoxetine, escitalopram, and sertraline was associated with a reduction in the severity of GAD symptoms for participants with CUD, AUD, cannabis use disorder (CaUD), and/or nicotine use disorder. However, clinicians must be careful about using SSRIs in these patients because stimulants (e.g., cocaine, 3,4-methylenedioxymethamphetamine [MDMA]), SSRIs, SNRIs, and many other medications are all serotonergic, increasing the risk of serotonin syndrome; this risk is highest with monoamine oxidase inhibitors.

## Stimulants and PTSD

PTSD is a known comorbidity of CUD. It may precede cocaine use to self-medicate symptoms, or cocaine use may lead to PTSD symptoms due to increased exposure to traumatic events. Not surprisingly, the severity of each disorder influences the other. One study found that improvement in PTSD symptoms was associated with decreased cocaine use. Conversely, a worsening of symptoms was associated with increased cocaine use (Back et al. 2006).

For adolescents, PTSD appears to increase the risk of developing subsequent stimulant use and use disorders and to worsen the progression. A longitudinal study of youth ages 11–21 years found a dose-response relationship between number of traumatic events experienced (e.g., neglect; abuse; threatened, witnessed, or experienced violence; parental incarceration; substance use) and degree of substance use in adolescence, emerging adulthood, and adulthood (Scheidell et al. 2018). Among juvenile offenders who used crack cocaine, PTSD was a risk factor for continued use into adulthood and subsequent health consequences (Wojciechowski 2018). In adults, comorbid PTSD and stimulant use disorders correlates with greater impairment and treatment needs. An RCT of 428 cocaine-dependent adults in outpatient treatment with and without PTSD found those with both disorders were generally more impaired and in greater need of dual-diagnosis treatment (Najavits et al. 2007).

Treatment options for comorbid PTSD and CUD necessitate concurrent psychotherapy. A study of outpatients with comorbid CUD and PTSD in which patients received imaginal and in vivo exposure therapy for PTSD and CBT for cocaine use, demonstrated significant reductions in depression on the Beck Depression Inventory and in psychiatric and cocaine use severity on the Addiction Severity Index. These improvements were consistent even at 6-month follow-up (Brady et al. 2001). Among the medications for CUD listed in Table 6–1, doxazosin and topiramate have evidence for PTSD. Doxazosin seems to target hyperarousal symptoms and nightmares, whereas topiramate targets reexperiencing symptoms such as intrusive memories, flashbacks, and nightmares. We recommend going low and slow with topiramate, starting at 25 mg and increasing weekly by 25 mg, to improve tolerability and decrease the likelihood of medication nonadherence.

# Tobacco

Tobacco is a leading cause of death worldwide, and its use is frequently comorbid in patients with other SUDs and mental health disorders. Tobacco use should be treated concurrently with these comorbid conditions because 1) roughly half of all patients with mental health disorders die from a condition related to tobacco use (Callaghan et al. 2014) and 2) concurrent abstinence from nicotine improves chances of abstinence from another substance while patients are in treatment (Prochaska et al. 2004). According to the 2001–2002 NESARC, although adults with a psychiatric disorder made up only 7.1% of the U.S. population, they consumed 31% of all cigarettes nationally (Grant et al. 2004). Despite these clear correlations to adverse outcomes, patients with SUDs and psychiatric conditions may be reluctant to stop their tobacco use because they often perceive other conditions as being more impairing. However, patients are usually interested in quitting, and on average, half have attempted to quit smoking in the past year (Stockings et al. 2013).

## Tobacco and Drug-Drug Interactions

Although nicotine is metabolized by the liver's CYP2D6 enzyme, tar and the polycyclic aromatic hydrocarbons in tobacco smoke can affect the metabolism of psychiatric medications by increasing their metabolic clearance rate via the liver's CYP1A2 isozyme. Consequently, nicotine replacement therapy (NRT) medications do not affect psychotropic medication levels. Smoking cessation can lead to increased psychotropic medication blood levels due to a slowing of activity of the CYP1A2 enzyme. Among psychotropic medications, this interaction affects duloxetine, mirtazapine, clozapine, and olanzapine levels. The clinician must adjust the dosage according to the patient's level of smoking. A patient taking clozapine and olanzapine may experience excessive sedation due to high blood levels. Conversely, if a patient resumes smoking after stabilizing with clozapine or olanzapine for psychosis or mood disorder, they may experience worsening psychiatric symptoms.

In general, tobacco and nicotine users consume more caffeine than nonusers to enhance the stimulant effects of nicotine. However, because smoking induces caffeine metabolism, smoking abstinence substantially increases caffeine blood levels. The combination of elevated caffeine levels and nicotine withdrawal can exacerbate anxiety and insomnia. Patients should be advised to reduce their caffeine use at the same time as quitting smoking.

## Tobacco and Mood Disorders

Tobacco is a leading cause of morbidity and mortality in the United States, and individuals with mental health disorders are more likely to consume tobacco products. A systematic review studying the longitudinal association between smoking and mental illness found evidence for a link between smoking and depression and vice versa but found no clear bidirectional relationship (Fluharty et al. 2017). A meta-analysis of 93 different studies found that individuals with depression who also smoke are motivated to quit and that smoking itself does not worsen symptoms of depression. Having a diagnosis of MDD also does not have a clear negative impact on smoking cessation outcomes (Morozova et al. 2015). However, the opposite holds true: Individuals who smoke have an 81% greater risk of death from suicide than those who never smoked, with some of the risk attributable to comorbid psychiatric disorders (Li et al. 2012). Other theories behind this association are that tobacco smokers have increased impulsivity and lower levels of monoamine oxidase enzyme related to hormonal stress response (Bohnert et al. 2014). Tobacco smoking is at least twice as common among people with bipolar disorder as in the general population, and these individuals tend to have lower quit rates than those without bipolar disorder (Thomson et al. 2015). With this lower quit rate, those with bipolar disorder may be more susceptible to the negative effects of tobacco smoking, such as suboptimal management of bipolar disorder symptoms due to smoking-induced metabolism of mood stabilizers leading to lower blood levels.

## Tobacco and Anxiety Disorders

Anxiety disorders and tobacco use disorder (TUD) are highly associated. On average, 15%–25% of smokers in the United States have one comorbid anxiety disorder, and people with anxiety disorders are 2–3 times more likely to smoke (Fluharty et al. 2017). Patients with both disorders face greater risk for the severity of the disease and for poor treatment response. For example, people with both TUD and anxiety disorders experience more severe withdrawal symptoms during smoking cessation compared with those without anxiety disorders, which can lead to return to use (Morissette et al. 2007). Likewise, patients with anxiety disorders are more at risk for developing TUDs at lower use levels (Kushner et al. 2012).

Smoking usually occurs during periods of emotional turmoil, which may be more common for people who experience anxiety. Except for social anxiety disorder, in which smoking follows the diagnosis, smoking tends to occur before the development of anxiety disorders (Battista et al. 2008). The anxiety sensitivity theory suggests that cognitive distortions around anxiety (i.e., fear of anxiety) increase smoking. In addition, more significant difficulty tolerating nicotine withdrawal symptoms creates negative reinforcement that leads to continued use. This translates to lower levels of abstinence in individuals with anxiety disorders, which has been reflected in studies showing that the recent decline in smoking rates among the general population is not seen in smokers with anxiety disorders (Cook et al. 2014).

As of July 2022, three pharmacological treatments for smoking cessation have FDA approval: varenicline, an $\alpha_4\beta_2$ nicotine receptor partial agonist; bupropion, a norepinephrine-dopamine reuptake inhibitor, and NRTs in various over-the-counter and prescription formulations (see Table 6–2). Current research indicates that patients with anxiety disorders tolerate each of these medications equally, but fewer studies have looked at how patients with comorbid anxiety disorders and TUD tolerate the medications. Findings also vary on the efficacy of these medications for patients who have comorbid anxiety disorders and TUD. A 2020 subgroup analysis of the Evaluating Adverse Events in a Global Smoking Cessation Study (EAGLES) trial revealed that people with anxiety disorders who smoke experienced more neuropsychiatric adverse events during smoking cessation than did those who smoked but had no anxiety disorders (approximately 6% vs. 2%). The group with anxiety disorders was also less likely to be abstinent during the final 3 weeks of a 12-week treatment phase (GAD OR 0.72; panic disorder OR 0.53) (Ayers et al. 2020). Conversely, an analysis of the NESARC found that anxiety disorders had no impact on lifetime smoking cessation rates (Lopez-Quintero et al. 2011). Another study of 1,504 people who smoked determined that the participants with a lifetime diagnosis of an anxiety disorder had no statistically significant response to either single or dual therapy with sustained-release bupropion and/or NRT (Piper et al. 2011).

## Varenicline

Before the 2016 removal of varenicline's black box warning about its potential effects on neuropsychiatric symptoms and suicidality, there was initial reservation about using it in patients with co-occurring psychiatric disorders. The research leading up to removal of the black box warning and since has largely supported the safety and efficacy of varenicline for smoking cessation in patients with anxiety and other neuropsychiatric disorders. A subgroup analysis in 2013 combining 17 RCTs ($N=8,027$) and observational data from a U.S. Department of Defense study ($N=35,800$) found varenicline did not worsen anxiety symptoms more than placebo for patients with or without a psychiatric disorder (Ayers et al. 2020).

### Nicotine Replacement Therapy

Nicotine, during both intoxication and withdrawal, can have an impact on different anxiety symptoms. Therefore, an important question arises about the effect of NRTs on chronic anxiety in individuals undergoing smoking cessation. A study that compared primary care patients without psychiatric disorders who successfully quit smoking using NRTs with patients who continued smoking revealed significant improvements in anxiety and mood levels after quitting with NRTs (Taylor et al. 2015). Regarding management of short-term withdrawal symptoms, buspirone, a serotonergic anxiolytic, reduces anxiety, nicotine cravings, restlessness, and irritability during periods of smoking cessation (Hilleman et al. 1992).

## Tobacco and Psychotic Disorders

Smoking tobacco is associated with a twofold risk of incident schizophrenia or psychosis more broadly. One cause might be genetic, with the existence of a single nucleotide polymorphism associated with nicotine use disorder (cholinergic receptor gene *CHRNA5*) that is also associated with schizophrenia (Chen et al. 2016). Other factors include prenatal maternal tobacco smoking, which increases the odds of tobacco use in the offspring during adolescence, and the thousands of chemicals in tobacco products that could have psychiatric effects (Scott et al. 2018).

People with psychosis are more prone to smoke tobacco products. Various theories have tried to explain this link, including self-medication for the dopamine blockade by antipsychotics or for negative symptoms of schizophrenia. A systematic review and meta-analysis of prospective, case control, and cross-sectional studies found that daily tobacco use is associated with an increased risk and earlier onset of psychosis. Notably, people who smoke daily develop psychotic illness on average 1 year earlier than nonsmokers (Gurillo et al. 2015).

When treating patients with psychosis using medications metabolized by the liver's CYP1A2 enzyme, keep in mind that polyaromatic hydrocarbons in tobacco smoke induce this enzyme, thereby increasing metabolic clearance of these medications. Conversely, smoking cessation can increase psychotropic medication blood levels because of a slowing of CYP1A2 enzyme activity. Antipsychotic medication levels (e.g., olanzapine, clozapine) must be monitored carefully as tobacco use changes.

## Tobacco and ADHD

Approximately 40% of people with ADHD smoke, a higher rate than that in the general population. They also initiate smoking tobacco products earlier and tend to use more regularly at higher amounts. Conversely, for those with comorbid ADHD and TUD, the number and severity of a person's ADHD symptoms are positively associated with the frequency of tobacco use over the past year (Upadhyaya and Carpenter 2008). Transitional-age youth with ADHD who are matriculating from high school to college are a population of interest because they are at increased risk of TUD, particularly in electronic cigarette form. Individuals with ADHD have poorer smoking cessation outcomes compared with those without the disorder. The literature supports incorporating tobacco prevention skills into treatment for youth with ADHD (Corona et al. 2020).

# Cannabis

No pharmacological treatments have been FDA-approved for the treatment of CaUD. RCTs examining pharmacological treatments for CaUD have identified N-acetylcysteine, an antioxidant that affects glutamatergic pathways, as an agent that could reduce marijuana use in adolescents (Sharma et al. 2022). Another RCT assessing gabapentin use in treatment found that participants who received gabapentin 1,200 mg/day reduced their weekly cannabis use (Mason et al. 2012). Dronabinol, a cannabinoid agonist, was found to reduce cannabis withdrawal symptoms and to positively affect treatment retention (Levin et al. 2016). Rimonabant, a cannabinoid type 1 ($CB_1$) receptor inverse agonist, reduced the pleasurable effects associated with use and reduced marijuana-associated tachycardia but increased suicidal ideation (Huestis et al. 2007). In terms of psychotherapy, CBT together with contingency management increased the odds of abstinence among substance users. Motivational enhancement therapy combined with these two therapy practices further improves outcomes (Kadden et al. 2007).

## Cannabis and Mood Disorders

Cannabis affects dopaminergic pathways, which affects mood and cognition. Depression is one of the most common psychiatric disorders worldwide, and individuals with MDD are more at risk of substance use. One meta-analysis found that cannabis use, particularly heavy use, is linked to depression. However, confounding factors prevent definitive conclusions about causality. Although MDD has been associated with increased incidence of cannabis use, future incidence of MDD is not significantly higher among cannabis users compared with nonusers (Feingold et al. 2015). Trials of CBT can be used to increase rates of cannabis abstinence and are most effective when combined with motivational enhancement therapy and contingency management in adults and youth (Kadden et al. 2007).

The lifetime prevalence of SUDs is 40% among individuals with bipolar I disorder; 20%–50% of those with bipolar disorder endorse cannabis-related problems (Cerullo and Strakowski 2007), and comorbid cannabis use and CaUD are independently associated with greater disability in individuals with bipolar disorder. These individuals may use cannabis to alleviate mood symptoms related to the manic, hypomanic, and depressive stages of the disorder. Similar to those with SUDs, they tend to score high on sensation-seeking domains (Bizzarri et al. 2007).

## Cannabis and Anxiety Disorders

The relationship between cannabis and anxiety disorders is not yet clear. The onset of anxiety frequently precedes CaUD in adults with comorbid conditions (Kedzior and Laeber 2014). On the other hand, anxiety often occurs during cannabis intoxication and withdrawal. Zvolensky et al. (2006) found that lifetime cannabis use was associated with an increased risk of lifetime panic attacks (OR 1.6), even after controlling for demographic differences and lifetime polysubstance use. Conversely, people with certain anxiety disorders such as panic disorder may be at increased risk of cannabis use, particularly at older ages. One study followed Australian adolescents who used cannabis daily over a 15-year period and found that they were more likely to develop an anxiety disorder (Feingold et al. 2016). However, two other studies suggested that cannabis users are not at increased risk of developing anxiety disorders longitudinally (Degenhardt et al. 2013; van Laar et al. 2007). Taken together, the literature has been conflicting about the link between cannabis use and anxiety disorders.

Regarding treatment, individuals with CaUD and elevated anxiety experience worse outcomes. Motivational enhancement therapy combined with CBT is effective for both CaUD and anxiety disorders and may be tailored to dual-diagnosis patients. Integrated cannabis and anxiety reduction treatment is a transdiagnostic process for the treatment of multiple anxiety disorders that has been demonstrated to result in greater cannabis abstinence (Buckner et al. 2016).

## Cannabis and PTSD

Cannabis is used for its calming effects to relieve PTSD symptoms such as flashbacks, nightmares, hyperarousal, and insomnia. Cannabinoid modulation affects concentrations of brain-derived neurotrophic factor in the amygdala and the hippocampus involved in memory consolidation and retrieval. Cannabinoids reduce responses to conditioned fear cues, impair retrieval of aversive memories, and trigger the extinction of unwanted memories (LaFrance et al. 2020). Empirically supported treatments exist for PTSD (cognitive processing therapy, prolonged exposure) and CaUD (CBT, motivational enhancement) separately, but no known framework is currently available for treatment integration.

Many individuals with PTSD tend to turn to cannabis use when psychological interventions are insufficient for symptom relief. Evidence is mixed for the safety and efficacy of medical cannabis. As of 2022, 36 U.S. states have approved medical cannabis for the treatment of PTSD. Studies of medical cannabis users with self-identified PTSD over a 31-month period revealed that acute cannabis intoxication provided relief from the PTSD-related symptoms of intrusion, flashbacks, irritability, and anxiety. Cannabis users dominantly using $\Delta$-9-tetrahydrocannabinol ($\Delta$-9 THC) exhibited a greater than twofold rate of remission from their PTSD diagnosis compared with control subjects by the 1-year follow-up assessment (Bonn-Miller et al. 2022). However, tolerance develops, and higher doses of medical cannabis are needed to manage anxiety in the long term, without any change in baseline severity of symptoms (LaFrance et al. 2020). Cannabis users generally view cannabis favorably for PTSD symptom relief. However, the only available high-quality RCT did not report a significant change in the severity of PTSD symptoms with cannabis use compared with the placebo for any cannabis preparation (i.e., high THC [12%] with <0.05% cannabidiol [CBD]; high CBD [11%] with 0.50% THC; or THC plus CBD [~7.9% THC and 8.1% CBD]) (Bonn-Miller et al. 2021). One important finding is that cannabis use doubles the likelihood of dropout from CBT and trauma-focused psychotherapy and the cessation of established pharmacological treatments for PTSD (Bedard-Gilligan et al. 2018). Because psychotherapy is the gold standard treatment for PTSD, this treatment dropout is highly concerning. We recommend that clinicians continually update their patients on the emerging evidence for the long-term impact of cannabis on PTSD (and other psychiatric conditions) and discuss engaging in evidence-based interventions.

## Cannabis and Psychotic Disorders

Cannabis use is a known risk factor for the development of psychotic symptoms, although neurobiological mechanisms and causality are still uncertain. Factors such as demographics, intrinsic genetic vulnerability, self-medication for mental health symptoms such as the negative symptoms of schizophrenia, and sequelae of intoxication episodes may all contribute to the association of cannabis use with schizophrenia. The literature suggests that cannabis use increases the risk of developing schizophrenia threefold, in a dose-response relationship (van Os et al. 2002). Questions remain with respect to the impact of use frequency. An 11-year study by the NESARC from 2002 to 2013 found that participants with any use of nonmedical cannabis and those with CaUD were at increased risk of self-reported psychosis compared with nonusers, regardless of the degree of use (Livne et al. 2022). Some of the neurobiological markers of chronic cannabis exposure (i.e., P300, synaptic vesicular density) overlap with those of psychotic disorders, making a causal relationship plausible (Ganesh and D'Souza 2022). It is important to provide adolescents with early education about the risks of cannabis use and psychosis, because they are more vulnerable than other groups to experiencing this outcome. Treatment involves cannabis abstinence and prescribing antipsychotics to anyone with a psychotic disorder.

### Case Example

A.B. is a 45-year-old white female with a history of problematic alcohol use, recent intermittent treatment for OUD, past military trauma exposure, and a vaguely reported history of recurring depression and anxiety. Because of changes in her insurance, she is now presenting to the clinic after being off medications for several months. In the past, she has tried naltrexone and "one of those psych drugs that messes with your sex drive." The naltrexone did not help with her cravings, and she acknowledges continued use of alcohol and opioids, given her ambivalence about sobriety. Similarly, she recalls stopping the antidepressant because of side effects. A.B.'s previous psychiatrist started her on buprenorphine maintenance. However, she has been inconsistent with appointments because of financial instability and abnormal work hours given her evening shifts. Work has become more overwhelming, and A.B. fears everything—her commute to work, interactions with others, daily chores, and being inefficient on the job. In the past, she has had intrusive thoughts and would become overstimulated in crowded settings. Now, getting through the day is difficult.

When her buprenorphine intake becomes irregular, A.B.'s mood swings worsen. When she cannot afford her buprenorphine prescription, she buys hydrocodone from her dealer and uses more than she intends. Last year, she unintentionally overdosed on opioids but was rescued by a friend at home with naloxone spray. Overdoses were not an issue when she used hydrocodone regularly. A.B. says she feels unmotivated for treatment. Upon further questioning, she attributes her lack of motivation to feeling sad and lethargic. She struggles to get out of bed, eat, and brush her teeth. She asks for recommendations on the next best step for treatment. Using active listening and motivational interviewing techniques, the clinician notes A.B.'s intense ambivalence and hopelessness about her ability to maintain sobriety.

The initial approach to treating A.B. is as follows:

1. Assess safety, including acute medical and psychiatric symptoms that may need to be stabilized (i.e., suicidal ideation, psychosis).
2. Screen for depression (bipolar vs. unipolar), PTSD, and anxiety disorders using validated instruments such as the Patient Health Questionnaire–2, the General Anxiety Disorder–7, and the Posttraumatic Stress Disorder Checklist for DSM-5.
3. Resume buprenorphine, which is a more feasible treatment than methadone because of her unpredictable work schedule. A.B.'s condition has not yet failed to respond to buprenorphine maintenance, nor has she experienced more severe, dangerous issues regarding her OUD. When she takes her buprenorphine regularly, her mood and behaviors are more stable. Buprenorphine has also been shown to have an antidepressant effect among patients with OUDs. Because she has difficulty affording buprenorphine, the clinician should consider patient assistance programs and brainstorm other options with her.
4. Prescribe naloxone for overdose rescue, especially given that this patient has needed this medication in the past.
5. Discuss the viability of A.B. attending an intensive outpatient program for OUD in a facility where buprenorphine is available. Discuss the option for residential rehabilitation if she has difficulty achieving stability.
6. Make a plan for A.B. to return to the next appointment and address any potential barriers.

A.B. is diagnosed with PTSD and MDD. In the follow-up visit, she hints that she might be using other substances. Therefore, the next steps are as follows:

1. Screen for benzodiazepines, given A.B.'s comorbid diagnoses of OUD and PTSD. She would be at risk of respiratory depression with these combinations.

2.  Recommend that the patient find a support group, peer recovery support specialist, or recovery case management program to help her stay active in her treatment. Co-occurring disorders with PTSD lead to higher rates of dropout.

3.  Discuss medications for PTSD and refer her to evidence-based psychotherapy. Recent data support integrated and simultaneous treatment for PTSD and SUD instead of stepwise treatment for only SUDs first.

4.  Explore dual-diagnosis programs. Consider residential rehabilitation if her depressive and/or PTSD symptoms hinder A.B. from engaging in care.

5.  In the future, if A.B.'s psychiatric symptoms do not improve, screen her for chronic pain and sleep disorders. Also screen her for intimate partner violence and other potential ongoing threats.

# Conclusion

Across populations, comorbid SUDs and psychiatric disorders are associated with higher resistance to treatment, greater attrition, and worse outcomes. We have found that dual-diagnosis treatment is the rule rather than the exception. With higher degrees of multi-substance use, our patients display more persistent and higher severity of psychiatric symptoms. In most cases, finalizing the diagnoses and treatment plan in one clinic visit can be challenging, if not impossible. Only after getting to know the patient over several visits can we understand the timeline of their life. Therefore, we recommend that clinicians and patients set small, attainable goals for each treatment encounter. For example, assessing and ensuring safety may be the primary concern of the first few appointments. Patients may reveal more about their lives as the relationship develops, providing information for other diagnoses. The clinician may feel a strong urge to warn and may provide unsolicited advice as a reaction to the patient's risky behaviors. However, this may elicit defensiveness from the patient. We recommend asking for permission before giving advice, using tact, and focusing on building rapport.

# References

Abrahamsson T, Berge J, Öjehagen A, et al: Benzodiazepine, z-drug and pregabalin prescriptions and mortality among patients in opioid maintenance treatment: a nation-wide register-based open cohort study. Drug Alcohol Depend 174(May):58–64, 2017 28315808

Ahmed S, Bachu R, Kotapati P, et al: Use of gabapentin in the treatment of substance use and psychiatric disorders: a systematic review. Front Psychiatry 10:228, 2019 31133886

American Psychiatric Association: Diagnostic and Statistical Manual of Mental Disorders, 4th Edition. Washington, DC, American Psychiatric Association, 1994

American Psychiatric Association: Diagnostic and Statistical Manual of Mental Disorders, 5th Edition. Arlington, VA, American Psychiatric Association, 2013

American Psychiatric Association: Diagnostic and Statistical Manual of Mental Disorders, 5th Edition, Text Revision. Washington, DC, American Psychiatric Association, 2022

Amiri S, Behnezhad S: Alcohol use and risk of suicide: a systematic review and meta-analysis. J Addict Dis 38(2):200–213, 2020 32469287

Anton RF, Latham P, Voronin K, et al: Efficacy of gabapentin for the treatment of alcohol use disorder in patients with alcohol withdrawal symptoms: a randomized clinical trial. JAMA Intern Med 180(5):728–736, 2020 32150232

Arunogiri S, Foulds JA, McKetin R, et al: A systematic review of risk factors for methamphetamine-associated psychosis. Aust N Z J Psychiatry 52(6):514–529, 2018 29338289

Ayers CR, Heffner JL, Russ C, et al: Efficacy and safety of pharmacotherapies for smoking cessation in anxiety disorders: subgroup analysis of the randomized, active- and placebo-controlled EAGLES trial. Depress Anxiety 37(3):247–260, 2020 31850603

Back SE, Brady KT, Jaanimägi U, et al: Cocaine dependence and PTSD: a pilot study of symptom interplay and treatment preferences. Addict Behav 31(2):351–354, 2006 15951125

Back SE, Flanagan JC, Jones JL, et al: Doxazosin for the treatment of co-occurring PTSD and alcohol use disorder: design and methodology of a randomized controlled trial in military veterans. Contemp Clin Trials 73(October):8–15, 2018 30145268

Barry DT, Beitel M, Cutter CJ, et al: An evaluation of the feasibility, acceptability, and preliminary efficacy of cognitive-behavioral therapy for opioid use disorder and chronic pain. Drug Alcohol Depend 194(January):460–467, 2019 30508769

Batki SL, Pennington DL, Lasher B, et al: Topiramate treatment of alcohol use disorder in veterans with posttraumatic stress disorder: a randomized controlled pilot trial. Alcohol Clin Exp Res 38(8):2169–2177, 2014 25092377

Battista SR, Stewart SH, Fulton HG, et al: A further investigation of the relations of anxiety sensitivity to smoking motives. Addict Behav 33(11):1402–1408, 2008 18691826

Bedard-Gilligan M, Garcia N, Zoellner LA, et al: Alcohol, cannabis, and other drug use: engagement and outcome in PTSD treatment. Psychol Addict Behav 32(3):277–288, 2018 29595297

Bernardy N, Montaño M: Opioid use among individuals with posttraumatic stress disorder. PTSD Research Quarterly, 30(1):1–3, 2019. Available at: https://www.ptsd.va.gov/publications/rq_docs/V30N1.pdf. Accessed February 23, 2023.

Bizzarri JV, Sbrana A, Rucci P, et al: The spectrum of substance abuse in bipolar disorder: reasons for use, sensation seeking and substance sensitivity. Bipolar Disord 9(3):213–220, 2007 17430295

Bohnert KM, Ilgen MA, McCarthy JF, et al: Tobacco use disorder and the risk of suicide mortality. Addiction 109(1):155–162, 2014 24134689

Bonn-Miller MO, Sisley S, Riggs P, et al: The short-term impact of 3 smoked cannabis preparations versus placebo on PTSD symptoms: a randomized cross-over clinical trial. PLoS One 16(3):e0246990, 2021 33730032

Bonn-Miller MO, Brunstetter M, Simonian A, et al: The long-term, prospective, therapeutic impact of cannabis on post-traumatic stress disorder. Cannabis Cannabinoid Res 7(2):214–223, 2022 33998874

Brady KT, Dansky BS, Back SE, et al: Exposure therapy in the treatment of PTSD among cocaine-dependent individuals: preliminary findings. J Subst Abuse Treat 21(1):47–54, 2001 11516926

Brady KT, Sonne S, Anton RF, et al: Sertraline in the treatment of co-occurring alcohol dependence and posttraumatic stress disorder. Alcohol Clin Exp Res 29(3):395–401, 2005 15770115

Brown HD, DeFulio A: Contingency management for the treatment of methamphetamine use disorder: a systematic review. Drug Alcohol Depend 216(Nov):108307, 2020 33007699

Buckner JD, Ecker AH, Beighley JS, et al: Integrated cognitive behavioral therapy for comorbid cannabis use and anxiety disorders. Clin Case Stud 15(1):68–83, 2016 28603457

Burnette EM, Nieto SJ, Grodin EN, et al: Novel agents for the pharmacological treatment of alcohol use disorder. Drugs 82(3):251–274, 2022 35133639

Callaghan RC, Veldhuizen S, Jeysingh T, et al: Patterns of tobacco-related mortality among individuals diagnosed with schizophrenia, bipolar disorder, or depression. J Psychiatr Res 48(1):102–110, 2014 24139811

Carroll KM, Nich C, Rounsaville BJ: Differential symptom reduction in depressed cocaine abusers treated with psychotherapy and pharmacotherapy. J Nerv Ment Dis 183(4):251–259, 1995 7714514

Castillo-Carniglia A, Keyes KM, Hasin DS, et al: Psychiatric comorbidities in alcohol use disorder. Lancet Psychiatry 6(12):1068–1080, 2019 31630984

Cerullo MA, Strakowski SM: The prevalence and significance of substance use disorders in bipolar type I and II disorder. Subst Abuse Treat Prev Policy 2(1):29, 2007

Chen J, Bacanu S-A, Yu H, et al: Genetic relationship between schizophrenia and nicotine dependence. Sci Rep 6(May):25671, 2016 27164557

Coffin PO, Santos G-M, Hern J, et al: Effects of mirtazapine for methamphetamine use disorder among cisgender men and transgender women who have sex with men: a placebo-controlled randomized clinical trial. JAMA Psychiatry 77(3):246–255, 2020 31825466

Conner KR, Bagge CL: Suicidal behavior: links between alcohol use disorder and acute use of alcohol. Alcohol Res 40(1):arcr.v40.1.02, 2019 31649836

Cook BL, Wayne GF, Kafali EN, et al: Trends in smoking among adults with mental illness and association between mental health treatment and smoking cessation. JAMA 311(2):172–182, 2014 24399556

Corona R, Dvorsky MR, Romo S, et al: Integrating tobacco prevention skills into an evidence-based intervention for adolescents with ADHD: results from a pilot efficacy randomized controlled trial. J Abnorm Child Psychol 48(11):1439–1453, 2020 32778992

Crits-Christoph P, Wadden S, Gaines A, et al: Symptoms of anhedonia, not depression, predict the outcome of treatment of cocaine dependence. J Subst Abuse Treat 92(Sept):46–50, 2018 30032944

Degenhardt L, Coffey C, Romaniuk H, et al: The persistence of the association between adolescent cannabis use and common mental disorders into young adulthood. Addiction 108(1):124–133, 2013 22775447

Department of Veterans Affairs, Department of Defense: VA/DOD Clinical Practice Guideline for the Management of Posttraumatic Stress Disorder and Acute Stress Disorder. Washington, DC, Department of Veterans Affairs, 2017. Available at: https://www.healthquality.va.gov/guidelines/MH/ptsd/VADoDPTSDCPGPocketCardFinal.pdf. Accessed February 23, 2023.

Ecker AH, Hundt N: Posttraumatic stress disorder in opioid agonist therapy: a review. Psychol Trauma 10(6):636–642, 2018 28758767

Ellis JD, Pasman E, Brown S, et al: An examination of correlates of simultaneous opioid and benzodiazepine use among patients in medication treatment for opioid use disorder in a small midwestern community. J Addict Dis 40(4):542–551, 2022 35285423

Farrell M, Martin NK, Stockings E, et al: Responding to global stimulant use: challenges and opportunities. Lancet 394(10209):1652–1667, 2019 31668409

Feingold D, Weiser M, Rehm J, et al: The association between cannabis use and mood disorders: a longitudinal study. J Affect Disord 172(Feb):211–218, 2015 25451420

Feingold D, Weiser M, Rehm J, et al: The association between cannabis use and anxiety disorders: results from a population-based representative sample. Eur Neuropsychopharmacol 26(3):493–505, 2016 26775742

Fluharty M, Taylor AE, Grabski M, et al: The association of cigarette smoking with depression and anxiety: a systematic review. Nicotine Tob Res 19(1):3–13, 2017 27199385

Frye MA, Salloum IM: Bipolar disorder and comorbid alcoholism: prevalence rate and treatment considerations. Bipolar Disord 8(6):677–685, 2006 17156154

Ganesh S, D'Souza DC: Cannabis and psychosis: recent epidemiological findings continuing the "causality debate." Am J Psychiatry 179(1):8–10, 2022 34974754

Glasner-Edwards S, Mooney LJ: Methamphetamine psychosis: epidemiology and management. CNS Drugs 28(12):1115–1126, 2014 25373627

Gomes T, Juurlink DN, Antoniou T, et al: Gabapentin, opioids, and the risk of opioid-related death: a population-based nested case-control study. PLoS Med 14(10):e1002396, 2017 28972983

Grant BF, Hasin DS, Chou SP, et al: Nicotine dependence and psychiatric disorders in the United States: results from the national epidemiologic survey on alcohol and related conditions. Arch Gen Psychiatry 61(11):1107–1115, 2004 15520358

Groenman AP, Oosterlaan J, Rommelse NNJ, et al: Stimulant treatment for attention-deficit hyperactivity disorder and risk of developing substance use disorder. Br J Psychiatry 203(2):112–119, 2013 23846996

Grunze H, Schaefer M, Scherk H, et al: Comorbid bipolar and alcohol use disorder: a therapeutic challenge. Front Psychiatry 12:660432, 2021 33833701

Guina J, Merrill B: Benzodiazepines I: upping the care on downers: the evidence of risks, benefits and alternatives. J Clin Med 7(2):17, 2018 29385731

Gurillo P, Jauhar S, Murray RM, et al: Does tobacco use cause psychosis? Systematic review and meta-analysis. Lancet Psychiatry 2(8):718–725, 2015 26249303

Heikkinen M, Taipale H, Tanskanen A, et al: Association of pharmacological treatments and hospitalization and death in individuals with amphetamine use disorders in a Swedish nationwide cohort of 13,965 patients. JAMA Psychiatry 80(1):31–39, 2022 36383348

Hilleman DE, Mohiuddin SM, Del Core MG, et al: Effect of buspirone on withdrawal symptoms associated with smoking cessation. Arch Intern Med 152(2):350–352, 1992 1739365

Hirschfeld RMA, Bowden CL, Gitlin MJ, et al: Practice Guideline for the Treatment of Patients With Bipolar Disorder, 2nd Edition. Arlington, VA, American Psychiatric Association, 2010. Available at: https://psychiatryonline.org/pb/assets/raw/sitewide/practice_guidelines/guidelines/bipolar-1410197656063.pdf. Accessed February 23, 2023.

Huang J, Zheng Y, Gao D, et al: Effects of exercise on depression, anxiety, cognitive control, craving, physical fitness and quality of life in methamphetamine-dependent patients. Front Psychiatry 10:999, 2020 32047445

Huestis MA, Boyd SJ, Heishman SJ, et al: Single and multiple doses of rimonabant antagonize acute effects of smoked cannabis in male cannabis users. Psychopharmacology (Berl) 194(4):505–515, 2007 17619859

Isenberg D, Wong SC, Curtis JA: Serotonin syndrome triggered by a single dose of suboxone. Am J Emerg Med 26(7):840.e3–840.e5, 2008 18774063

Jones CM, Mack KA, Paulozzi LJ: Pharmaceutical overdose deaths, United States, 2010. JAMA 309(7):657–659, 2013 23423407

Jones JL, Mateus CF, Malcolm RJ, et al: Efficacy of ketamine in the treatment of substance use disorders: a systematic review. Front Psychiatry 9:277, 2018 30140240

Kadden RM, Litt MD, Kabela-Cormier E, et al: Abstinence rates following behavioral treatments for marijuana dependence. Addict Behav 32(6):1220–1236, 2007 16996224

Kedzior KK, Laeber LT: A positive association between anxiety disorders and cannabis use or cannabis use disorders in the general population: a meta-analysis of 31 studies. BMC Psychiatry 14(May):136, 2014 24884989

Kosten TR, Morgan C, Kosten TA: Depressive symptoms during buprenorphine treatment of opioid abusers. J Subst Abuse Treat 7(1):51–54, 1990 2313769

Koyuncu A, İnce E, Ertekin E, et al: Comorbidity in social anxiety disorder: diagnostic and therapeutic challenges. Drugs Context 8(April):212573, 2019 30988687

Kushner MG, Abrams K, Borchardt C: The relationship between anxiety disorders and alcohol use disorders: a review of major perspectives and findings. Clin Psychol Rev 20(2):149–171, 2000 10721495

Kushner MG, Menary KR, Maurer EW, et al: Greater elevation in risk for nicotine dependence per pack of cigarettes smoked among those with an anxiety disorder. J Stud Alcohol Drugs 73(6):920–924, 2012 23036209

LaFrance EM, Glodosky NC, Bonn-Miller M, et al: Short and long-term effects of cannabis on symptoms of post-traumatic stress disorder. J Affect Disord 274(Sept):298–304, 2020 32469819

Latif Z-E-H, Benth JS, Solli KK, et al: Anxiety, depression, and insomnia among adults with opioid dependence treated with extended-release naltrexone vs buprenorphine-naloxone: a randomized clinical trial and follow-up study. JAMA Psychiatry 76(2):127–134, 2019 30566177

Lembke A: Time to abandon the self-medication hypothesis in patients with psychiatric disorders. Am J Drug Alcohol Abuse 38(6):524–529, 2012 22924576

Levin FR, Mariani JJ, Pavlicova M, et al: Dronabinol and lofexidine for cannabis use disorder: a randomized, double-blind, placebo-controlled trial. Drug Alcohol Depend 159(Feb):53–60, 2016 26711160

Li D, Yang X, Ge Z, et al: Cigarette smoking and risk of completed suicide: a meta-analysis of prospective cohort studies. J Psychiatr Res 46(10):1257–1266, 2012 22889465

Liu Z, Zhang Y, Yuan T-F: Prevalence and risk factors for depressive symptom in methamphetamine use disorder. Stress Brain 1(2):160–172, 2021

Livne O, Shmulewitz D, Sarvet AL, et al: Association of cannabis use-related predictor variables and self-reported psychotic disorders: U.S. adults, 2001–2002 and 2012–2013. Am J Psychiatry 179(1):36–45, 2022 34645275

Longo LP, Campbell T, Hubatch S: Divalproex sodium (Depakote) for alcohol withdrawal and relapse prevention. J Addict Dis 21(2):55–64, 2002 11916372

Lopez-Quintero C, Hasin DS, de Los Cobos JP, et al: Probability and predictors of remission from life-time nicotine, alcohol, cannabis or cocaine dependence: results from the National Epidemiologic Survey on Alcohol and Related Conditions. Addiction 106(3):657–669, 2011 21077975

Madison CA, Eitan S: Buprenorphine: prospective novel therapy for depression and PTSD. Psychol Med 50(6):881–893, 2020 32204739

Mariani JJ, Levin FR: Treatment strategies for co-occurring ADHD and substance use disorders. Am J Addict 16(Suppl 1):45–54, 2007 17453606

Mason BJ, Crean R, Goodell V, et al: A proof-of-concept randomized controlled study of gabapentin: effects on cannabis use, withdrawal and executive function deficits in cannabis-dependent adults. Neuropsychopharmacology 37(7):1689–1698, 2012 22373942

McCance-Katz EF, Sullivan LE, Nallani S: Drug interactions of clinical importance among the opioids, methadone and buprenorphine, and other frequently prescribed medications: a review. Am J Addict 19(1):4–16, 2010 20132117

McKetin R, McLaren J, Lubman DI, et al: The prevalence of psychotic symptoms among methamphetamine users. Addiction 101(10):1473–1478, 2006 16968349

Menkes DB, Herxheimer A: Interaction between antidepressants and alcohol: signal amplification by multiple case reports. Int J Risk Saf Med 26(3):163–170, 2014 25214162

Mohammadi M, Kazeminia M, Abdoli N, et al: The effect of methadone on depression among addicts: a systematic review and meta-analysis. Health Qual Life Outcomes 18(1):373, 2020 33225933

Morissette SB, Tull MT, Gulliver SB, et al: Anxiety, anxiety disorders, tobacco use, and nicotine: a critical review of interrelationships. Psychol Bull 133(2):245–272, 2007 17338599

Morozova M, Rabin RA, George TP: Co-morbid tobacco use disorder and depression: a re-evaluation of smoking cessation therapy in depressed smokers. Am J Addict 24(8):687–694, 2015 26354720

Na PJ, Ralevski E, Jegede O, et al: Depression and/or PTSD comorbidity affects response to antidepressants in those with alcohol use disorder. Front Psychiatry 12(Jan):768318, 2022 35058816

Najavits LM, Harned MS, Gallop RJ, et al: Six-month treatment outcomes of cocaine-dependent patients with and without PTSD in a multisite national trial. J Stud Alcohol Drugs 68(3):353–361, 2007 17446974

Niciu MJ, Luckenbaugh DA, Ionescu DF, et al: Clinical predictors of ketamine response in treatment-resistant major depression. J Clin Psychiatry 75(5):e417–e423, 2014 24922494

Nunes EV, Weiss RD: Co-occurring mood and substance use disorders, in The ASAM Principles of Addiction Medicine, 6th Edition. Edited by Miller SC, Fiellin DA, Rosenthal RN, et al. Philadelphia, PA, Wolters Kluwer, 2019, pp 3181–3244

Papatheofani I, Kollia E, Panagouli E, et al: Possible correlations between cocaine use, generalized anxiety and panic disorders in adolescents and young adults: a review of the literature. Developmental and Adolescent Health 1(4):15–25, 2021

Petrakis I, Ralevski E, Nich C, et al: Naltrexone and disulfiram in patients with alcohol dependence and current depression. J Clin Psychopharmacol 27(2):160–165, 2007 17414239

Pettinati HM, Oslin DW, Kampman KM, et al: A double-blind, placebo-controlled trial combining sertraline and naltrexone for treating co-occurring depression and alcohol dependence. Am J Psychiatry 167(6):668–675, 2010 20231324

Piper ME, Cook JW, Schlam TR, et al: Anxiety diagnoses in smokers seeking cessation treatment: relations with tobacco dependence, withdrawal, outcome and response to treatment. Addiction 106(2):418–427, 2011 20973856

Poling J, Oliveto A, Petry N, et al: Six-month trial of bupropion with contingency management for cocaine dependence in a methadone-maintained population. Arch Gen Psychiatry 63(2):219–228, 2006 16461866

Prochaska JJ, Delucchi K, Hall SM: A meta-analysis of smoking cessation interventions with individuals in substance abuse treatment or recovery. J Consult Clin Psychol 72(6):1144–1156, 2004 15612860

Ralevski E, Olivera-Figueroa LA, Petrakis I: PTSD and comorbid AUD: a review of pharmacological and alternative treatment options. Subst Abuse Rehabil 5(Mar):25–36, 2014 24648794

Randall CL, Thomas S, Thevos AK: Concurrent alcoholism and social anxiety disorder: a first step toward developing effective treatments. Alcohol Clin Exp Res 25(2):210–220, 2001 11236835

Sansone RA, Whitecar P, Wiederman MW: The prevalence of childhood trauma among those seeking buprenorphine treatment. J Addict Dis 28(1):64–67, 2009 19197597

Saunders JB, Schuckit MA, Sirovatka P, et al: Diagnostic Issues in Substance Use Disorders: Refining the Research Agenda for the DSM-V. Washington, DC, American Psychiatric Publishing, 2007

Scheidell JD, Quinn K, McGorray SP, et al: Childhood traumatic experiences and the association with marijuana and cocaine use in adolescence through adulthood. Addiction 113(1):44–56, 2018 28645136

Schuckit MA: Comorbidity between substance use disorders and psychiatric conditions. Addiction 101(Suppl 1):76–88, 2006 16930163

Scott JG, Matuschka L, Niemelä S, et al: Evidence of a causal relationship between smoking tobacco and schizophrenia spectrum disorders. Front Psychiatry 9(Nov):607, 2018 30515111

Sharma R, Tikka SK, Bhute AR, et al: N-acetyl cysteine in the treatment of cannabis use disorder: a systematic review of clinical trials. Addict Behav 129(June):107283, 2022 35189496

Shoptaw SJ, Kao U, Ling W: Treatment for amphetamine psychosis. Cochrane Database Syst Rev 2009(1):CD003026, 2009 19160215

Stockings E, Bowman J, McElwaine K, et al: Readiness to quit smoking and quit attempts among Australian mental health inpatients. Nicotine Tob Res 15(5):942–949, 2013 23089486

Substance Abuse and Mental Health Services Administration: Key Substance Use and Mental Health Indicators in the United States: Results From the 2020 National Survey on Drug Use and Health. Rockville, MD, Substance Abuse and Mental Health Services Administration, 2021, p 156. Available at: https://www.samhsa.gov/data/sites/default/files/reports/rpt35325/NSDUHFFRPDFWHTMLFiles2020/2020NSDUHFFR1PDFW102121.pdf. Accessed February 15, 2023.

Taylor G, Girling A, McNeill A, et al: Does smoking cessation result in improved mental health? A comparison of regression modelling and propensity score matching. BMJ Open 5(10):e008774, 2015 26490099

Thomson D, Berk M, Dodd S, et al: Tobacco use in bipolar disorder. Clin Psychopharmacol Neurosci 13(1):1–11, 2015 25912533

Torrens M, Fonseca F, Mateu G, et al: Efficacy of antidepressants in substance use disorders with and without comorbid depression: a systematic review and meta-analysis. Drug Alcohol Depend 78(1):1–22, 2005 15769553

Upadhyaya HP, Carpenter MJ: Is attention deficit hyperactivity disorder (ADHD) symptom severity associated with tobacco use? Am J Addict 17(3):195–198, 2008 18463996

van Laar M, van Dorsselaer S, Monshouwer K, et al: Does cannabis use predict the first incidence of mood and anxiety disorders in the adult population? Addiction 102(8):1251–1260, 2007 17624975

van Os J, Bak M, Hanssen M, et al: Cannabis use and psychosis: a longitudinal population-based study. Am J Epidemiol 156(4):319–327, 2002 12181101

Varma A, Moore MB, Miller CWT, et al: Topiramate as monotherapy or adjunctive treatment for posttraumatic stress disorder: a meta-analysis. J Trauma Stress 31(1):125–133, 2018 29388709

Williams NR, Heifets BD, Blasey C, et al: Attenuation of antidepressant effects of ketamine by opioid receptor antagonism. Am J Psychiatry 175(12):1205–1215, 2018 30153752

Wojciechowski TW: Developmental trajectories of cocaine/crack use among juvenile offenders: PTSD as a risk factor. J Drug Issues 48(1):50–66, 2018

Yoon G, Petrakis IL, Krystal JH: Association of combined naltrexone and ketamine with depressive symptoms in a case series of patients with depression and alcohol use disorder. JAMA Psychiatry 76(3):337–338, 2019 30624551

Zvolensky MJ, Bernstein A, Sachs-Ericsson N, et al: Lifetime associations between cannabis, use, abuse, and dependence and panic attacks in a representative sample. J Psychiatr Res 40(6):477–486, 2006 16271364

# 11

# HIV and Substance Use Disorders

Richa Vijayvargiya, M.D.
Thanh Thuy Truong, M.D.

*Those who* treat substance use disorders (SUDs) are likely to encounter patients with HIV and vice versa. Approximately 37 million people live with HIV worldwide, with approximately 1.8 million new infections occurring in 2017. Hazardous substance use is a risk factor for HIV acquisition. The direct consequences of behaviors related to substance use, such as sharing needles used in injection drug use (IDU), and the indirect consequences, such as unsafe sexual practices while intoxicated, contribute to the elevated risk of HIV transmission in this population. Approximately 20% of HIV infections can be attributed to IDU (Chilunda et al. 2019). The use of psychoactive substances to enhance one's sexual experience, commonly known as chemsex, is also becoming increasingly common and is associated with high-risk sexual behaviors and transmission of HIV and other sexually transmitted infections.

Substance use is common in the HIV population. In an epidemiological study of HIV-positive adults (2,248 men who have sex with men [MSM], 373 heterosexual men, 637 women) performed in the United Kingdom from 2011 to 2012, half of MSM reported recreational drug use, and 25% used at least three types of drugs simultaneously. In addition to being a risk factor for HIV, substance use is a driver of poor health outcomes among people living with HIV (PLWH). Patients with active substance use are more likely to miss health care appointments, adhere poorly to antiretroviral therapy (ART), and experience the direct negative pathophysiological consequences of illicit substances on the course and progression of HIV infection. The rate of mental illness is disproportionately high in the HIV population; this represents both a risk factor for HIV acquisition and a consequence of it because of the shame and stigma associated with an HIV diagnosis. The heavy burden of mental illness among PLWH is thought to be a driver of further substance use and to be related to other health-related risk factors, such as obesity, smoking, social isolation, and homelessness, leading to a vicious circle of suffering, unhealthy lifestyle behaviors, and poor health (McGowan et al. 2017; Speakman et al. 2013). The American Academy of HIV Medicine (www.aahivm.org) has several up-to-date resources for patients and providers.

# Impact of Substance Use on HIV Outcomes

Active substance use is associated with worse HIV outcomes as a result of HIV-related treatment nonadherence and accelerated disease progression independent of adherence. ART adherence is crucial to achieving optimal viral suppression, preserving immune function, and preventing virus transmission to HIV seronegative sexual partners. Literature reviews consistently show that hazardous substance use is associated with reduced ART adherence, leading to lower cluster of differentiation 4 (CD4) T cell counts, lower HIV viral suppression, and higher rates of AIDS-defining complications. Many studies have examined the role of individual substances in perpetuating ART nonadherence. A negative effect on adherence has been consistently demonstrated for each class of illicit substance. Moreover, depression has been hypothesized to be a factor linking substance use with ART nonadherence. Misconceptions surrounding treatment, such as the belief that combining alcohol or other drugs with HIV medication will have a toxic mixing effect, may also contribute. Substance users who are cognizant of the possible drug interactions between ART and specific substances may avoid ART while using. Studies are ongoing to identify other causal factors behind decreased adherence in this population. Interventions designed to promote adherence among the substance use population improve patient outcomes independent of general substance use treatment (Gonzalez et al. 2011).

Studies have examined various indicators of HIV disease progression in the substance use population. In the Johns Hopkins HIV clinical practice cohort, one study examined the incidence of AIDS-defining illnesses (ADI) in IDU compared with non-IDU in the highly active antiretroviral therapy (HAART) and post-HAART eras. The amount of decrease in ADI from the

HAART era to the post-HAART era was significantly lower among individuals with IDU, with 45% greater relative incidence of ADI in the IDU group. This finding persisted after controlling for antiretroviral medication regimen characteristics, baseline CD4 count, baseline HIV viral load, and significantly lower rates of sustained viral suppression among the IDU population (Moore et al. 2004). In the Concerted Action on Seroconversion to AIDS and Death in Europe (CASCADE) collaboration, the magnitude of decrease in progression to AIDS and rates of mortality from the pre-HAART era to the HAART era was less in the IDU population, who had a 2 times faster rate of AIDS progression and a more than 4 times higher mortality rate (Porter et al. 2003).

Faster rates of progression to AIDS have also been seen in substance users with IDU. In a study that followed 961 females after the initiation of HAART, current substance users (noninjection use of cocaine, crack, or heroin) had a greater likelihood of developing an ADI (hazard ratio [HR] 1.49) and more significant AIDS-related mortality (HR 2.35) (Anastos et al. 2005). These results were noted after controlling for HAART medication, nadir CD4 count, peak HIV viral load, presence of AIDS diagnosis prior to starting HAART, HAART nonadherence, age, income, depression, and cigarette smoking. In a study of 1,686 females in the Women's Interagency HIV Study (WIHS), persistent crack cocaine users had a higher risk of ADI (HR 1.65) and 3 times greater AIDS-related mortality (HR 3.61). Persistent crack cocaine users also had more rapid decreases in CD4+ count below 200 cells/$\mu$L and increased HIV viral load higher than 100,000 copies/mL. Intermittent crack cocaine users also had faster rates of decrease in CD4+ cell count and increased HIV viral load regardless of whether they were actively using at the time. The adverse effects of crack cocaine use on HIV progression were also supported by a study of 222 HIV-positive substance users in Miami, Florida. In that study, crack cocaine use was associated with a faster decline to a CD4+ count of 200 cells/$\mu$L or less, even after controlling for ART adherence and baseline CD4+ count (HR 2.14; 95% CI 1.08–4.25) (Baum et al. 2009).

HIV is associated with detrimental effects on the CNS, mediated through multiple mechanisms. Toxic effects of HIV in the CNS are thought to contribute to developing HIV-associated neurocognitive disorders (HANDs). The most severe form of HAND, HIV-associated dementia, is now much less common in the ART era; however, milder forms persist, even in the presence of viral suppression in the peripheral blood from adequate ART treatment. HANDs are estimated to occur among 15%–55% of PLWH. Substance use combined with HIV infection was associated with greater CNS neuroinflammation and burden of HIV CNS disease in a handful of studies. HIV appears to enter the CNS via transmigration of infected monocytes across the blood-brain barrier. These monocytes differentiate into long-lived HIV-infected macrophages and serve as reservoirs of HIV within the CNS. One study reported increased monocyte activation in the periphery of infected substance users with adequate viral suppression independent of ART adherence. This activation of monocytes in the periphery may be due to increased immune cell entry into the CNS, leading to neuroinflammation. Many substances of abuse are also associated with increased leakiness of the blood-brain barrier, thought to be associated with increased permeability to activated immune cells into the CNS (Chilunda et al. 2019).

# General Approach to Treatment

Effective treatment of PLWH who also have SUD involves a multidisciplinary approach incorporating medical, psychiatric, and addiction care. Conceptualizing care through a long-term chronic disease model may alleviate frustrations from the clinical team. This involves recognizing that the illness will have periods of recovery and recurrence. Rather than failure, recurrences are framed as part of trial and error in achieving an effective care regimen. Some individuals may not be able to achieve abstinence despite treatment; thus, a harm reduction approach may consist of reducing their frequency and severity of use and improving their overall functioning. An interdisciplinary team that supports PLWH may consist of psychiatry, primary care, social work, substance use counselors, case management, and peer recovery.

Barriers to care should be discussed during the first appointment—many PLWH struggle with homelessness, lack of transportation, and food and financial instability. Social work and case management may connect patients with local resources. The care team's understanding of the patient's goals and needs strengthens the therapeutic alliance. In the clinic, tests for HIV/AIDS, hepatitis B and C, tuberculosis, and other infectious diseases should be readily available (ideally on-site). A comprehensive psychiatric evaluation would elucidate primary psychiatric disorders alongside SUD. Medications and psychotherapy or referrals should be offered.

The clinician may match the patient to the appropriate level of care based on the acuity of symptoms, medical conditions, readiness for change, and social support. The American Society of Addiction Medicine criteria are a valuable tool for matching patients with the appropriate level of care. In general, inpatient treatment is recommended if patients are a danger to themselves or to others because of intoxication or acute psychiatric symptoms (e.g., suicidal ideation, psychosis), need intensive withdrawal management, or have a life-threatening medical condition. Residential treatment programs may be considered for those who need a highly structured and supportive environment but are not experiencing acute complications. Partial hospitalization and intensive outpatient programs are appropriate for patients who are transitioning out of a residential or hospital setting to a lower level of care but still need support for recurrence prevention; these programs are also appropriate for patients who can tolerate outpatient withdrawal management, abstain from substance use, and have high motivation and social support. General outpatient management is appropriate for patients who are in the later stages of their recovery and have been stable for a sustained amount of time (e.g., continued stability after completing an intensive outpatient program).

# Special Considerations in the Treatment of Substance Use Disorders and HIV

## Overview of Antiretroviral Therapy

The precipitous development of HIV pharmacotherapy, known as HAART, is one of the most noteworthy achievements of modern medicine. Zidovudine, a nucleoside reverse transcriptase inhibitor (NRTI), was the first drug developed in 1987. It soon became clear that HIV was more optimally treated with a combination of antiretrovirals rather than with a single agent. Standard ART regimens now include the combination of a base of two NRTIs with one additional agent from a different class, most commonly a non-nucleoside reverse transcriptase inhibitor (NNRTI), a protease inhibitor typically boosted with ritonavir, or an integrase inhibitor. Alternatives to this regimen are used in patients with intolerable side effects of viral resistance.

Antiretroviral medications work at various stages in the viral replication process of HIV. Reverse transcriptase is an enzyme that produces viral DNA by copying viral RNA. NRTIs are nucleoside analogs that insert themselves into the elongating DNA strand, blocking further transcription of DNA, whereas NNRTIs bind directly to the reverse transcriptase enzyme. Protease inhibitors inhibit the function of the enzyme protease, which cleaves portions of produced protein material, producing mature viral proteins necessary for propagation and responsible for the virus's detrimental effects on the host.

Finally, integrase inhibitors block the integration of viral DNA into the human genome of the infected individual.

## Drug Interactions With Antiretroviral Therapy

Substances of abuse and medications used in the treatment of SUDs interact with ART through a number of mechanisms. Antiretroviral medications vary in their pharmacodynamic and pharmacokinetic properties, with certain patterns roughly shared among medications within a class. Antiretrovirals are especially prone to drug-drug interactions because two medications with potent cytochrome P450 (CYP) 3A4 inhibition, ritonavir and cobicistat, are specifically used in HAART regimens as boosters to enhance the effect of protease inhibitors, which are predominantly metabolized by this enzyme. Integrase inhibitors are also CYP3A4 inhibitors, whereas NNRTIs are CYP3A4 inducers. Drug-drug interactions involving ART may also occur via the effect on drug transporters, such as p-glycoprotein (Desai et al. 2020; Hakkola et al. 2020; Pau and George 2014). Finally, some ART medications are known to cause false positives on urine drug testing (e.g., efavirenz for cannabis and benzodiazepines). These considerations are discussed in detail in Chapter 4, "Laboratory Testing."

## Opioids

Problematic opioid use has become a national epidemic and significant public health concern, with misuse of prescription opioid medications and illicit use of heroin and fentanyl occurring in about 11 million people in the United States. About 20%–50% of PLWH are prescribed opioids, and evidence suggests an increased risk of developing an opioid use disorder in this population (Chilunda et al. 2019). Opioid use is associated with the acquisition of HIV through sharing of IDU equipment and risky sexual behaviors. HIV can survive in a used syringe for 42 days, and an individual without HIV has a 1:160 chance of seroconversion after using a syringe previously used by someone with HIV. Evidence suggests that people who misuse prescription opioids are also at higher risk of HIV acquisition because of their having higher rates of condomless sex and multiple sexual partners (Substance Abuse and Mental Health Services Administration 2020).

Medications for opioid use disorder, including methadone and buprenorphine, are associated with greater rates of abstinence as well as prevention of recurrence, as discussed in other chapters of this book. Methadone and buprenorphine treatment is associated with a decreased rate of HIV transmission and greater rates of initiation and compliance with ART (Woody et al. 2014). Not surprisingly, ART is increasingly being implemented in methadone clinics to improve patient outcomes. When prescribing methadone or buprenorphine, a clinician should be mindful of the potential for drug interactions with ART, which are mediated by both pharmacokinetic and pharmacodynamic mechanisms. It is sometimes difficult to predict the possibility of drug-drug interactions, so it is important to assess patients clinically for the advent of adverse effects, namely, opioid withdrawal, toxicities from the opioid medications or antiretrovirals, and ART treatment failure due to inadequate medication exposure (McCance-Katz 2005).

## Methadone and Buprenorphine

Methadone and buprenorphine are metabolized significantly by the hepatic CYP450 enzymes, most notably CYP3A4. Many ART medications are substrates of CYP3A4 and inhibit or induce this enzyme, leading to drug-drug interactions with opioids. In clinical practice, drug-drug interactions may not always follow a predictable pattern, despite in vitro studies showing CYP450 enzyme induction or inhibition of ART agents. Interactions may also be challenging to study because ART contains many different combinations of medications, and it may not always be clear which drug is responsible for adverse effects. Existing knowledge, therefore, relies on studies examining interactions between opioids and single antiretroviral agents used as monotherapy. Here we briefly review some drug-drug interactions that have been reported in the literature.

In general, methadone, a medication older than buprenorphine, has been studied more extensively for drug-drug interactions with ART. Although additional studies are needed to clarify the interactions between buprenorphine and ART, buprenorphine seems to have fewer interactions than methadone. Among NRTIs, zidovudine was the first to be studied for drug interactions with methadone. Although zidovudine is unlikely to alter concentrations of methadone, buprenorphine, or naltrexone, methadone has been shown to inhibit the glucuronidation of zidovudine, thus leading to increased plasma levels and a greater likelihood of zidovudine toxicity. Didanosine and stavudine levels are decreased with methadone because reduced bioavailability from slowed gastrointestinal transit leads to decreased absorption due to longer exposure to digestive enzymes and gastric acid. An enteric-coated formulation of didanosine has been developed to ameliorate this problem. Neither didanosine nor stavudine is associated with altered levels of methadone. Lamivudine plus zidovudine is not associated with altered methadone levels, whereas abacavir is associated with increased methadone clearance but does not require adjustment of methadone dosage.

Protease inhibitors have the potential for drug-drug interactions due to their CYP3A4 inhibition. This led the manufacturers of ART to become concerned about the possibility of opioid-related toxicity. However, in vivo studies have shown that many protease inhibitors actually decrease methadone levels. Nelfinavir has been found to decrease methadone levels; however, this effect appears to be offset by competition between nelfinavir and methadone for protein binding, which actually results in an increase in free methadone concentrations. This competition decreases the likelihood of clinically significant opioid withdrawal with this combination. Ritonavir plus saquinavir induces methadone metabolism; however, this combination affects the inactive form of methadone (*S*-methadone) more strongly than the active form (*R*-methadone) and thus is not associated with opioid withdrawal or the need to adjust methadone dosage. Amprenavir plus abacavir is associated with opioid withdrawal because both medications can reduce the plasma levels of methadone. Lopinavir plus ritonavir is associated with decreased levels of methadone, even though ritonavir modestly increases methadone levels. When this combination is prescribed with methadone, it is important to monitor patients clinically for opioid withdrawal and possibly increase their methadone dosage. As a class, NNRTIs are associated with significant drug interactions with methadone. Nevirapine is a CYP3A4 inducer associated with decreased methadone levels, which can lead to opioid withdrawal. Efavirenz is similarly associated with increased methadone clearance and opioid withdrawal because it is both an inducer and substrate of CYP3A4. On the other hand, delavirdine has been found to decrease methadone elimination, which may result in opioid toxicity.

Buprenorphine confers the advantage of being an office-based intervention. Like methadone, it is primarily metabolized by CYP3A4, which converts buprenorphine to norbuprenorphine via *N*-demethylation. Fewer drug interactions are known to be associated with buprenorphine compared with methadone. Decreased pharmacodynamic interactions are thought to be related to buprenorphine's high affinity to the μ opioid receptor and slow dissociation from the receptor. Norbuprenorphine is an active metabolite that also agonizes the μ opioid receptor. When taken with the NNRTI efavirenz, buprenorphine and norbuprenorphine levels are decreased; however, this effect is not associated with opioid withdrawal, and adjustments of buprenorphine dosage have not been required (Desai et al. 2020; Pau and George 2014).

# Stimulants

Stimulants such as cocaine and methamphetamine have been used to enhance sexual activity since the 1970s. They contribute to risky sexual behaviors that increase the risk of HIV infection. Among PLWH, stimulant use is associated with an increase in mortality because of risky behaviors leading to concomitant infections such as hepatitis C, medication nonadherence, and direct effects of stimulants on immunity. In vitro studies have shown that cocaine enhances the infection of stimulated lymphocytes (Adams et al. 2018). Long-term use of cocaine is associated with coronary artery disease, which may compound with the side effects of certain ART medications. It may also exacerbate dyslipidemia and hepatic and myocardial toxicities of protease inhibitors (Lai et al. 2017; Li et al. 2018).

Pharmacotherapy for stimulant use disorders is discussed in more detail in Chapter 6, "Stimulants and Co-occurring Substance Use." For PLWH, considerations may be made for medications that can also be helpful for other symptoms:

- *Mirtazapine:* Clinicians should consider mirtazapine for PLWH who also have depression, insomnia, and low appetite.
- *Doxazosin:* Given the high rate of trauma and PTSD in this patient population, clinicians should consider doxazosin for PLWH who also have cocaine use disorder, trauma-related nightmares, and hyperarousal.
- *Stimulants:* Methylphenidate has been studied for HIV-related cognitive symptoms. Extended-release formulations are preferred because of lower risk of misuse. Atomoxetine may also be considered if cognitive symptoms are prominent.
- *Topiramate:* Cognitive side effects of topiramate may worsen in PLWH, so we recommend a slow titration and lowest effective dosage.
- *Bupropion:* Although commonly used for stimulant use disorder, bupropion should be avoided in PLWH who have anorexia and associated electrolyte abnormalities because of increased risk of seizures. As discussed in Chapter 6, combination of bupropion and naltrexone injection may be more effective for methamphetamine use disorder than either alone, but naltrexone is not an option for patients taking opioids.

# Cannabis

The availability and use of cannabis products have rapidly increased in recent years because of legalization and perceived lower risk. A study of 226 PLWH from Canada found that 97.7% reported recreational cannabis use and 21.8% reported use for stress, anorexia, nausea, and pain. Although the participants reported more perceived benefits than negative consequences, cannabis use was associated with high-risk behaviors such as driving under the influence, other substance use, and paranoia (Harris et al. 2014). Cannabis use among PLWH is also associated with significantly more significant cognitive impairment. Because data on cannabis safety in PLWH are inconclusive, we recommend discouraging use and offering alternative interventions for various concerns such as appetite, anxiety, and sleep. No studies have examined pharmacotherapy for cannabis use disorder in PLWH. Among potentially effective medications, gabapentin may be considered for patients with comorbid neuropathic pain.

# Tobacco

Rates of cigarette smoking among PLWH vary from 34% to 70%, much higher than in the general population. Smoking is associated with worse outcomes, including a reduced life expectancy, lung cancer and other respiratory illnesses, lower CD4 counts, higher viral loads, and lower quality of life. Lung cancer is the leading cause of cancer death among PLWH receiving ART. PLWH who smoke are more likely to engage in risky substance use and have decreased adherence to ART. Some people report smoking to self-medicate emotional distress (e.g., depression, anxiety), improve concentration, control weight, and socialize. Tobacco cessation among PLWH decreases the risk of *Pneumocystis* pneumonia, cardiovascular disease, and cancer mortality. PLWH who successfully quit using tobacco also report a higher quality of life, with reduced mental and physical symptom burden (Ledgerwood and Yskes 2016; Reddy et al. 2022).

Several interventions exist that can help PLWH reduce or quit smoking. Studies have shown that Screening, Brief Intervention, and Referral to Treatment (SBIRT) and a single session of motivational interviewing are effective to reduce the number of cigarettes smoked per day among PLWH. Pharmacotherapy using FDA-approved methods such as nicotine replacement therapy, bupropion, and varenicline has shown efficacy in reducing tobacco use among PLWH (detailed in Chapter 6). However, study results suggest that abstinence rates are modest. Novel technology-based interventions are emerging as accessible and practical options for people with or without HIV who smoke (Reddy et al. 2022). Quitlines provide free and effective coaching to help people quit smoking. In the United States, the number 1-800-QUIT-NOW connects callers with their state quitline. Various smartphone applications provide a platform to monitor use, cravings, and progress toward their goals. QuitGuide and QuitStart are free applications from by Smokefree.gov, which has many other resources to help people quit smoking.

# Approaches to Reducing HIV Transmission

## Pre-exposure Prophylaxis

Pre-exposure prophylaxis (PrEP) is an intervention that involves taking daily oral antiretroviral medication to reduce the risk of acquiring HIV. It can be helpful in populations at higher risk of HIV infection, such as injection drug users, binge drinkers, recreational drug users, and MSM. PrEP is about 99% effective at preventing HIV transmission with proper adherence. Significant treatment barriers may exist obtaining for PrEP, including reduced awareness of its availability, cost limitations, lack of transportation to care providers, lack of insurance coverage, underestimation of HIV infection risk, and concern for side effects. Interventions to enhance PrEP utilization include text check-in reminders, group therapy, and integration of PrEP prescriptions with HIV testing centers, pharmacies, and methadone maintenance clinics.

## Syringe Services Programs

Syringe services programs (SSPs) are efforts to decrease the rate of infectious diseases related to IDU via preventive measures such as distribution of sterile syringes and IDU-related equipment, education, and coordination of mental health care and substance use treatment. The efficacy of SSPs in decreasing the rate of infectious disease transmissions, such as HIV and the hepatitis C virus, has been extensively supported in the literature. SSPs are associated with decreased self-reported syringe sharing and substance use frequency and decreased HIV incidence. SSPs have been used successfully in both urban and rural settings to address new outbreaks.

## Contingency Management

Contingency management is a behavior therapy that uses motivational rewards and tangible reinforcers to promote a given behavior. With this therapy, people are offered rewards such as vouchers that they can exchange for money or items or opportunities to earn prizes when they have negative drug screen results or they adhere to certain desired behaviors, such as attending appointments. Contingency management is limited in application as a result of financial limitations because insurance may not compensate providers for the rewards. The Department of Health and Human Services Office of the Inspector General formerly enforced a rule that the Centers for Medicare and Medicaid Services cannot reimburse more than $75 annually or $15 per individual appointment for rewards. However, recent advocacy has pushed the Office of the Inspector General to endorse higher amounts (Knopf 2022). Regarding HIV transmission, contingency management has been associated with a reduction in self-reported risky sexual behaviors and drug use behaviors that increase risk of HIV (e.g., IDU, syringe sharing), reduced viral load, and greater ART adherence (Haug and Sorensen 2006).

## Chemsex

Chemsex can be fatal when multiple chemicals with compounding side effects, including cardiac and respiratory depression, are combined. Phosphodiesterase type 5 inhibitors (e.g., sildenafil, tadalafil, vardenafil) that are used in combination with sedating drugs can lead to dangerous drops in blood pressure, which can result in strokes or myocardial infarction. Chemsex is increasingly common among the MSM population, especially individuals who are HIV positive, because the illicit chemicals are taken to counteract the impotence-inducing effects of certain ART medications (Giorgetti et al. 2017). Many patients experience shame when discussing chemsex; thus, the clinician should initiate conversations about sexual behaviors and sexual concerns as part of a thorough assessment. Distinguishing between different types of sexual dysfunction, whether it is ART induced or results from other causes (e.g., trauma, other psychological barriers), is necessary to direct the patient to appropriate treatment and interventions.

# Conclusion

Substance use significantly increases HIV transmission, morbidity, and mortality. Given the high association of substance use and HIV infection, all at-risk patients should be routinely screened and tested for both. Treatment for either condition improves outcomes for the other, including increased adherence to life-saving ART, lower risk of acquiring other infections, and higher quality of life. With the many challenges that PLWH face, clinicians would work best within a multidisciplinary team that includes providers from internal medicine, general and addiction psychiatry, case management, social work, and peer support. All patients should receive education on measures to reduce harm and risk of HIV infection.

# References

Adams JW, Bryant KJ, Edelman EJ, et al: Association of cannabis, stimulant, and alcohol use with mortality prognosis among HIV-infected men. AIDS Behav 22(4):1341–1351, 2018 28887669

Anastos K, Schneider MF, Gange SJ, et al: The association of race, sociodemographic, and behavioral characteristics with response to highly active antiretroviral therapy in women. J Acquir Immune Defic Syndr 39(5):537–544, 2005 16044004

Baum MK, Rafie C, Lai S, et al: Crack-cocaine use accelerates HIV disease progression in a cohort of HIV-positive drug users. J Acquir Immune Defic Syndr 50(1):93–99, 2009 19295339

Chilunda V, Calderon TM, Martinez-Aguado P, et al: The impact of substance abuse on HIV-mediated neuropathogenesis in the current ART era. Brain Res 1724(Dec):146426, 2019 31473221

Desai N, Burns L, Gong Y, et al: An update on drug-drug interactions between antiretroviral therapies and drugs of abuse in HIV systems. Expert Opin Drug Metab Toxicol 16(11):1005–1018, 2020 32842791

Giorgetti R, Tagliabracci A, Schifano F, et al: When "chems" meet sex: a rising phenomenon called "chemsex." Curr Neuropharmacol 15(5):762–770, 2017 27855594

Gonzalez A, Barinas J, O'Cleirigh C: Substance use: impact on adherence and HIV medical treatment. Curr HIV/AIDS Rep 8(4):223–234, 2011 21858414

Hakkola J, Hukkanen J, Turpeinen M, et al: Inhibition and induction of CYP enzymes in humans: an update. Arch Toxicol 94(11):3671–3722, 2020 33111191

Harris GE, Dupuis L, Mugford GJ, et al: Patterns and correlates of cannabis use among individuals with HIV/AIDS in maritime Canada. Can J Infect Dis Med Microbiol 25(1):e1–e7, 2014 24634690

Haug NA, Sorensen JL: Contingency management interventions for HIV-related behaviors. Curr HIV/AIDS Rep 3(4):154–159, 2006 17032574

Knopf A: OIG for first time endorses more than $75 a year for contingency management. Alcohol Drug Abuse Wkly 34(10):1–4, 2022

Lai S, Gerstenblith G, Moore RD, et al: Cocaine use may modify HIV/ART-associated myocardial steatosis and hepatic steatosis. Drug Alcohol Depend 177(Aug):84–92, 2017 28578226

Ledgerwood DM, Yskes R: Smoking cessation for people living with HIV/AIDS: a literature review and synthesis. Nicotine Tob Res 18(12):2177–2184, 2016 27245237

Li J, Lai H, Chen S, et al: Impact of cocaine use on protease inhibitor-associated dyslipidemia in HIV-infected adults. Int J STD AIDS 29(8):781–789, 2018 29471762

McCance-Katz EF: Treatment of opioid dependence and coinfection with HIV and hepatitis C virus in opioid-dependent patients: the importance of drug interactions between opioids and antiretroviral agents. Clin Infect Dis 41(Suppl 1):S89–S95, 2005 16265622

McGowan JA, Sherr L, Rodger AJ, et al: Age, time living with diagnosed HIV infection, and self-rated health. HIV Med 18(2):89–103, 2017 27385511

Moore RD, Keruly JC, Chaisson RE: Differences in HIV disease progression by injecting drug use in HIV-infected persons in care. J Acquir Immune Defic Syndr 35(1):46–51, 2004 14707791

Pau AK, George JM: Antiretroviral therapy: current drugs. Infect Dis Clin North Am 28(3):371–402, 2014 25151562

Porter K, Babiker A, Bhaskaran K, et al: Determinants of survival following HIV-1 seroconversion after the introduction of HAART. Lancet 362(9392):1267–1274, 2003 14575971

Reddy KP, Kruse GR, Lee S, et al: Tobacco use and treatment of tobacco dependence among people with human immunodeficiency virus: a practical guide for clinicians. Clin Infect Dis 75(3):525–533, 2022 34979543

Speakman A, Rodger A, Phillips AN, et al: The "Antiretrovirals, Sexual Transmission Risk and Attitudes" (ASTRA) study: design, methods and participant characteristics. PLoS One 8(10):e77230, 2013 24143214

Substance Abuse and Mental Health Services Administration: Prevention and Treatment of HIV Among People Living With Substance Use and/or Mental Disorders. Rockville, MD, Substance Abuse and Mental Health Services Administration, 2020. Available at: https://store.samhsa.gov/sites/default/files/SAMHSA_Digital_Download/PEP20-06-03-001.pdf. Accessed November 19, 2022.

Woody GE, Bruce D, Korthuis PT, et al: HIV risk reduction with buprenorphine-naloxone or methadone: findings from a randomized trial. J Acquir Immune Defic Syndr 66(3):288–293, 2014 24751432

# 12

# Substance Use Disorders in Pregnancy

Andres Ojeda, M.D.
Claire K. Morice, M.D.
Thanh Thuy Truong, M.D.

*According* to the 2019 National Survey on Drug Use and Health (NSDUH; Substance Abuse and Mental Health Services Administration 2020), 9.5% of pregnant people reported past-month use of alcohol; rates were 9.6% for the use of tobacco products and 5.8% for illicit drug use (Center for Behavioral Health Statistics and Quality 2020). Actual percentages are thought to be higher because of patients' tendency to underreport, likely because of stigma surrounding substance use disorders (SUDs) in pregnancy, and patients' fears of legal involvement (Bishop et al. 2017; Ondersma et al. 2019). SUD in pregnancy is associated with increased suicidality: 28% of reproductive-age females who completed suicide met criteria for an SUD at the time of death, and 9.3% of perinatal people with SUD have suicidal ideation or parasuicidal behaviors (Forray and Yonkers 2021). Fortunately, pregnancy is an opportune time to intervene, given patients' increased contact with medical professionals; in 2016, an estimated 77% of pregnant individuals received prenatal care in the first trimester (Osterman and Martin 2018). Moreover, concern for their infant's health is a strong motivating factor for pregnant individuals to seek treatment (Frazer et al. 2019). Given the high prevalence, associated risks, and possibility for medical intervention during this period, it is vital to examine treatment options for SUDs in this unique population.

The greatest difficulty for determining the safety and efficacy of medications for SUD in pregnancy is the lack of robust clinical trials in this population. We examined current (albeit often limited) evidence and how the agents are used in clinical practice. A risk-benefit analysis conducted with the patient should direct treatment, but anecdotal evidence suggests that the absence of clear guidelines and directives for SUD treatment in the peripartum period often influences a lack of frank discussions about treatment options. Clincians should especially be mindful of the risks of *not* treating the illness and inform patients of such. Special considerations may apply to transgender individuals, and a detailed overview of treatment perspectives in that group is presented in Chapter 14, "Substance Use Disorders in the LGBTQ+ Population."

# Alcohol Use Disorder

## Epidemiology

Unfortunately, alcohol use during pregnancy is not uncommon, and rates appear to be rising. The global prevalence of alcohol use during pregnancy is estimated to be 9.8%. From 2011 to 2018, rates of drinking in pregnancy in the United States increased from 9.2% to 11.3%, and rates of binge drinking in pregnancy increased from 2.5% to 4.0% (Popova et al. 2017).

## Risks of Not Treating

One of the biggest concerns about alcohol consumption during pregnancy is the risk of fetal alcohol spectrum disorder (FASD). Features of FASD include growth restriction, craniofacial abnormalities, neurological deficits (ranging from fine motor deficits to major malformations), and various neuropsychiatric impairments, including decreased intellectual ability, sleep disorders, executive functioning deficits (e.g., ADHD, oppositional defiant disorder), and increased rates of depression, anxiety, and suicidality (Kingdon et al. 2016; Lange et al. 2018b; Oei 2020). Alcohol use during pregnancy is the leading preventable cause of intellectual disability in the offspring in the United States (Lee et al. 2021). An estimated 1 in every 67 people who drink during pregnancy deliver a child with fetal alcohol syndrome (Popova et al. 2017). Alcohol use disorder (AUD) in pregnancy can also raise risk of maternal infection after cesarean section, chorioamnionitis, premature delivery, and impaired immune function in the neonate (de Wit et al. 2013; Gauthier 2015).

## Pharmacological Treatment

The three FDA-approved medications for maintenance treatment of AUD in the general population are naltrexone (oral and intramuscular formulations), disulfiram, and acamprosate (Table 12–1).

### Naltrexone

***Mechanism.*** Naltrexone (available in oral and intramuscular form) is a nonselective opioid receptor antagonist that is FDA-approved for both AUD and opioid use disorder (OUD).

***Current Evidence.*** Animal studies with naltrexone have had varied results. Many murine models showed no adverse maternal or congenital outcomes, but other studies showed decreased spontaneous motor activity in chicken embryos and altered pain response in rodents (Jones et al. 2012). In their prospective cohort study, Towers et al. (2020) evaluated naltrexone's safety in pregnant patients ($n=230$) for treatment of OUD. Oral naltrexone 50 mg/day was compared with opioid agonist treatment (OAT; buprenorphine or methadone). The naltrexone group had no incidents of spontaneous abortion or stillbirth and no increase in birth anomalies relative to the opioid agonist group. Obstetric outcomes in the naltrexone group (percentage of vaginal deliveries, preterm births, average gestational age at delivery) were comparable with national averages (Martin et al. 2021). In a smaller retrospective cohort study, neonates exposed to implant naltrexone ($n=68$) for maternal treatment of OUD were smaller in size (3,137.1 g vs. 3,378.0 g) and had longer hospital stays (5.5 days vs. 4.3 days), but there were no differences in rates of congenital anomalies, stillbirths, or neonatal mortality from the control group (Kelty and Hulse 2017).

***Clinical practice.*** Oral naltrexone 50 mg/day may be a reasonable choice, especially in pregnant individuals with high-risk alcohol use. Monthly intramuscular naltrexone has not been studied. We recommend avoiding the use of naltrexone in patients with liver impairment.

### Disulfiram

***Mechanism.*** Disulfiram is an aldehyde dehydrogenase inhibitor that increases levels of the toxic metabolite acetaldehyde in the presence of alcohol, producing an aversive reaction (Suh et al. 2006). In addition, it blocks dopamine β-hydroxylase, which inhibits the conversion of dopamine to norepi-

**Table 12–1. Treatment of alcohol use disorder (maintenance) during pregnancy**

| Medication | Recommendation and strength | Known effects on obstetrical outcomes | Known effects on fetal outcomes | Quality of evidence | Contraindications |
|---|---|---|---|---|---|
| Naltrexone (oral) | First line, 50 mg/day | No increase in preterm births or obstetrical complications | No increase in birth anomalies, stillbirths, or mortality | Low | Liver impairment |
| Acamprosate | First line, 666 mg PO tid | None known | None known; in animal studies, may mitigate brain damage with alcohol exposure | Low | Adjust to 333 mg tid if creatinine clearance is 30–50; avoid if <30. |
| Topiramate | Avoid using during pregnancy | None known | 2–5 times increased risk of cleft palate; 2 times increased risk of low birth weight | Strong | Relative contraindications: nephrolithiasis, use with other carbonic anhydrase inhibitors, angle-closure glaucoma (Janssen Pharmaceuticals 2022) |
| Gabapentin | Second line, 400 mg PO tid | Preterm birth | Cardiac malformations, small for gestational age | Low | Renal impairment |
| Disulfiram | Discontinue during pregnancy and switch to another agent | Disulfiram reaction causes hypotension, vomiting | Can cause copper deficiency, fetal alcohol spectrum disorder risk with alcohol use | Strong | |

nephrine. A subsequent increase in dopamine levels may counter the loss of dopaminergic surge in recently abstinent individuals with AUD.

***Current evidence.*** Based on a limited number of reported cases of disulfiram use in pregnancy, the absence of an increase in birth defects after disulfiram exposure suggests that the drug has no definitive teratogenic effect (Briggs and Freeman 2015b). However, a major cause for concern is the risk of a disulfiram-alcohol reaction to maternal and fetal health, including sequelae of tachycardia, vomiting, and hypotension. Second, disulfiram is a copper chelating agent, which may lead to copper deficiency in the neonate. Copper deficiency in pregnancy is associated with congenital deficits and risk of perinatal mortality (Kelty et al. 2021). Third, in utero exposure to acetaldehyde can also contribute to FASD, making the benefit-risk ratio of disulfiram low (Lui et al. 2014).

***Clinical practice.*** Disulfiram is an unfavorable medication choice for AUD in pregnancy because of the risks of acetaldehyde exposure and sequelae of a disulfiram reaction. Even in patients in remission from AUD, because of the risk of copper deficiency, we recommend discontinuing disulfiram in patients who become pregnant and switching to another agent such as naltrexone or acamprosate.

### Acamprosate

***Mechanism.*** Acamprosate is FDA-approved for AUD in nonpregnant patients. It is thought to reduce excitatory glutamate transition and to increase inhibitory GABA neurotransmission, an imbalance that occurs after cessation of chronic heavy alcohol use (Kalk and Lingford-Hughes 2014).

***Current evidence.*** Preclinical animal studies have been promising overall, with no teratogenic effect observed. In fact, use of acamprosate in pregnant hamsters and rats who were also exposed to alcohol actually reduced the risk of fetal brain damage. In clinical research, one small retrospective cohort study compared pregnant individuals with AUD treated with acamprosate ($n=54$) with matched comparison groups (Kelty et al. 2019). Those treated with acamprosate had lower rates of hospitalization than nontreated patients with AUD. No differences were seen in neonatal outcomes (birth weight, congenital abnormalities).

***Clinical practice.*** Limited data show acamprosate appears to be unharmful in pregnancy, although the sample size was small. Therefore, in cases in which the severity of maternal alcohol consumption is high, the benefits of acamprosate use likely outweigh the risks. It may also be a good choice in patients with comorbid nicotine use disorder on the basis of its efficacy in animal models.

## Topiramate

**Mechanism.**    Topiramate is a monosaccharide D-fructose analog commonly used as an antiepileptic drug and frequently used off-label to treat AUD in the general population (Hernández-Díaz et al. 2012). Topiramate blocks sodium channels, potentiates GABA, and antagonizes α-amino-3-hydroxy-5-methyl-4-isoxazolepropionic acid (AMPA) glutamate receptors, reducing neuronal excitability (Guglielmo et al. 2015).

**Current evidence.**    The safety of topiramate in pregnant patients has been studied predominantly at higher doses used for treatment of epilepsy. Topiramate use in the first trimester increases the risk of oral cleft development by 2–5 times. However, at dosages below 100 mg/day, the relative risk decreases to 1.64 (Hernández-Díaz et al. 2018). Fetal topiramate exposure also more than doubles the risk of low birth weight (Hernández-Díaz et al. 2014).

**Clinical practice.**    Although dosages of topiramate used off-label for AUD may often not exceed 100 mg/day, we still recommend avoiding it in pregnancy entirely.

## Gabapentin

**Mechanism.**    Gabapentin binds to $\alpha_2\delta$ subunits on voltage-gated calcium channels to decrease excitability, reduces glutamate release, and indirectly increases GABA activity. Gabapentin can help mild withdrawal symptoms, particularly anxiety and insomnia. It is used off-label in the general population for alcohol maintenance, although studies have shown it is primarily efficacious only for reducing the frequency of heavy drinking (Kranzler et al. 2019; Modesto-Lowe et al. 2019).

**Current evidence.**    In animal studies, gabapentin has been associated with delayed bone ossification and hydronephrosis when given at supratherapeutic doses (Briggs and Freeman 2015c). A large population-based cohort study compared more than 6,000 pregnant subjects exposed to gabapentin with a nonexposed reference group. Neonates born in the gabapentin-exposed group tended to have greater risk of cardiac malformations (adjusted RR 1.12). Maternal use of gabapentin in late pregnancy (after 20 weeks gestational age) led to a 20%–30% increased risk of preterm birth, a 30%–40% increased risk of delivering neonates who were small for gestational age, and a 35% increased risk of neonates requiring ICU admission at birth (Patorno et al. 2020). In a smaller prospective cohort study that compared pregnancy outcomes among participants with and without gabapentin exposure ($n=223$ for each group), the drug did not appear to cause major malformations. However, this study also showed a 4.8% increase in the rate of preterm births and a risk of birth weight below 2,500 g in the gabapentin group (Fujii et al. 2013).

***Clinical practice.*** Given limited data in pregnancy, we recommend oral gabapentin 400 mg three times daily as a second-line agent for alcohol maintenance and mild withdrawal symptoms.

## Alcohol and Benzodiazepine Withdrawal

Given that alcohol and benzodiazepine withdrawal syndromes have a shared underlying pathophysiology, the treatment options explored here apply to both (Table 12–2).

### Risks of Not Treating

Loss of GABA-mediated inhibition with abrupt alcohol cessation can cause autonomic instability and withdrawal seizures, which are associated with increased risk of mortality (McDonald et al. 2018). Additional risks in pregnancy include placental abruption, preterm labor, and fetal distress (McDonald et al. 2018). If a patient does not undergo alcohol withdrawal during their pregnancy, alcohol withdrawal syndrome (AWS) can occur in the neonate after birth (Kelty et al. 2021). Symptoms of neonatal AWS include tremors, hypertonia, restlessness, and reflex abnormalities.

### Benzodiazepines

***Current evidence.*** Benzodiazepines are used for first-line treatment of alcohol withdrawal in nonpregnant patients. However, benzodiazepine exposure in the first trimester has an unclear risk of fetal harm. Four meta-analyses revealed no increased risk of major fetal malformations, with some exceptions (Dolovich et al. 1998; Enato et al. 2011; Grigoriadis et al. 2019; National Collaborating Centre for Mental Health 2014). Data from one analysis of case control studies indicated an 80% increased risk of cleft palate in offspring with first-trimester exposure to benzodiazepines (Dolovich et al. 1998). However, this was not seen in a more recent meta-analysis, and pooled data from cohort studies showed no increased risk of cleft palate (National Collaborating Cen-

**Table 12–2.** Treatment of alcohol and benzodiazepine withdrawal during pregnancy

| Medication | Recommendation and strength | Known effects on obstetric outcomes | Known effects on fetal outcomes | Quality of evidence |
|---|---|---|---|---|
| Benzodiazepines | First line (strong) at lowest possible amount; diazepam and chlordiazepoxide often used | With chronic use, risk of preterm birth, cesarean delivery, and spontaneous abortion | Unclear, but minimal if used sparingly | Low (World Health Organization 2014) |
| Valproic acid | Discontinue during pregnancy; avoid prescribing to those of childbearing age (strong) | No significant findings | Known teratogen; 10–20 times increased risk of neural tube defects and cleft palate | Strong (World Health Organization 2014) |
| Carbamazepine | Avoid using specifically for withdrawal (strong) | No significant findings | 2.6 times increased risk of neural tube defects | Strong |

tre for Mental Health 2014). When used in conjunction with antidepressants, benzodiazepines have been associated with major malformations (Grigoriadis et al. 2019). Delivery outcomes also may be affected by benzodiazepine use, including an 86% increased risk of spontaneous abortion, 96% increased risk of preterm birth, 161% increased risk of neonatal ICU admission, 119% increased risk of low Apgar scores, and some increased risk of cesarean delivery (absolute risk increase 33 per 1,000 deliveries) (Grigoriadis et al. 2020).

***Clinical practice.*** Given the risks of untreated alcohol withdrawal and the lack of significant harm from short-term benzodiazepine use, international guidelines for the treatment of alcohol withdrawal in pregnancy strongly recommend inpatient hospitalization and administration of a long-acting benzodiazepine, such as diazepam or chlordiazepoxide, titrated to the severity of withdrawal. The Clinical Institute Withdrawal Assessment (CIWA) protocol helps with determining the intensity of the AWS and avoiding giving an excess amount of benzodiazepines (Thibaut et al. 2019).

### Other Agents

Nonbenzodiazepine anticonvulsants are sometimes utilized in nonpregnant populations to manage AWS (Minozzi et al. 2010). Reviews of these agents, such as gabapentin, carbamazepine, and valproic acid, describe varying levels of success (Farheen et al. 2021).

In the general population, carbamazepine has been shown to be as effective as benzodiazepines in treating mild to moderate withdrawal symptoms and perhaps superior to lorazepam at reducing anxiety and insomnia (Malcolm et al. 2002). However, carbamazepine in pregnancy more than doubles the risk of spina bifida, likely via folate antagonism (Jentink et al. 2010). Carbamazepine has a relative risk of 2.7 for major malformations and has been associated with cardiovascular and urinary tract deficits (Briggs and Freeman 2015a). Therefore, carbamazepine for AWS should be avoided.

Studies of valproic acid for alcohol withdrawal have been mixed, and positive studies demonstrated only small clinical significance (Lum et al. 2006). Moreover, in pregnancy strong evidence indicates that valproic acid increases the risk of major congenital malformations in the offspring (risk difference 20 more per 1,000), with an estimated event rate of 6.7%–9.7%. Valproic acid has a significant association with cleft lip and palate (absolute risk difference 11 more per 1,000) and neural tube defects (absolute risk difference 10 more per 1,000) (National Collaborating Centre for Mental Health 2014). Given the low benefit-risk ratio and known teratogenic effect, valproic acid should be discontinued as soon as a patient becomes pregnant. Administration of high doses of folic acid (4–5 mg/day) has not been shown to prevent malformations from valproic acid exposure (Ornoy et al. 2018).

## Additional Concerns

In all pregnant patients, supplementation with thiamine (vitamin $B_1$) 1.4 mg/day is recommended because of a 30% increase in metabolic demands (Institute of Medicine Food and Nutrition Board 1998). Furthermore, heavy alcohol consumption is a leading cause of thiamine deficiency (Johnson 2020). Thiamine deficiency can cause Wernicke-Korsakoff syndrome in the pregnant person and can negatively affect fetal development, leading to language impairment, intrauterine growth restriction, and encephalopathy (Kloss et al. 2018). In treating alcohol withdrawal, intravenous or intramuscular thiamine 100 mg/day for 3–5 days should be provided prior to giving intravenous glucose to prevent Wernicke encephalopathy.

Folic acid, the dietary supplement version of folate (vitamin $B_9$), reduces the risk of maternal anemia and fetal neural tube and congenital heart defects and potentially reduces preterm birth (Greenberg et al. 2011). Folic acid supplementation of 600 µg/day is recommended for individuals who are trying to conceive and those who are pregnant (Bibbins-Domingo et al. 2017). Ethanol impairs folic acid absorption and increases its excretion (Shrestha and Singh 2013). Furthermore, heavy alcohol use decreases folic acid transport across the placenta to the fetus, making folate supplementation particularly important in AUD in pregnancy. Decreased fetal folate may play a role in the development of FASD (Hutson et al. 2012). We recommend supplementation with folic acid 1 mg/day.

## Summary

- First-line agents for treating AUD in pregnancy are acamprosate (in animal models it reduces fetal brain damage with alcohol exposure and helps with nicotine use) and oral naltrexone.
- We recommend *discontinuing* disulfiram upon conception.
- Treatment of AWS should be performed inpatient with administration of the shortest effective course of benzodiazepines. Intravenous thiamine and folic acid should be administered.
- Because of high teratogenicity, valproic acid is *not* recommended for pregnant patients.

# Opioid Use Disorder

OUD is a global public health crisis with significant effects on individuals' lives and functioning. Among the 67,387 drug overdoses in the United States in 2018, 70% involved an opioid (Centers for Disease Control and Prevention 2021). OUDs are particularly dangerous during pregnancy, and opioid use has become increasingly prevalent. In the United States, the prevalence of OUD in pregnancy is estimated to have more than quadrupled from 1999 to 2014 (Haight et al. 2018). According to commercial insurance and Medicaid claims, in 2019, 6.6% of female patients reported the use of prescription opioid pain medications during pregnancy; 20% of these patients reported misuse of prescription opioids, and 27.1% described wanting to cut down or stop using (Maeda et al. 2014).

## Risks of Not Treating

Untreated OUDs during pregnancy can be detrimental to the fetus because repeated withdrawal periods can affect placental function and increase the risk of preterm labor and even fetal death (Kaltenbach et al. 1998). Opioid use is also associated with a sixfold increase in obstetric complications. Opioid use in pregnancy causes increased neonatal mortality, increased risk of sudden infant death syndrome, postnatal growth deficiencies, neurobehavioral problems, and microcephaly (Mozurkewich and Rayburn 2014). Neonates face the risk of neonatal opioid withdrawal syndrome (NOWS), also known as neonatal abstinence syndrome, a condition that increased n occurrece sevenfold from 2000 to 2016. NOWS occurs following chronic exposure to opiates and is associated with a wide range of symptoms, including CNS irritability (tremors, increased muscle tone, seizures), autonomic nervous system activation (sweating, increased respirations, fever), and gastrointestinal dysfunction (difficulty feeding, vomiting, watery stools) (Patrick et al. 2020). NOWS is thought to be multifactorial, related to duration and type of opioid exposure, maternal and infant metabolism, and exposure to other substances, including benzodiazepines and nicotine. Each of these factors may be potential targets for treatment.

## Comparison of Treatment Options

As of 2022, the three FDA-approved medications for maintenance treatment of OUD in the general population are naltrexone (an opioid antagonist), methadone (a full μ opioid agonist), and buprenorphine (a partial μ opioid agonist, formulated with or without the opioid antagonist naloxone) (Table 12–3). This group of medications is collectively called medication treatment for opioid use disorder (MOUD). OAT is defined as MOUD with the opioid agonists buprenorphine and methadone; this term excludes the opioid antagonist naltrexone. In pregnant patients, OAT with methadone or buprenorphine has the best evidence of safety and efficacy. OAT is the standard of care per guidelines from the American College of Obstetricians and Gynecologists, the American Society of Addiction Medicine, and the Substance Abuse and Mental Health Services Administration (Committee on Obstetric Practice American Society of Addiction Medicine 2017; Crotty et al. 2020). In the following paragraphs we compare methadone and buprenorphine and discuss their superiority to naltrexone and medication-assisted withdrawal.

### Methadone Versus Buprenorphine

Historically, methadone was the gold standard treatment for OUD in pregnancy, even after buprenorphine entered the market in 2002. However, over the past two decades, a greater percentage of pregnant individuals have been treated with buprenorphine, in part because of the ease of prescribing it outside of an opioid treatment program (OTP). Several studies have compared outcomes of pregnant patients with OUD treated with buprenorphine versus those treated with methadone. The Maternal Opioid Treatment: Human Experimental Research (MOTHER) trial established that neonates of mothers treated with buprenorphine—compared with those of mothers treated with methadone—required less morphine for NOWS treatment, had shorter hospital stays, and had shorter durations of treatment (Jones et al. 2010). A meta-analysis affirmed these findings, also establishing that although methadone is associated with higher treatment retention for females with SUDs, buprenorphine prescriptions during pregnancy decreased NOWS incidence by 10% (Brogly et al. 2014). A systematic review of three randomized controlled trials (RCTs; $n=223$) and 15 observational cohort studies ($n=1,923$) identified no difference in spontaneous fetal death or congenital anomalies (evidence grade: low). Compared with methadone, buprenorphine had a decreased risk of preterm birth, higher birth weights, and a larger neonatal head circumferences (evidence grade: moderate) (Zedler et al. 2016). No differences in obstetric outcomes between buprenorphine/naloxone, buprenorphine, and methadone have been reported, including rates of cesarean sections, analgesia during delivery, medical complications at delivery, and length of maternal hospital stay (Lund et al. 2013). A Cochrane review of four RCTs ($n=271$)

**Table 12–3. Comparison of treatment options for OUD in pregnancy**

| | Methadone | Buprenorphine | Naltrexone |
|---|---|---|---|
| Efficacy | Lower dropout rates than buprenorphine; decreases opioid use, number of overdose deaths, and mortality risk | Decreases opioid use, number of overdose deaths, and mortality risk | Similar to methadone and buprenorphine, but more studies are needed; in nonpregnant populations, generally less effective |
| Safety profile for fetus | Greater risk of preterm birth and low birth weight than buprenorphine | Potentially fewer preterm births and higher birth weight than methadone | Similar to methadone and buprenorphine, but more studies needed |
| NOWS risk | Highest | Moderate | Lowest |
| Breastfeeding | Recommended; <1% crosses to breast milk | Recommended; <1% crosses to breast milk | Not contraindicated; <1% crosses to breast milk |
| Drawbacks | Distribution through an OTP Risk of QTc prolongation | May not be as effective in patients with more severe OUD (e.g., heroin users) | Requires full withdrawal management (usually 1 week) |
| | Greatest risk of overdose and diversion | Risk of precipitated withdrawal | May interfere with pain management after cesarean section |

*Note.* NOWS=neonatal opioid withdrawal syndrome; OTP=opioid treatment program; OUD=opioid use disorder.

stated buprenorphine versus methadone showed no difference in recurrence rates, birth weights, Apgar scores, rates of NOWS, or mothers with serious adverse events (Minozzi et al. 2020). However, the quality of evidence was deemed low to moderate given small sample sizes, high dropout rates (30%–40%), and inconsistencies in results. The authors concluded there was insufficient evidence to recommend one agonist treatment over the other. In summary, methadone and buprenorphine have similar efficacy and safety profiles when looking at maternal treatment and delivery outcomes, but the quality of evidence varies.

### Buprenorphine With Naloxone

The combined formulation of buprenorphine with naloxone has also been compared with buprenorphine monoproduct (brand name Subutex) in pregnancy. Previously, buprenorphine/naloxone was discouraged in pregnancy because of a lack of data on the safety of the naloxone component (Poon et al. 2014). However, the latest evidence suggests buprenorphine/naloxone is not harmful to fetal health (Substance Abuse and Mental Health Services Administration 2018b). A review by Lund et al. (2013) showed no differences in outcomes among the two treatments, including rates of cesarean section, medical complications, length of stay, rates of NOWS or duration of treatment required, preterm birth rates, and gestational age at delivery, with a few notable exceptions. Compared with buprenorphine monotherapy, the buprenorphine/naloxone group had shorter neonatal lengths and lower Apgar scores at 5 minutes; however, measurements were still within normal limits. Overall, it is no longer recommended that a pregnant patient already taking buprenorphine/naloxone transition to buprenorphine alone.

### Naltrexone

Naltrexone, a competitive antagonist at the μ opioid receptor, blocks the euphoric effects of other opiates. As previously discussed in the section "Alcohol Use Disorder," Towers et al. (2020) conducted a nonrandomized prospective cohort study of pregnant women treated with oral naltrexone ($n=121$) compared with OAT (buprenorphine or methadone, $n=109$). No differences were seen in obstetric outcomes, birth anomalies, or fetal heart tracings among the three groups. One advantage of treatment with naltrexone was much lower rates of NOWS in newborns (8.4% in the naltrexone group vs. 75.2% in the opioid agonist group). Patients who received naltrexone up until the day of delivery had no newborns with NOWS. Unfortunately, because naltrexone can cross the placenta, it requires full withdrawal management and abstinence from opiates for 7 days prior to induction to prevent fetal withdrawal in utero. This mandatory abstinence period can be challenging for patients and increases the likelihood of returning to using opiates (Tran et al. 2017). Furthermore, naltrexone's rapid clearance also increases the odds of returning to use if a patient suddenly stops taking it (Towers et al. 2020). An additional concern is the potential interference of an opioid antagonist with postoperative pain management in the event of a cesarean delivery. Given these challenges, naltrexone works best for the subset of patients who have successfully withdrawn from opiates or who were already taking naltrexone prior to their pregnancy.

## Opioid Withdrawal

Tapering pregnant patients off of opiates prior to delivery using medically assisted withdrawal (e.g., symptomatic management with clonidine, loperamide) should be avoided. Withdrawal increases the risk of returning to opiate use at an average rate of 48%. Data are inconsistent regarding whether withdrawal worsens or has no impact on fetal stress (Jones et al. 2017). Medically assisted withdrawal does not seem to reduce the risk of NOWS. Given these limitations, OAT is instead the preferred method of treatment for OUD in pregnancy.

## Prescribing Opioid Agonists in Clinical Practice

We recommend starting pregnant patients on opioid agonists in an inpatient setting, especially given the risk of precipitated withdrawal with buprenorphine. Obstetric monitoring of the fetal heart rate via a nonstress test is key for the safety of both the mother and fetus (Table 12–4).

### Buprenorphine

Buprenorphine is a $\mu$ opioid receptor partial agonist used to manage withdrawal symptoms in acute-phase opioid cravings in the maintenance phase. Because of its high binding affinity, buprenorphine outcompetes and displaces other opiates at the opioid receptor. Formulations include a sublingual film, sublingual tablet, subdermal implant, and extended-release monthly injection, although only the sublingual formulations have been studied in pregnancy (Indivior 2022).

To prevent precipitated withdrawal, buprenorphine should not be started until 6 hours after use of a short-acting opioid and 24–48 hours after use of a

**Table 12–4.**  Opioid use disorder treatment in pregnancy

| Medication | Dosing | Additional comments |
|---|---|---|
| Buprenorphine | 4–8 mg/day starting dosage | May need to increase dosage by 20% or split dosage to twice daily during the third trimester |
| Clonidine | 0.1 mg every 4–6 hours prn; can use 0.025–0.05 mg depending on blood pressure | Target blood pressure > 100/60 mm Hg |
| Acetaminophen | 650–1,000 mg every 4–6 hours prn analgesia | Limited use of nonsteroidal anti-inflammatory drugs, concern for closure of ductus arteriosus<br><br>Maximum 4,000 mg/day |
| Hydroxyzine | 25–50 mg every 4–6 hours prn anxiety and insomnia | |
| Diphenhydramine | 25–50 mg nightly prn insomnia, anxiety, and nausea | |
| Ondansetron | 4–8 mg every 12 hours prn nausea | Preferred to promethazine<br><br>Maximum 16 mg/day<br><br>Risk of QTc prolongation<br><br>Mixed outcomes on fetal risk; absolute risk low (Erick et al. 2018) |
| Trazodone | 50–100 mg nightly prn insomnia | |
| Loperamide | 4 mg followed by 2 mg after each loose stool | Maximum 16 mg/day |

long-acting opioid. Physicians should administer the initial dose of buprenorphine at 2–4 mg for moderate withdrawal symptoms. During initiation in the first and second trimesters of pregnancy, buprenorphine is dosed at a daily maximum of between 4 mg and 8 mg. During the third trimester, the dosage should be increased by 20% daily because of increased glomerular filtration rate and volume of distribution. The medication can be titrated up or down according to the patient response, balancing control of withdrawal symptoms as scored by the Clinical Opiate Withdrawal Scale (COWS) with the risk of overmedication. Generally, patients who use opiates intravenously may require higher doses of opioid replacement.

### Methadone

A long-acting μ opioid full receptor agonist, methadone is intended to mitigate withdrawal and to reduce opioid cravings through opioid replacement. Given the risk of overdose with a full agonist, methadone is prescribed only on an outpatient basis through an OTP, which initially requires daily administration of the medication from the clinic. Methadone can also be initiated within a hospital setting with the assurance that the patient is able to participate in a long-term methadone OTP.

Upon initiation, methadone should be started at a dose of 30 mg, with an additional 5–10 mg if withdrawal symptoms continue after 1 hour (Levounis et al. 2016). The first dose should not exceed 30 mg, and the total dosage the first day should not exceed 40 mg. Methadone generally takes 5 days to achieve steady state and is prone to more clinically significant drug-drug interactions than buprenorphine because of its metabolism through the liver's cytochrome P450 (CYP) 3A4 enzyme (Substance Abuse and Mental Health Services Administration 2018a). Clinicians should also be mindful of polysubstance use in patients, given that methadone taken with alcohol, benzodiazepines, or other CNS depressants can result in respiratory depression.

During pregnancy, methadone is metabolized more quickly, with one model estimating a reduction in half-life from 22–24 hours to 8.1 hours (Swift et al. 1989). As a result, clinicians may consider splitting the methadone dosing (i.e., prescribing half the dose in the morning and half in the evening), although this can pose logistical challenges when considering administration via an OTP. Increased total body fluid and blood volume throughout pregnancy create a dilutional effect; therefore, pregnant patients often require increased doses of methadone in the third trimester (Shiu and Ensom 2012).

*Adjunct Medications for Managing Withdrawal*

Clonidine, an $\alpha_2$ adrenergic agonist, reduces autonomic symptoms of opioid withdrawal. Dosing should begin with 0.1 mg every 4–6 hours and can be increased by 0.1–0.2 mg/day to a maximum of 1.2 mg/day. Clonidine dosing may be titrated lower to 0.05 mg/day or 0.025 mg/day if appropriate, particularly during the second trimester when blood pressures rates are lower. Blood pressure monitoring is recommended because of the risks posed by hypotension; blood pressure should be kept above 100 mm Hg systolic and 60 mm Hg diastolic to prevent hypoperfusion (Kleber 2007). Clonidine may be tapered toward the end of treatment to prevent rebound hypertension.

For pain management, acetaminophen should be used instead of nonsteroidal anti-inflammatory drugs, which are discouraged in the third trimester because of the risk of premature closure of the ductus arteriosus (Aker et al. 2015). This risk increases after 28 weeks of gestation and with increasing maternal age. Other medications that could be helpful to manage withdrawal symptoms are loperamide for gastrointestinal motility, ondansetron for nausea, trazodone for insomnia, hydroxyzine for anxiety, and diphenhydramine for anxiety or insomnia.

## Barriers to Treatment

Despite the positive impact of pharmacotherapy for maintenance treatment of OUD in pregnancy, pregnant individuals still struggle to obtain treatment. A cross-sectional study using the national census data system Treatment Episode Data Set: Admissions (1996–2014) found that nearly half of pregnant individuals with OUD treated at publicly funded centers were not receiving MOUD (Short et al. 2018). One reason for this may be the medical complexity of OUD treatment in pregnant individuals, including an increased risk of obstetric complications. During the induction phase of OAT, close monitoring in an inpatient setting is preferred, especially given the risk of precipitated withdrawal. Other medications prescribed for withdrawal management may also require greater patient observation. Moreover, adult females have a different opioid binding capacity than adult males, such that dose changes such as elevation and splitting must be made to account for hormonal enzyme induction (Unger et al. 2010). Additionally, co-occurring psychiatric conditions such as mood disorders may make treatment planning more challenging for a nonpsychiatric SUD treatment provider. Stigma surrounding treatment can limit both the number of available treatment programs and the number of individuals willing to engage in treatment. A published study of pregnant females with OUDs showed that this population already feels internal stigma related to self-perceptions of being a substance user. They also encounter external stigma from others, such as medical care staff (Howard 2015). With hormonal changes in pregnancy, the greater chance of mood instability, and increased stigma, it may be more challenging to retain pregnant individuals in treatment for OUD than the general population.

## Summary

- OAT with methadone, buprenorphine monoproduct, or buprenorphine/ naloxone is the standard of care for treating OUD in pregnancy.
- Opioid agonists have similar safety profiles. The choice of medication should be determined in a collaborative manner that accounts for the patient's individual needs.
- Medication-assisted opioid withdrawal should be avoided because of poor fetal and maternal outcomes.
- We recommend starting an opioid agonist in an inpatient setting to provide close fetal monitoring.
- Starting doses of buprenorphine tend to be lower in pregnancy.
- In the third trimester, patients may require dose increases or split dosing to account for increased fluid volume and rapid metabolism in pregnancy.

# Tobacco or Nicotine Use Disorder

## Epidemiology

Use of tobacco products, including cigarette smoking, smokeless tobacco, and electronic (e-)cigarettes, during pregnancy is associated with several adverse maternal and fetal outcomes. The global prevalence of smoking during pregnancy is estimated to be 1.7%. This prevalence varies between countries; in the United States in 2016, the estimated prevalence of peripartum smoking was 7.2%, being highest for females between the ages of 20 and 24 (10.7%) and declining with age. Among females who smoke daily, an average of 52.9% continue smoking during pregnancy (Lange et al. 2018a).

## Risks of Not Treating

Smoking during pregnancy is associated with complications such as ectopic pregnancy, placental abruption, placenta previa, preeclampsia, and higher medical expenditure. Numerous adverse health outcomes to the fetus include low birth weight, increased fetal mortality, stillbirth, and major birth malformations such as craniosynostosis, gastroschisis, and oral clefts. Evidence suggests that the impact extends to later in life, with behavioral and intellectual functioning impairments (U.S. Department of Health and Human Services 2014). Noncombustible tobacco products (smokeless tobacco) demonstrate similar adverse maternal and fetal health effects. Smokeless tobacco exposure during pregnancy increases risks of abnormal fetal autonomic cardiac regulation and nicotine withdrawal in neonates, which are similar to those in females who smoke tobacco. Vape products are often seen as being safer than cigarettes, but combustion of the vape liquid produces harmful chemicals such as formaldehyde, benzene, and toluene. In animal studies, e-cigarettes appear to have similar consequences on lung development and health compared with cigarette smoking (American College of Obstetricians and Gynecologists 2020).

## Treatment Options

### Screening, Brief Intervention, and Referral to Treatment

Screening, Brief Intervention, and Referral to Treatment (SBIRT) is an approach that applies to alcohol and tobacco use. The brief interventions are counseling sessions during routine clinical care that last less than 20 minutes. Repeated sessions with a trusted provider are more effective than single sessions with an unfamiliar provider. Referral to treatment may involve quitlines and additional psychiatric and/or SUD treatment. Cochrane reviews on brief interventions for alcohol use and cigarette smoking during pregnancy support the effectiveness of brief interventions for increasing abstinence, reducing peripartum alcohol use and cigarette smoking, and improving obstetric outcomes (Chamberlain et al. 2017). The World Health Organization recommends the 5A's approach, which parallels the counseling and intervention aspects of the SBIRT model:

1. *Ask* about all types of tobacco and nicotine use.
2. *Advise* to quit through clear messages about risks of continued use.
3. *Assess* willingness to quit. Use motivational interviewing to strengthen intrinsic desire for change.
4. *Assist* quit attempt by providing pregnancy-specific resources.
5. *Arrange* follow-up visits to continue providing support and track patient progress.

## Pharmacological Treatment

*Nicotine replacement therapy.*    The FDA-approved medications for smoking cessation include nicotine replacement therapy (NRT), bupropion, and varenicline, all of which have limited data regarding their effects in pregnancy. Thus, any pharmacotherapy intervention must be viewed on a risk-benefit continuum, with tobacco exposure having more probable harm. NRT is the medication option used most often, but it has not demonstrated strong efficacy for smoking cessation. Exposure to NRT is not known to cause congenital anomalies. However, it may increase the risk of later-life adverse events, such as infantile colic at 6 months and ADHD. More data are needed to determine whether these associations are from direct NRT exposure or other factors, such as genetic vulnerability (Blanc et al. 2021).

*Varenicline and bupropion.*    Studies suggest that, compared with NRT, varenicline and bupropion may be more effective at helping pregnant women stop smoking. Bupropion doubles the rate of smoking abstinence in nonpregnant smokers. However, a small RCT showed bupropion reduced use, nicotine cravings, and withdrawal but did not increase abstinence rates relative to placebo (Nanovskaya et al. 2017). These results contradict an earlier observational study showing that bupropion increased abstinence, but that study included only 22 participants in each arm (Chan et al. 2005). Data on varenicline effectiveness in pregnancy are limited, but a population-based cohort study in Australia suggested that it may be more effective than NRT. The authors found that pregnant patients receiving varenicline were 3 times more likely to quit smoking than those receiving NRT (Choi et al. 2021).

Bupropion and varenicline both appear to be safer than ongoing tobacco use. A 2019 systematic review and meta-analysis of 18 low-quality studies on bupropion and varenicline did not indicate negative or positive effects on fetal outcomes, including congenital anomalies, birth weights, and premature birth (Turner et al. 2019). Bupropion used as an antidepressant causes no known congenital anomalies and has inconsistent data regarding cardiovascular malformations. Fewer data on varenicline are available, but it did not show teratogenicity in animal studies. Two extensive population-based cohort studies from Australia, Denmark, and Sweden did not find an increased risk of congenital abnormalities or other adverse birth outcomes with bupropion ($n=330$) and varenicline ($n=1,057$ in one study and 335 in the other). Varenicline-exposed participants were *less likely* than NRT-exposed participants to have an adverse perinatal event. Varenicline-exposed infants were *less likely* to be premature, to be small for gestational age, and to have severe neo-natal complications. Given the known risks of ongoing tobacco use exposure, these data question the preference for using NRT and bupropion over vareni-cline (Pedersen et al. 2020; Tran et al. 2020).

## Clinical Practice

Based on the available data on risks of treating versus not treating tobacco use disorder (TUD), we recommend using all available options to aid in reduc-tion or cessation. Pregnant females with a mild TUD may respond to SBIRT alone, whereas those with ongoing daily smoking are likely to need pharma-cotherapy. Recent data suggest varenicline outperforms bupropion and NRT for efficacy, but safety data remain the most robust for NRT. We recommend starting with NRT, then switching to varenicline within a few weeks of treat-ment if NRT is insufficient, especially if the patient smokes heavily (i.e., more than 20 cigarettes per day). Consider bupropion in females with comorbid depression. Pregnant patients prescribed these medications should be coun-seled on the risks, benefits, and potential adverse outcomes for them and their infants.

## Summary

- Benefits of treatment for TUD outweigh the risks of not treating.
- SBIRT should be used routinely for every pregnant patient.
- NRT, bupropion, and varenicline are effective interventions that have no known significant harm to the mother or the fetus.
- Bupropion and varenicline may be more effective than NRT for smoking cessation.

# Stimulant Use Disorder

## Epidemiology

Stimulants such as cocaine, methamphetamine, and (misuse of) prescription stimulants are the second most used substance in pregnancy. Methamphet-amine use has been increasing in the past few decades, with prevalence rang-ing from 0.7% to 4.8% in highly endemic areas. On the other hand, cocaine use has decreased in the same period. From 1988 to 2004, nearly a quarter-million pregnant females received methamphetamine treatment at federally funded treatment centers in the United States. Notably, females seem to experience a telescoping phenomenon in which the progression from first exposure to addiction is much faster than it is in males (Smid et al. 2019).

## Risks of Not Treating

Pregnant females are at higher risk of cocaine-induced cardiovascular toxicity, even at low doses. This observation may be due to increased progesterone concentrations sensitizing cardiac muscle to cocaine. Both cocaine and methamphetamine can lead to hypertension, myocardial infarction and ischemia, hyperthermia, seizures, preeclampsia, placental abruption, and maternal death. Risks to the fetus include preterm delivery, growth restriction, and fetal hypoxia from vasoconstriction. Illicit stimulant use is also associated with risky behavior that increases the likelihood of acquiring blood-borne illnesses such as HIV and hepatitis B and C. Cognitive impairment and psychiatric symptoms such as insomnia, depression, and psychosis lead to poor follow-up and unhealthy lifestyle choices that exacerbate adverse outcomes. Available data on prescription stimulants in pregnancy were acquired from studying females with ADHD, and misuse was not assessed. The safety data of prescription stimulants are mixed, with some studies showing a small increased risk of preeclampsia and preterm birth. In contrast, others found that females with ADHD with or without prescription stimulant use had similar rates of adverse outcomes (Smid et al. 2019; Wright et al. 2015). These findings are interpreted cautiously because the studies did not differentiate between amphetamines and methylphenidate. A separate review and meta-analysis of methylphenidate exposure in early pregnancy revealed a small, but significantly increased, risk of cardiac malformations (Koren et al. 2020).

## Treatment

### *Nonpharmacological Interventions*

Nonpharmacological interventions are first-line treatment. Pregnant women who cannot abstain from stimulant use should be referred to a higher level of care, such as a residential treatment program. If this is not feasible, clinicians should consider referral to an intensive outpatient program that follows the Matrix Model for stimulant use disorders. The Matrix Model combines a variety of therapeutic interventions, including family education, 12-step support, cognitive-behavioral therapy, and motivational enhancement therapy, to increase rates of abstinence. Contingency management for stimulant use disorder has also been shown to be effective in nonpregnant populations. Extrapolating from data on TUD, contingency management is also effective in pregnant females.

### Pharmacotherapy

As detailed in Chapter 6, "Stimulants and Co-occurring Substance Use," no medications have shown consistent efficacy for stimulant use disorder. Data are even sparser on efficacy in pregnancy. A case report was published suggesting potential benefit of contingency management combined with lisdexamfetamine in a patient with HIV and methamphetamine use. This patient was able to stop methamphetamine use and adhere to antiretroviral therapy (Turner et al. 2022).

## Clinical Practice

The benefits may outweigh the risks of trialing certain medications in pregnant patients if behavioral interventions are insufficient, especially for individuals with a severe stimulant use disorder. Medications may also increase retention in treatment and alleviate symptoms such as ADHD, depression, and cognitive impairment. Note that pharmacotherapy should be combined with nonpharmacological interventions. On the basis of the available data, bupropion and naltrexone have not been known to cause significant adverse fetal or maternal outcomes. However, it is unclear whether this combination would lead to different outcomes in pregnant individuals. If medications are prescribed, we recommend starting with bupropion and then adding naltrexone if stimulant use continues. Bupropion may also decrease tobacco use, which is frequently comorbid in patients with stimulant use disorder. Atomoxetine may be the next safest option because it has not been demonstrated to increase maternal or fetal complications in animal studies or in two small human studies (Organization of Teratology Information Specialists 1994). For patients who have significantly impairing ADHD symptoms, it would be reasonable to consider prescribing atomoxetine first. Although prescription stimulants are not without risk, they may be safer than illicit stimulants. If the previous interventions are ineffective, clinicians should consider switching the patient to a long-acting prescription stimulant, such as lisdexamfetamine, using the lowest effective dosage. Informed consent with counseling about the risks, benefits, and potential side effects must be obtained from the patient for each medication.

## Summary

- Illicit stimulant use is rising in prevalence among pregnant females.
- Nonpharmacological interventions are first-line treatment, including referral to a residential treatment program if the patient is unable to stop use.
- No pharmacological interventions have been proven to be consistently effective for stimulant use disorder in nonpregnant populations, and data on efficacy in pregnant females is scarce. However, the benefits of some medications may outweigh the risks.

# Conclusion

Pregnant females with SUD experience significant barriers to care, including stigma within and outside the medical community. Although we continue to acquire data about the safety and efficacy of medications for various SUDs in pregnancy, the literature remains minimal. Nevertheless, for some recommended medications, we extrapolated efficacy data from the general population and safety data from other analyses in pregnant patients. Although not ideal, this approach must be balanced with the risks of not treating. The high rate of substance use in pregnancy indicates an urgent need for more studies to inform treatment further.

# References

Aker K, Brantberg A, Nyrnes SA: Prenatal constriction of the ductus arteriosus following maternal diclofenac medication in the third trimester. BMJ Case Rep 2015(Oct):bcr2015210473, 2015 26427495

American College of Obstetricians and Gynecologists: Tobacco and nicotine cessation during pregnancy. Obstet Gynecol 135(5):e221–e229, 2020 32332417

Bibbins-Domingo K, Grossman DC, Curry SJ, et al: Folic acid supplementation for the prevention of neural tube defects: US Preventive Services Task Force recommendation statement. JAMA 317(2):183–189, 2017 28097362

Bishop D, Borkowski L, Couillard M, et al: Pregnant Women and Substance Use: Overview of Research and Policy in the United States. Washington, DC, Jacobs Institute of Women's Health at George Washington University, 2017. Available at: https://publichealth.gwu.edu/sites/default/files/downloads/JIWH/Pregnant_Women_and_Substance_Use_updated.pdf. Accessed February 13, 2022.

Blanc J, Tosello B, Ekblad MO, et al: Nicotine replacement therapy during pregnancy and child health outcomes: a systematic review. Int J Environ Res Public Health 18(8):4004, 2021 33920348

Briggs GG, Freeman RK: Carbamazepine, in Drugs in Pregnancy and Lactation: A Reference Guide to Fetal and Neonatal Risk, 10th Edition. Philadelphia, PA, Lippincott Williams & Wilkins, 2015a, pp 197–202

Briggs GG, Freeman RK: Disulfiram, in Drugs in Pregnancy and Lactation: A Reference Guide to Fetal and Neonatal Risk, 10th Edition. Philadelphia, PA, Lippincott Williams & Wilkins, 2015b, pp 420–421

Briggs GG, Freeman RK: Gabapentin, in Drugs in Pregnancy and Lactation: A Reference Guide to Fetal and Neonatal Risk, 10th Edition. Philadelphia, PA, Lippincott Williams & Wilkins, 2015c, pp 602–604

Brogly SB, Saia KA, Walley AY, et al: Prenatal buprenorphine versus methadone exposure and neonatal outcomes: systematic review and meta-analysis. Am J Epidemiol 180(7):673–686, 2014 25150272

Center for Behavioral Health Statistics and Quality: 2019 National Survey on Drug Use and Health. Rockville, MD, Substance Abuse and Mental Health Services Administration, 2020. Available at: https://www.samhsa.gov/data/report/2019-nsduh-women. Accessed January 8, 2022.

Centers for Disease Control and Prevention: Opioid Overdose: Understanding the Epidemic. Atlanta, GA, Centers for Disease Control and Prevention, 2021. Available at: https://www.cdc.gov/drugoverdose/epidemic/index.html. Accessed January 12, 2023.

Chamberlain C, O'Mara-Eves A, Porter J, et al: Psychosocial interventions for supporting women to stop smoking in pregnancy. Cochrane Database Syst Rev 2(2):CD001055, 2017 28196405

Chan B, Einarson A, Koren G: Effectiveness of bupropion for smoking cessation during pregnancy. J Addict Dis 24(2):19–23, 2005 15784520

Choi SKY, Tran DT, Kemp-Casey A, et al: The comparative effectiveness of varenicline and nicotine patches for smoking abstinence during pregnancy: evidence from a population-based cohort study. Nicotine Tob Res 23(10):1664–1672, 2021 34398235

Committee on Obstetric Practice American Society of Addiction Medicine: Committee Opinion No. 711: opioid use and opioid use disorder in pregnancy. Obstet Gynecol 130(2):e81–e94, 2017 28742676

Crotty K, Freedman KI, Kampman KM: Executive summary of the focused update of the ASAM National Practice Guideline for the Treatment of Opioid Use Disorder. J Addict Med 14(2):99–112, 2020 32209915

de Wit M, Goldberg A, Chelmow D: Alcohol use disorders and hospital-acquired infections in women undergoing cesarean delivery. Obstet Gynecol 122(1):72–78, 2013 23743466

Dolovich LR, Addis A, Vaillancourt JMR, et al: Benzodiazepine use in pregnancy and major malformations or oral cleft: meta-analysis of cohort and case-control studies. BMJ 317(7162):839–843, 1998 9748174

Enato E, Moretti M, Koren G: The fetal safety of benzodiazepines: an updated meta-analysis. J Obstet Gynaecol Can 33(1):46–48, 2011 21272436

Erick M, Cox JT, Mogensen KM: ACOG Practice Bulletin No. 189: nausea and vomiting of pregnancy. Obstet Gynecol 131(5):935, 2018 29683896

Farheen SA, Chhatlan A, Tampi RR: Anticonvulsants for alcohol withdrawal: a review of the evidence. Curr Psychiatr 20(2): 2021

Forray A, Yonkers KA: The collision of mental health, substance use disorder, and suicide. Obstet Gynecol 137(6):1083–1090, 2021 33957654

Frazer Z, McConnell K, Jansson LM: Treatment for substance use disorders in pregnant women: motivators and barriers. Drug Alcohol Depend 205(Dec):107652, 2019 31704383

Fujii H, Goel A, Bernard N, et al: Pregnancy outcomes following gabapentin use: results of a prospective comparative cohort study. Neurology 80(17):1565–1570, 2013 23553472

Gauthier TW: Prenatal alcohol exposure and the developing immune system. Alcohol Res 37(2):279–285, 2015 26695750

Greenberg JA, Bell SJ, Guan Y, Yu Y-H: Folic acid supplementation and pregnancy: more than just neural tube defect prevention. Rev Obstet Gynecol 4(2):52–59, 2011 22102928

Grigoriadis S, Graves L, Peer M, et al: Benzodiazepine use during pregnancy alone or in combination with an antidepressant and congenital malformations: systematic review and meta-analysis. J Clin Psychiatry 80(4):1845, 2019 31294935

Grigoriadis S, Graves L, Peer M, et al: Pregnancy and delivery outcomes following benzodiazepine exposure: a systematic review and meta-analysis. Can J Psychiatry 65(12):821–834, 2020 32148076

Guglielmo R, Martinotti G, Quatrale M, et al: Topiramate in alcohol use disorders: review and update. CNS Drugs 29(5):383–395, 2015 25899459

Haight SC, Ko JY, Tong VT, et al: Opioid use disorder documented at delivery hospitalization—United States, 1999–2014. MMWR Morb Mortal Wkly Rep 67(31):845–849, 2018 30091969

Hernández-Díaz S, Smith CR, Shen A, et al: Comparative safety of antiepileptic drugs during pregnancy. Neurology 78(21):1692–1699, 2012 22551726

Hernández-Díaz S, Mittendorf R, Smith CR, et al: Association between topiramate and zonisamide use during pregnancy and low birth weight. Obstet Gynecol 123(1):21–28, 2014 24463659

Hernández-Díaz S, Huybrechts KF, Desai RJ, et al: Topiramate use early in pregnancy and the risk of oral clefts: a pregnancy cohort study. Neurology 90(4):e342–e351, 2018 29282333

Howard H: Reducing stigma: lessons from opioid-dependent women. J Soc Work Pract Addict 15(4):418–438, 2015

Hutson JR, Stade B, Lehotay DC, et al: Folic acid transport to the human fetus is decreased in pregnancies with chronic alcohol exposure. PLoS ONE 7(5):e38057, 2012 22666445

Indivior: Suboxone [package insert]. Chesterfield, VA, Indivior PLC, June 2022. Available at: https://www.suboxone.com/pdfs/prescribing-information.pdf. Accessed February 12, 2022.

Institute of Medicine Food and Nutrition Board: Dietary Reference Intakes: A Risk Assessment Model for Establishing Upper Intake Levels for Nutrients. Washington, DC, National Academies Press, 1998

Janssen Pharmaceuticals: Topamax [package insert]. Beerse, Belgium, Janssen Pharmaceuticals, October 2022. Available at: https://www.janssenlabels.com/package-insert/product-monograph/prescribing-information/TOPAMAX-pi.pdf. Accessed February 6, 2022.

Jentink J, Dolk H, Loane MA, et al: Intrauterine exposure to carbamazepine and specific congenital malformations: systematic review and case-control study. BMJ 341:c6581, 2010 21127116

Johnson LE: Thiamin deficiency: nutritional disorders, in Merck Manuals, Professional Edition. Rahway, NJ, Merck & Co, 2020. Available at: https://www.merckmanuals.com/professional/nutritional-disorders/vitamin-deficiency,-dependency,-and-toxicity/thiamin-deficiency. Accessed February 13, 2022.

Jones HE, Kaltenbach K, Heil SH, et al: Neonatal abstinence syndrome after methadone or buprenorphine exposure. N Engl J Med 363(24):2320–2331, 2010 21142534

Jones HE, Heil SH, Baewert A, et al: Buprenorphine treatment of opioid-dependent pregnant women: a comprehensive review. Addiction 107(Suppl 1):5–27, 2012 23106923

Jones HE, Terplan M, Meyer M: Medically assisted withdrawal (detoxification): considering the mother-infant dyad. J Addict Med 11(2):90–92, 2017 28079573

Kalk NJ, Lingford-Hughes AR: The clinical pharmacology of acamprosate. Br J Clin Pharmacol 77(2):315–323, 2014 23278595

Kaltenbach K, Berghella V, Finnegan L: Opioid dependence during pregnancy: effects and management. Obstet Gynecol Clin North Am 25(1):139–151, 1998 9547764

Kelty E, Hulse G: A retrospective cohort study of obstetric outcomes in opioid-dependent women treated with implant naltrexone, oral methadone or sublingual buprenorphine, and non-dependent controls. Drugs 77(11):1199–1210, 2017 28536980

Kelty E, Tran D, Lavin T, et al: Prevalence and safety of acamprosate use in pregnant alcohol-dependent women in New South Wales, Australia. Addiction 114(2):206–215, 2019 30152012

Kelty E, Terplan M, Greenland M, et al: Pharmacotherapies for the treatment of alcohol use disorders during pregnancy: time to reconsider? Drugs 81(7):739–748, 2021 33830479

Kingdon D, Cardoso C, McGrath JJ: Research review: executive function deficits in fetal alcohol spectrum disorders and attention-deficit/hyperactivity disorder: a meta-analysis. J Child Psychol Psychiatry 57(2):116–131, 2016 26251262

Kleber HD: Pharmacologic treatments for opioid dependence: detoxification and maintenance options. Dialogues Clin Neurosci 9(4):455–470, 2007 18286804

Kloss O, Eskin NAM, Suh M: Thiamin deficiency on fetal brain development with and without prenatal alcohol exposure. Biochem Cell Biol 96(2):169–177, 2018 28915355

Koren G, Barer Y, Ornoy A: Fetal safety of methylphenidate: a scoping review and meta analysis. Reprod Toxicol 93(Apr):230–234, 2020 32169555

Kranzler HR, Feinn R, Morris P, et al: A meta-analysis of the efficacy of gabapentin for treating alcohol use disorder. Addiction 114(9):1547–1555, 2019 31077485

Lange S, Probst C, Rehm J, et al: National, regional, and global prevalence of smoking during pregnancy in the general population: a systematic review and meta-analysis. Lancet Glob Health 6(7):e769–e776, 2018a 29859815

Lange S, Rehm J, Anagnostou E, et al: Prevalence of externalizing disorders and autism spectrum disorders among children with fetal alcohol spectrum disorder: systematic review and meta-analysis. Biochem Cell Biol 96(2):241–251, 2018b 28521112

Lee K, Cascella M, Marwaha R: Intellectual disability, in StatPearls. Treasure Island, FL, StatPearls Publishing, 2021. Available at: https://www.ncbi.nlm.nih.gov/books/NBK547654. Accessed February 24, 2023.

Levounis P, Zerbo E, Aggarwal R, et al (eds): Pocket Guide to Addiction Assessment and Treatment. Washington, DC, American Psychiatric Association Publishing, 2016

Lui S, Jones RL, Robinson NJ, et al: Detrimental effects of ethanol and its metabolite acetaldehyde, on first trimester human placental cell turnover and function. PLoS One 9(2):e87328, 2014 24503565

Lum E, Gorman SK, Slavik RS: Valproic acid management of acute alcohol withdrawal. Ann Pharmacother 40(3):441–448, 2006 16507623

Lund IO, Fischer G, Welle-Strand GK, et al: A comparison of buprenorphine + naloxone to buprenorphine and methadone in the treatment of opioid dependence during pregnancy: maternal and neonatal outcomes. Subst Abuse 7:61–74, 2013 23531704

Maeda A, Bateman BT, Clancy CR, et al: Opioid abuse and dependence during pregnancy: temporal trends and obstetrical outcomes. Anesthesiology 121(6):1158–1165, 2014 25405293

Malcolm R, Myrick H, Roberts J, et al: The differential effects of medication on mood, sleep disturbance, and work ability in outpatient alcohol detoxification. Am J Addict 11(2):141–150, 2002 12028744

Martin JA, Hamilton BE, Osterman MJK, et al: Births: final data for 2019. Natl Vital Stat Rep 70(2):1–51, 2021 33814033

McDonald PLL, Jia L, Vipler S: Alcohol withdrawal management and relapse prevention in pregnancy. Can J Addict 9(4):32–41, 2018

Minozzi S, Amato L, Vecchi S, et al: Anticonvulsants for alcohol withdrawal. Cochrane Database Syst Rev (3):CD005064, 2010 20238337

Minozzi S, Amato L, Jahanfar S, et al: Maintenance agonist treatments for opiate-dependent pregnant women. Cochrane Database Syst Rev 11(11):CD006318, 2020 33165953

Modesto-Lowe V, Barron GC, Aronow B, et al: Gabapentin for alcohol use disorder: a good option, or cause for concern? Cleve Clin J Med 86(12):815–823, 2019 31821139

Mozurkewich EL, Rayburn WF: Buprenorphine and methadone for opioid addiction during pregnancy. Obstet Gynecol Clin North Am 41(2):241–253, 2014 24845488

Nanovskaya TN, Oncken C, Fokina VM, et al: Bupropion sustained release for pregnant smokers: a randomized, placebo-controlled trial. Am J Obstet Gynecol 216(4):420.e1–420.e9, 2017 27890648

National Collaborating Centre for Mental Health: Antenatal and Postnatal Mental Health: Clinical Management and Service Guidance, Updated Edition. London, British Psychological Society, 2014

Oei JL: Alcohol use in pregnancy and its impact on the mother and child. Addiction 115(11):2148–2163, 2020 32149441

Ondersma SJ, Chang G, Blake-Lamb T, et al: Accuracy of five self-report screening instruments for substance use in pregnancy. Addiction 114(9):1683–1693, 2019 31216102

Organization of Teratology Information Specialists: Atomoxetine (Strattera®). MotherToBaby Fact Sheet. Brentwood, TN, Organization of Teratology Information Specialists, 1994. Available at: https://www.ncbi.nlm.nih.gov/books/NBK582587. Accessed January 13, 2023.

Ornoy A, Koren G, Yanai J: Is post exposure prevention of teratogenic damage possible: studies on diabetes, valproic acid, alcohol and anti folates in pregnancy: animal studies with reflection to human. Reprod Toxicol 80(Sept):92–104, 2018 29859881

Osterman MJK, Martin JA: Timing and adequacy of prenatal care in the United States, 2016. Natl Vital Stat Rep 67(3):1–14, 2018 29874159

Patorno E, Hernandez-Diaz S, Huybrechts KF, et al: Gabapentin in pregnancy and the risk of adverse neonatal and maternal outcomes: a population-based cohort study nested in the US Medicaid Analytic eXtract dataset. PLOS Med 17(9):e1003322, 2020 32870921

Patrick SW, Barfield WD, Poindexter BB, et al: Neonatal opioid withdrawal syndrome. Pediatrics 146(5):e2020029074, 2020 33106341

Pedersen L, Petronis KR, Nørgaard M, et al: Risk of adverse birth outcomes after maternal varenicline use: a population-based observational study in Denmark and Sweden. Pharmacoepidemiol Drug Saf 29(1):94–102, 2020 31713302

Poon S, Pupco A, Koren G, et al: Safety of the newer class of opioid antagonists in pregnancy. Can Fam Physician 60(7):631–632, e348–e349, 2014 25022635

Popova S, Lange S, Probst C, et al: Estimation of national, regional, and global prevalence of alcohol use during pregnancy and fetal alcohol syndrome: a systematic review and meta-analysis. Lancet Glob Health 5(3):e290–e299, 2017 28089487

Shiu JR, Ensom MH: Dosing and monitoring of methadone in pregnancy: literature review. Can J Hosp Pharm 65(5):380–386, 2012 23129867

Short VL, Hand DJ, MacAfee L, et al: Trends and disparities in receipt of pharmacotherapy among pregnant women in publically funded treatment programs for opioid use disorder in the United States. J Subst Abuse Treat 89(June):67–74, 2018 29706175

Shrestha U, Singh M: Effect of folic acid in prenatal alcohol induced behavioral impairment in Swiss albino mice. Ann Neurosci 20(4):134–138, 2013 25206036

Smid MC, Metz TD, Gordon AJ: Stimulant use in pregnancy: an under-recognized epidemic among pregnant women. Clin Obstet Gynecol 62(1):168–184, 2019 30601144

Substance Abuse and Mental Health Services Administration: Chapter 3B: methadone, in Medications for Opioid Use Disorder: For Healthcare and Addiction Professionals, Policymakers, Patients, and Families (Treatment Improvement Protocol [TIP] Series 63). Rockville, MD, Substance Abuse and Mental Health Services Administration, 2018a.

Substance Abuse and Mental Health Services Administration: Clinical Guidance for Treating Pregnant and Parenting Women With Opioid Use Disorder and Their Infants (HHS Publ No SMA-18-5054). Rockville, MD, Substance Abuse and Mental Health Services Administration, 2018b

Substance Abuse and Mental Health Services Administration: 2019 National Survey on Drug Use and Health. Rockville, MD, Substance Abuse and Mental Health Services Administration, 2020. Available at: https://www.samhsa.gov/data/report/2019-nsduh-women. Accessed February 11, 2022.

Suh JJ, Pettinati HM, Kampman KM, et al: The status of disulfiram: a half of a century later. J Clin Psychopharmacol 26(3):290–302, 2006 16702894

Swift RM, Dudley M, DePetrillo P, et al: Altered methadone pharmacokinetics in pregnancy: implications for dosing. J Subst Abuse 1(4):453–460, 1989 2485290

Thibaut F, Chagraoui A, Buckley L, et al: WFSBP and IAWMH guidelines for the treatment of alcohol use disorders in pregnant women. World J Biol Psychiatry 20(1):17–50, 2019 30632868

Towers CV, Katz E, Weitz B, et al: Use of naltrexone in treating opioid use disorder in pregnancy. Am J Obstet Gynecol 222(1):83.e1–83.e8, 2020 31376396

Tran DT, Preen DB, Einarsdottir K, et al: Use of smoking cessation pharmacotherapies during pregnancy is not associated with increased risk of adverse pregnancy outcomes: a population-based cohort study. BMC Med 18(1):15, 2020 32019533

Tran TH, Griffin BL, Stone RH, et al: Methadone, buprenorphine, and naltrexone for the treatment of opioid use disorder in pregnant women. Pharmacotherapy 37(7):824–839, 2017 28543191

Turner E, Jones M, Vaz LR, et al: Systematic review and meta-analysis to assess the safety of bupropion and varenicline in pregnancy. Nicotine Tob Res 21(8):1001–1010, 2019 29579233

Turner S, Nader M, Lurie E: A contingency management approach for treatment of methamphetamine use disorder and human immunodeficiency virus antiretroviral treatment adherence in pregnancy to prevent mother-to-child transmission: a case report. J Med Case Rep 16(1):165, 2022 35473945

Unger A, Jung E, Winklbaur B, et al: Gender issues in the pharmacotherapy of opioid-addicted women: buprenorphine. J Addict Dis 29(2):217–230, 2010 20407978

U.S. Department of Health and Human Services: The Health Consequences of Smoking—50 Years of Progress: A Report of the Surgeon General. Washington, DC, U.S. Department of Health and Human Services, 2014. Available at: https://www.hhs.gov/sites/default/files/consequences-smoking-exec-summary.pdf. Accessed February 24, 2023.

World Health Organization: Guidelines for the Identification and Management of Substance Use and Substance Use Disorders in Pregnancy. Geneva, World Health Organization, 2014

Wright TE, Schuetter R, Tellei J, et al: Methamphetamines and pregnancy outcomes. J Addict Med 9(2):111–117, 2015 25599434

Zedler BK, Mann AL, Kim MM, et al: Buprenorphine compared with methadone to treat pregnant women with opioid use disorder: a systematic review and meta-analysis of safety in the mother, fetus and child. Addiction 111(12):2115–2128, 2016 27223595

# 13

# Addictive Disorders in Adolescents

Crystal Obiozor, M.D.
Edore Onigu-Otite, M.D.

*Addictive* disorders are an ongoing public health concern, and substance use among adolescents is a significant cause of mortality and morbidity. By the time adolescents become adults in the United States, almost half of them will have tried an illicit drug, and more than 80% will have used alcohol (Blanco et al. 2018). Most use by adolescents will attenuate over time, but many individuals experience adverse health and social consequences (Chen and Kandel 1995). Some adolescents advance to levels of use and consequences that meet criteria for substance use disorders (SUDs) and are at high risk for the continuation of substance use in adulthood. The cognitive, behavioral, and physiological symptoms linked to substance use are particularly damaging to the developing brain. Substance use at an earlier age at onset is significantly associated with an increased risk of developing an SUD in adult life (Volkow and Wargo 2022).

## Adolescent Consent to Treatment

Adolescence poses unique challenges in consent. In the United States, parents are legally responsible for an adolescent until the appropriate "adult" age, except in specific circumstances (e.g., emancipated minor). However, the adolescent may disagree with the parent's wishes for treatment or nontreatment. Unsurprisingly, adolescents may feel reluctant to seek help if they are not assured confidentiality about specific topics. Many U.S. states responded to this issue by enacting laws allowing adolescents to consent to counsel and treatment for sensitive and private conditions, such as reproductive health, sexually transmitted diseases, substance use treatment, and suicide. However, laws vary among states on various matters such as the age of consent, consent sufficiency with only the minor versus either the parent or minor, inpatient versus outpatient treatment, and substance use versus mental health. Clinicians must review their state's adolescent consent laws before providing treatment.

# Epidemiology

The National Epidemiologic Survey on Alcohol and Related Conditions (NESARC) found that more than 50% of substance use initiation occurs between the ages of 15 and 19 years (Blanco et al. 2018). Advances have been made in recent years in several regards. Survey results have shown a decrease among high school students reporting substance use in the United States. According to the Monitoring the Future survey, the lifetime prevalence of using any illicit drug among eighth, tenth, and twelfth grade students was 27% in 2021. This is a relative decline of 22% from 2020. However, although this decline may appear to be positive, these findings overlap with the coronavirus SARS-CoV-2 disease (COVID-19) pandemic shutdown, which resulted in limited socialization among peers, increased parental supervision, and changes in perceived availability (Johnston et al. 2022).

Although the prevalence of substance use has declined overall in recent years from historical highs, alcohol use, binge drinking, tobacco use and cigarette smoking, and the use of other substances continue to rise. The rapid rise of adolescents using electronic nicotine and cannabis delivery systems (vaping) has become increasingly troubling. Although this trend recently has slowed, the rates remain significant. In 2019, 25% of U.S. twelfth graders and 20% of tenth graders reported vaping nicotine in the past 30 days. The use of illicit opioids (e.g., heroin) is less common because of perceived high risk by youth, but this risk perception declines for prescription opioids such as oxycodone and acetaminophen/hydrocodone. Opioids continue to cause significant harm and fatality by overdose, although data indicate that most of the increased use in the current opioid epidemic occurs among adults and not adolescents (Johnston et al. 2022; Miech et al. 2021). Nevertheless, most adults treated for an opioid use disorder (OUD) were younger than 25 when they first used opioids.

The potential for overdose in adolescents remains high, as indicated by data from 2018 showing that unintentional deaths in adolescents and young adults due to poisoning, including opioid-related deaths, surpassed those due to motor vehicle accidents (Lee and Mannix 2018). Another consideration includes access to treatment for OUD. Compared with adults, adolescents are less likely to receive medications for treatment of opioid use in a timely manner. Moreover, behavioral treatment is usually initiated only after a formal diagnosis of a use disorder has been established and the adolescent is willing to enter treatment, both of which may be delayed. Intentional overdoses contribute to the death toll, exemplified by studies indicating that as many as 30% of opioid overdoses may be suicide attempts (Volkow 2019). The COVID-19 pandemic further complicated entry into treatment and treatment availability among youth.

Alcohol, illicit substance use, and other risk-taking behaviors such as risky sexual behavior emerge in adolescence and tend to cluster together. They are associated with increased health risk behaviors, increased burden of disease, premature death, diminished work capacity, and poorer socioeconomic outcomes (Marshall 2014). Early identification of adolescent risk factors may help prevent or attenuate risk.

# Substances Commonly Used

The substances most used by adolescents include alcohol, tobacco, and cannabis, whereas opioids are used less. The prevalence of lifetime substance use among adolescents in 2018 was 26.3% for alcohol, 15.4% for cannabis, and 13.4% for tobacco. Nationally representative data from 2015 to 2018 showed that 10.7% of adolescents developed an SUD within 12 months of initiating cannabis use, and 20.1% developed an SUD within 36 months of initiating prescription drug misuse. These figures were higher than those for young adults, supporting the association between an earlier onset of drug use and faster progression to an SUD (Volkow et al. 2021). Adolescents also often use multiple substances, sometimes without meeting the criteria for an SUD. The individual substances used appears to be interrelated, such that cannabis use is more frequent in among adolescents who smoke than among those who do not, and those who smoke score significantly higher on the Alcohol Use Disorders Identification Test (AUDIT) than nonsmokers. Table 13–1 summarizes recent data on substance use in this population.

**Table 13–1.  Data from the 2021 Monitoring the Future survey**

| | Alcohol | Cigarettes | Marijuana | Amphetamine | Narcotics other than heroin | Inhalants | Vaping* |
|---|---|---|---|---|---|---|---|
| **Lifetime prevalence** | | | | | | | |
| Eighth graders | 21.7 | 7 | 10.2 | 5.8 | – | 11.3 | 17.5 |
| Tenth graders | 34.7 | 10 | 22 | 5.2 | – | 7.2 | 29.7 |
| Twelfth graders | 54.1 | 17.8 | 38.6 | 4.9 | 2.3 | 5 | 40.5 |
| **Perceived availability** | | | | | | | |
| Eighth graders | 47.9 | 38 | 26.7 | 11.4 | 6.0 | – | 37.8 |
| Tenth graders | 60.2 | 48 | 47.5 | 16.4 | 9.8 | – | 54.6 |
| Twelfth graders | 76.8 | 57.9 | 69.6 | 29.4 | 18.7 | – | 71.5 |

*Note.*   All values are percentages; – = not reported.

*For lifetime prevalence, vaping refers to vaping of any kind, whereas for perceived availability, vaping specifically refers to a vaping device.

*Source.*   Johnston et al. 2022

# Effects of Substance Use on the Adolescent Brain

Various factors increase the risk of substance use initiation in adolescents, including brain developmental changes, reward sensitivity, risk taking, peer influence, and decreased adult supervision within a period of increasing social autonomy. Adolescents vary in their ability to consistently regulate impulses, which contributes to variability in risk. Insights into brain development provide a more profound understanding of the neurocognitive underpinnings of adolescent behavior related to addiction. A growing body of research shows that adolescent substance use is associated with cognitive and learning difficulties, particularly when use is frequent and heavy (Chambers et al. 2003). Knowledge of the specifics of adolescent brain development is vital to understanding adolescents' increased risk of substance use and the effect of substances on their developing brains.

## Adolescent Brain Development

Adolescence is a critical time for brain maturation. The hallmark of this period is the profound reorganization of brain regions necessary for adaptive cognitive and executive function, working memory, decision-making, reward processing, emotional regulation, and motivated behavior. This remodeling occurs in gray matter, white matter, and related neurochemical systems, resulting in an experience-dependent loss of synapses and the simultaneous strengthening of remaining connections. These adaptive changes are geared toward optimal neurocognitive performance associated with the initiation of substance use (Dumontheil 2016).

The prefrontal cortex, in particular, is prominently remodeled, which results in development of a more efficient executive functioning system. This higher-order control system regulates the efficiency and accuracy with which information is attended to, processed, and used to inform goal-directed, future-oriented behaviors. These changes stimulate further cognitive development, allowing adolescents to perform more complex executive functioning tasks and ramp up emotionally driven responses around reward sensitivity, all within a psychosocial environment that allows for increased social interaction with peers and the influence this confers, including the initiation and continuation of drug use. These factors result in adolescents being much more powerfully motivated by reward than by negative reinforcement (Spear 2000). As such, they are more likely to take high-risk behaviors with little attention paid to the downsides.

In addition to this structural remodeling, the adolescent brain experiences considerable neurochemical maturation. The dopaminergic system undergoes an extensive reorganization that is likely critical for developing motivated behaviors and associative learning. During adolescence, alterations in dopamine firing activity have been shown to induce structural and functional changes in mesocortical pathways, which affects reward sensitivity and corresponding reward-driven behaviors (Grace et al. 2007; O'Donnell 2010). Animal studies, which provide valuable insights into human behavior, show that adolescents differ from adults in response to nearly all drugs of abuse studied, including nicotine, cannabis, and stimulants (Schepis et al. 2008).

## Alcohol

Alcohol is the substance most used by youth, yet alcohol use disorder (AUD) and its impact are often overlooked in adolescents. Adolescence is marked by progressive hippocampus development, which is central to memory formation and recall. Hippocampal volumes have been found to be significantly smaller in adolescents with AUD than in those without AUD. Moreover, the total hippocampal volume correlated positively with the age at onset of AUD and negatively with the duration of the AUD. Increased severity of AUD was associated with increased hippocampal asymmetry (Medina et al. 2007).

The age at drinking onset has important implications for ensuing cognitive and neurobiological abnormalities. Adolescents who had an earlier onset of weekly drinking performed poorer on measures of cognitive inhibition and working memory than those who had a later onset. An earlier age at drinking onset predicted worse psychomotor speed and visual attention functioning (Nguyen-Louie et al. 2017). Sex differences have also been found. The functional impact of AUD indicates that female adolescents with AUD show greater abnormalities in activation patterns than male adolescents with AUD, increasing their risk of behavioral deficits. Furthermore, female adolescents with AUD may be especially vulnerable to abnormal activity patterns. Studies suggest that they have greater compensatory activation in the temporal areas for a reduced frontal and cingulate response to the spatial working memory task (Caldwell et al. 2005).

Cognitive changes have been noted to persist in adolescents who drink alcohol. Adolescents with AUD in early remission had poorer performance on verbal and nonverbal memory tasks than a control group with no history of

AUD. Adolescents who drink alcohol have poorer working and verbal memory (Hanson et al. 2011). However, overall memory-related outcomes tend to improve with abstinence. Adolescent alcohol drinking appears to alter the developmental trajectory of impulsivity; impulsivity is linked with a faster escalation of drinking and heavy drinking. Adolescents with heavy drinking also had a stronger attentional bias for alcohol-related cues compared with those with light drinking (Field et al. 2007). Activation differences in the frontal, temporal, and parietal regions may predate and contribute to the initiation of alcohol use. Neural vulnerabilities in brain regions implicated in inhibitory control may predict alcohol use, and heavy drinking subsequently may lead to additional alterations (Wetherill et al. 2013).

## Nicotine

Adolescent brains are particularly vulnerable to the harmful effects of tobacco and nicotine, which activate the nicotinic acetylcholine receptors (nAChRs). Neuronal nAChRs show patterns of expression paralleling important developmental events within the cholinergic system and are critical modulators of brain maturation from prenatal development through adolescence. Neuronal nAChRs have a central role in regulating neurophysiology and signaling in addiction pathways (Dwyer et al. 2009). Studies indicate that the effects of nicotine are highly dependent on the timing of exposure, with a dynamic interaction of nAChRs with dopaminergic, endocannabinoid, and opioidergic systems that enhances overall drug reward and reinforcement. Disruption of nAChR development with early nicotine use may affect the functioning and pharmacology of the receptor subunits and alter the regulation of reward-related neurotransmitters, including acetylcholine, dopamine, GABA, serotonin, and glutamate.

Functional MRI (fMRI) studies have shown that adolescents who smoke experience higher novelty seeking and greater reward delay discounting compared with those who do not. In a large group of 14-year-old patients with matched comparisons from the IMAGEN study, fMRI studies showed that the adolescents who smoked had significantly higher delay discounting rates than their nonsmoking counterparts, preferring smaller and sooner rewards over larger and later rewards (Peters et al. 2011; Schumann et al. 2010).

## Cannabis

The major psychoactive cannabinoid in cannabis, Δ-9-tetrahydrocannabinol (Δ-9 THC), affects the endocannabinoid system, which plays a key role in the development of the brain and other organs. Cannabinoid receptors $(CB_1)$ are widely distributed throughout the brain and are involved in neurotransmitter release and concentrations across neural systems (excitatory and inhibitory). The genetic expression of cannabis-related receptors is increased during adolescence. Disruptions in brain development related to the neurotoxic effects of regular cannabis use could significantly alter neurodevelopmental trajectories. Alteration of the endocannabinoid system during this vulnerable period may result in a cascade of neurochemical and neurostructural aberrations, with cognitive and emotional outcomes that last into adulthood (Rubino and Parolaro 2008). Adolescents who engage in heavy cannabis use frequently show decrements in neurocognitive performance, macro- and microstructural brain development changes, and brain functioning alterations (Meier et al. 2018).

# Co-occurring Disorders

Studies have shown high rates of co-occurring mental health conditions in adolescents with SUD. Epidemiological studies estimate that 22% of adolescents in the United States have a mental health disorder (Winstanley et al. 2012). On the basis of regional studies, between 13% and 32% of adolescents are estimated to have a mental health disorder, and 9%–13% of adolescents have a serious emotional disturbance (Williams et al. 2018). The National Survey on Drug Use and Health (NSDUH) used a nationally representative sample and found that 4.6% of adolescents met criteria for an SUD. Among treatment-seeking adolescents, about two-thirds in community-based SUD treatment programs also meet diagnostic criteria for another mental illness. Rates of co-occurring mental health disorders among adolescents with SUDs range from 50% to 71% (Substance Abuse and Mental Health Services Administration 2021). Some research found that mental health conditions may precede the onset of substance use, suggesting that improved diagnosis in youth may reduce comorbid substance abuse (Goldstein and Bukstein 2010; O'Neil et al. 2011).

## Attention-Deficit/Hyperactivity Disorder

Adolescents with ADHD were 7 times more likely to have an SUD and were 5 times more likely to have alcohol abuse compared with control subjects. Childhood ADHD is associated with nicotine use by middle adolescence and with alcohol and drug use disorders in adulthood (OR 2.36). ADHD is a risk factor in smoking initiation and nicotine use disorder (Charach et al. 2011).

However, studies on the potential for smoking to affect the trajectory and symptomatology of ADHD in adolescents are conflicting.

Studies indicate that pharmacotherapy status is an essential modifier of the ADHD-SUD association. Pharmacotherapy for ADHD did not predict an increased risk for adolescent SUD. Rather, several studies have determined that pharmacological treatment of children with ADHD decreased the risk of a later SUD. More specifically, pharmacotherapy for ADHD delays the onset of SUDs in affected adolescents compared with those whose ADHD is untreated (Biederman 2003). Furthermore, a study found that early initiation of ADHD treatment before age 9 and a longer duration of treatment decreased the risk of adolescent SUD to match that of the general population. For every year older an adolescent was at the initiation of stimulant use, risk increased by a factor of 1.46 for SUD in adulthood (Dalsgaard et al. 2014; McCabe et al. 2016). Contrasting these findings are the results of the Multimodal Treatment of Attention-Deficit/Hyperactivity Disorder study, one of the largest longitudinal studies on ADHD. In the originally randomized treatment groups (mean age 17 years), medication for ADHD did not protect from or contribute to the risk of substance use or SUD at 8-year follow-up or earlier. Importantly, neither medication at follow-up (mostly stimulants) nor cumulative stimulant treatment was positively correlated with adolescent substance use or SUD (Molina et al. 2013). We interpret this cumulative information to mean that, at best, stimulants may reduce the risk of SUD in adolescents with ADHD and, at worst, they have minimal to no effect.

Other risk modifiers for the ADHD-SUD association include the presence of conduct disorder. Comorbid conduct disorder in childhood is associated with later substance abuse, increasing the risk of SUD in adulthood by almost 4 times. A naturalistic study showed that female sex, conduct disorder in childhood, and older age at initiation of stimulant treatment were associated with an increased risk of later SUD and alcohol abuse. Compared with young males with ADHD, young females with ADHD have been found to be at higher risk of both alcohol use and SUD (Dalsgaard et al. 2014). A follow-up study of females with ADHD into adolescence found an increased risk of SUD similar to that of males with ADHD (Disney et al. 1999).

## Depression and Anxiety

Co-occurring depressive conditions in adolescents with SUD include major depressive disorder, disruptive mood dysregulation disorder, persistent depressive disorder, and a variety of conditions related to adjustment difficulties. Youth with SUDs are 3 times more likely to be depressed and 4 times more likely to attempt suicide. When compared with adolescent males in the context of substance use, adolescent females had a greater degree of internalizing symptoms (e.g., depression, anxiety). Depression is common, but the association may be stronger between SUD and other disorders (e.g., bipolar disorder, ADHD, trauma and PTSD, specific anxiety disorders) (Crum et al. 2008).

The prevalence of anxiety symptoms and disorders among adolescents with SUD is high. About 67% of adolescents in inpatient drug treatment, 33% in inpatient psychiatric facilities, and 33% in community-based psychiatric facilities for comorbid substance use and psychiatric diagnoses had anxiety disorders. Common co-occurring anxiety conditions in adolescents with SUD include panic disorder, social anxiety, and trauma- and stressor-related conditions. In treatment-seeking youth with SUD and anxiety, alcohol and marijuana were the most frequently used substances (Deas-Nesmith et al. 1998).

## Trauma and PTSD

Adolescents with a history of trauma are at higher risk of substance use initiation and progression. However, an SUD increases the risk of further trauma because of the effects of the substance itself and the psychosocial factors surrounding obtaining and maintaining use. Adolescents who have experienced physical abuse or sexual abuse or assault are 3 times more likely to report past or current substance use. Up to 60% of adolescents with PTSD subsequently develop substance use problems. In turn, more than 70% of youth receiving treatment for substance use have a history of trauma exposure. Common conditions related to trauma- and stressor-related disorders among adolescents with substance use include adverse childhood experiences, acute stress disorder and PTSD, adjustment disorders, changes in family structure, loss, and traumatic grief (Langlois et al. 2021).

## Psychosis

A substantial body of evidence associates tobacco smoking during adolescence and young adulthood with an increased risk for psychosis and schizophrenia. This increased risk is more prominent among individuals with heavy smoking and initiation of smoking during early adolescence compared with later adolescence (McGrath et al. 2016). Cannabis use has also been correlated with an increased risk for later-life psychosis (Griffith-Lendering et al.

Table 13–2. Risk factors for adolescent substance use

| Domain | Examples |
|---|---|
| Individual | Genetic predisposition, prenatal drug exposure, neural disinhibition, mental health condition, emotional dysregulation, adverse childhood experiences, trauma history, high aggressivity, low risk perception |
| Family | Parent, sibling, or other household member with active substance use; permissive parenting; low parental involvement; poor parental supervision; parental hostility; parent-child conflict |
| School and peers | Substance-using partner, association with deviant peers, peer involvement in substance use, peer rejection or alienation, school failure, low school engagement |
| Neighborhood and community | High community violence, accessibility and availability of illegal substances, low community cohesion |

2013). This relationship is thought to be bidirectional, with cannabis use predicting psychosis vulnerability and vice versa in adolescents.

# Clinical Features of Specific Substances

The symptoms of SUD often result in dysfunction that trails into adulthood. Adolescents often initiate drug use by experimentation. They engage in intermittent use in the earlier stages, often with peers. As the disease progresses, using alone becomes more prominent, and drug use may become more hidden. The signs of intoxication vary and depend on the substance or combination of substances used. Particularly for alcohol, adolescents may not readily acknowledge intoxication states such as blackouts. Generally, primarily for nicotine, alcohol, and cannabis, adolescents consistently report fewer withdrawal symptoms than adults (McNeill et al. 1986), which partly contributes to a limited recognition of their need for treatment. The risk factors for adolescent substance abuse can involve individual, family, peer, and community elements (Table 13–2).

## Alcohol

Alcohol use in adolescents often involves binge drinking, generally defined as consuming the amount of alcohol needed to increase the blood alcohol

Table 13–3.  Binge drinking among adults compared with
            adolescents

| Category | Age, years | Drinks in a row, N |
|---|---|---|
| Adult males | ≥18 | ≥5 |
| Adult females | ≥18 | ≥4 |
| Adolescent males | 16–17 | 5 |
|  | 14–15 | 4 |
|  | 9–13 | 3 |
| Adolescent females | 9–17 | 3 |

*Note.*  *Binge drinking* is defined as consuming the amount of alcohol needed to raise blood
alcohol level above 80 mg/dL.

level (BAL) above 80 mg/dL. On the basis of age and sex, BALs rise higher
in adolescents than in adults for the same amount of alcohol consumed. Table 13–3 shows the approximate number of drinks needed to raise the BAL
above 80 mg/dL. In 2011, of the drug abuse–related emergency department
visits made by patients ages 20 and younger, more than 40% involved alcohol
(Substance Abuse and Mental Health Services Administration 2021).

Alcohol alters the neural transmission of the inhibitory neurotransmitter
GABA and the excitatory neurotransmitter glutamate. A correlational study
revealed neurocognitive deficits in attention, memory, information processing, and executive functioning in adolescents using alcohol compared with
nonusing control subjects (Quigley and Committee on Substance Use and
Prevention 2019). The sequelae observed with chronic alcohol use in adults,
such as Korsakoff's syndrome, Wernicke's aphasia, and cirrhosis of the liver,
are rarely observed in adolescents.

## Nicotine

Nicotine is known to be highly addictive. It acts on cholinergic receptors and
enhances acetylcholine, serotonin, and β-endorphin release. Nicotine withdrawal can cause depressed mood, anxiety, irritability, sleep disturbances, and
poor concentration. Exposure can be via cigarettes, smokeless tobacco (e.g.,
chewing tobacco, snuff, snus, dissolvable tobacco products), vaping, or a combination. In 2020, among individuals ages 12–20, 11.8% (4.4 million) used tobacco products, an electronic cigarette, or another vaping device to consume
nicotine in the past month. Within this age group, 7.7% (2.9 million) vaped
nicotine, 6.7% (2.5 million) used tobacco products, and 4.1% (1.5 million)

smoked cigarettes during that period (Substance Abuse and Mental Health Services Administration 2021). Smokeless tobacco is more commonly used by males than females and frequently leads to cigarette smoking in youth. Adolescents who use vapor liquids with a high nicotine concentration are at a higher risk of progressing to higher frequency and intensity of combustible and vaping use in the future relative to adolescents who do not engage in vaping or who vape at lower nicotine concentrations (Goldenson et al. 2017). Some studies have found that adolescents who vape nicotine have significantly higher levels of cotinine, a metabolite of nicotine, compared with adolescents who use combustible nicotine (Boykan et al. 2019).

## Cannabis

Cannabis has remained one of the most-used illicit substances in adolescence for almost 50 years, per the Monitoring the Future survey results. Despite legalization in some states and perceived low health risk of cannabis use by the general public, there is increasing clinical awareness about the spectrum of behavioral and neurobiological disturbances associated with cannabis use, including anxiety, depression, psychosis, cognitive deficits, social impairments, and addiction (Chadwick et al. 2013).

Cannabis can be smoked (including concentrated forms, e.g., hashish and honey oil), taken orally (mixed with food or drink), or vaped, a more recent method. Its active ingredient, THC, has several short-term effects, including memory and learning impairment, diminished problem-solving ability, apathy, distorted perception, and anxiety. A withdrawal syndrome has been reported in adolescents following abrupt cessation of heavy cannabis use that involves insomnia, irritability, restlessness, and cravings followed by anxiety, tremors, nausea, muscle twitches, increased sweating, myalgia, and general anxiety malaise (Chung et al. 2008). Withdrawal typically begins 24 hours after last cannabis use, peaks at 2–4 days, and resolves after 2 weeks. The risks of chronic cannabis use include impaired respiratory function, an increased risk of cardiovascular disease, and the potential increased risk of developing psychotic symptoms or disorders. A study published in 2018 that included 3,720 adolescents demonstrated a significant association of cannabis use frequency with increased psychotic symptoms (Bourque et al. 2018).

## Opioids

The term *opioids* serves as a hypernym that comprises both natural alkaloid compounds (e.g., morphine, codeine, thebaine) and semisynthetic and synthetic compounds (e.g., oxycodone, hydromorphone, heroin, fentanyl). Opioids are powerful pain relievers. They are notable for their rapid progression to physiological use disorder with tolerance and withdrawal and other addiction symptoms. Almost 50% of youth who misuse prescription opioids report getting them from friends or relatives. In a recent study examining the association between parent and adolescent medical prescription opioid use and misuse, parental use of prescription opioids in the prior 12 months was associated with adolescent use and misuse (Griesler et al. 2021).

Use in adolescence is thought to follow a pattern that maximizes drug bioavailability and effect, beginning with oral prescription opioids and then progressing to inhaled (smoking or nasal snorting) prescription opioids, inhaled heroin, and, finally, intravenous heroin use. As tolerance builds, heroin also becomes a more convenient choice because of its lower cost and higher potency. Within a few months after their first substance use, adolescents can progress to complete OUD, with a course of use that is often shorter than that of adults. It is worth noting that death via overdose does not require an OUD, and adolescents can overdose their first time trying opioids. The classic triad of opioid overdose is obtundation, pinpoint pupils, and respiratory depression. If it is not treated in time, respiratory depression will lead to full respiratory arrest and death.

A CDC study showed youth prescription opioid misuse was associated with high-risk behaviors. Adolescents with OUD were 2.8 times more likely to not use their seatbelt while riding in vehicles and to ride with an intoxicated driver, 3.9 times more likely to have first sexual intercourse before age 13, 2 times more likely not to use a condom before sexual intercourse, 4 times more likely to have engaged in physical fights in the past year, and 5 times more likely to have ever attempted suicide and to have carried a gun in the past 30 days (Bhatia et al. 2020).

## Cocaine

Cocaine is a tropane alkaloid derived from the leaves of two species of coca plants and exerts its stimulant effects via neurotransmission of primarily dopamine but also serotonin and norepinephrine. The 2019 NSDUH estimated past cocaine use among adolescents was 0.4%, a number that had decreased from 2.1% in 2002. Cocaine use occurs across all demographic and socioeconomic groups. Intoxication leads to euphoria, increased energy, alertness, increased sociability, and decreased appetite and need for sleep. Prolonged use and higher doses eventually lead to anxiety, irritability, restlessness, agitation, and psychosis. In addition, younger age is an independent risk factor for developing psychotic symptoms (Ryan 2019).

## Hallucinogens

Hallucinogens comprise two groups of substances, classic hallucinogens and dissociative agents. *Club drugs* are a group of substances used frequently by adolescents and young adults, mainly at rave parties, bars, nightclubs, music festivals, and concerts and include classic hallucinogens such as lysergic acid diethylamide (LSD), 3,4-methylenedioxymethamphetamine (MDMA), γ-hydroxybutyrate (GHB), flunitrazepam (Rohypnol), and methamphetamine. Dissociative agents are a group of substances that cause users to feel disconnected from themselves and their surroundings; these include phencyclidine (PCP) and ketamine. GHB, flunitrazepam, and ketamine are also colloquially known as "date rape" or predatory drugs because of their facilitation of rape or sexual assault on the often unsuspecting consumer. LSD and MDMA were among the most used substances in this category for twelfth graders, with an annual prevalence of 3.2% and 2.2%, respectively, in 2018. GHB had the smallest use, with a prevalence of 0.3% for twelfth graders in 2018 (Johnston et al. 2022). The use of methamphetamine generally increases with age. Despite club drugs having some unique characteristics (Table 13–4), there is much symptom overlap among them. It is also common for club drug users to take multiple substances concurrently, obscuring the overall clinical presentation.

## Over-the-Counter Drugs

### Dextromethorphan

Dextromethorphan is a semisynthetic morphine derivative with limited affinity with and effect on the μ opioid receptors. It is an active ingredient in more than 100 over-the-counter (OTC) cough and cold medications. In 2020, 3.7% of adolescents used dextromethorphan-containing cough medicines to get high, which was an increase from 2019 (Johnston et al. 2022). The route of administration is oral via tablet or liquid. Dextromethorphan has multiple mechanisms of action with sedative, dissociative, and stimulant properties. Symptoms of intoxication include alertness, euphoria, and laughing at lower doses, whereas hallucinations, a dreamlike state, and mild disassociation can be achieved with higher doses. Dissociative effects similar to those of PCP and ketamine occur when it is consumed in doses much higher

**Table 13–4.** Hallucinogens and other party drugs

| Drug | Symptoms of intoxication and withdrawal and physical signs | Additional notes |
|---|---|---|
| Flunitrazepam (Rohypnol) | *Intoxication:* low doses have alcohol-like effects, with decreased anxiety, muscle relaxation, disinhibition, drowsiness, slurred speech, psychomotor slowing; high doses cause confusion, loss of muscle control, loss of consciousness, amnesia<br><br>*Withdrawal:* restlessness, anxiety, headache, myalgia, photosensitivity, numbness, and increased seizure potential<br><br>*Physical signs:* mydriasis, variable pupil size, injected watery eyes; with high doses, bradycardia and respiratory depression | Benzodiazepine is 10 times more potent than diazepam<br><br>Standard protocol for treating benzodiazepine acute intoxication and withdrawal applies<br><br>Odorless and tasteless; causes anterograde amnesia<br><br>OOA: 30 minutes<br><br>DOA: 8–12 hours<br><br>ROA: oral (tablet, dissolved), snort, inject, smoke/vape[a] |
| GHB | *Intoxication:* euphoria; disinhibition; sedation; enhanced sexual performance; toxicity triad of coma, bradycardia, and myoclonus<br><br>*Withdrawal:* resembles that of alcohol, including nausea, vomiting, diaphoresis, insomnia, restlessness, irritability, anxiety, tremor, and delirium, which occurs 1–6 hours after last use and lasts 9–14 days<br><br>*Physical signs:* mydriasis or miosis, nystagmus | Anesthetic properties<br><br>Regular use leads to mild to moderate symptoms of anxiety, irritability, mood swings, aggression, insomnia, and hallucinations<br><br>Tolerance and use disorder can develop quickly<br><br>OOA: 10–20 minutes<br><br>DOA: 2–6 hours<br><br>ROA: oral (tablet, liquid, dissolved)[a] |

**Table 13–4. Hallucinogens and other party drugs (*continued*)**

| Drug | Symptoms of intoxication and withdrawal and physical signs | Additional notes |
|---|---|---|
| Ketamine | *Intoxication:* perceptual distortions of sound and sight, hallucinations, altered perception of time, relaxed sense of detachment or disconnection from one's surroundings and body<br><br>*Physical signs:* mydriasis; may appear catatonic with rigid posturing and flat facies along with a fixed, sightless stare | Dissociative anesthetic<br>Prolonged use can lead to tolerance, use disorder, memory impairment, confusion, word blocking<br>Odorless; causes amnesia and can be ingested unknowingly<br>OOA: 2–15 minutes<br>DOA: several hours<br>ROA: oral (tablet, liquid), snort, inject, smoke/vape[b] |
| LSD | *Intoxication:* perceptual experience depends on user's personality, mood, expectations, and setting. Pleasant response includes mentally stimulating visual distortions of shapes and movements; synesthesia is common. Unpleasant response can include thoughts of despair, nightmare-like sensations of doom, anxiety, panic, fears of losing control, insanity, and death<br><br>*Physical signs:* mydriasis, tachycardia, dizziness, sweating, nausea, fine tremor | Induces perceptual distortions of real stimuli, making it a true illusionogenic<br>Two long-term sequelae: persistent psychosis and hallucinogen persisting perception disorder<br>OOA: 30–90 minutes<br>DOA: up to 12 hours<br>ROA: oral (tablet, liquid, blotting paper)[c] |

**Table 13–4. Hallucinogens and other party drugs** *(continued)*

| Drug | Symptoms of intoxication and withdrawal and physical signs | Additional notes |
|------|-----------------------------------------------------------|------------------|
| MDMA | *Intoxication:* general sense of well-being, emotional warmth, empathy, decreased anxiety, mental simulation, perceptual distortion, alertness<br><br>*Withdrawal:* fatigue, difficulty concentrating, anorexia, depression<br><br>*Physical signs:* mydriasis, tachycardia, hypertension, bruxism, muscle aches, rigidity, spasms | Commonly known as Ecstasy or Molly<br><br>Potentiates serotonin and norepinephrine release, producing both psychedelic and stimulant effects<br><br>Extended intense physical activity while intoxicated (e.g., dancing) may lead to fatal dehydration, hyperthermia, rhabdomyolysis, or kidney failure<br><br>OOA: 20–60 minutes<br><br>DOA: 2–3 hours<br><br>ROA: oral (tablet, liquid), smoke/vape, snort[d] |
| Methamphetamine | *Intoxication:* increased awareness, alertness, and energy; euphoria; hallucinations<br><br>*Withdrawal:* irritability, fatigue, somnolence, depression<br><br>*Physical signs:* tachycardia, hypertension | Synthetic stimulant<br><br>Exerts effects via dopamine neurotransmission<br><br>Prolonged use can lead to executive function impairments and increased depression and anxiety in adolescents (Basedow et al. 2021) |

**Table 13–4. Hallucinogens and other party drugs** *(continued)*

| Drug | Symptoms of intoxication and withdrawal and physical signs | Additional notes |
|---|---|---|
| Methamphetamine *(continued)* | | OOA: depends on route of administration. Smoking or injection: seconds to a few minutes; snorting: 3–5 minutes; ingestion 15–30 minutes<br><br>DOA: 8–12 hours, sometimes longer<br><br>ROA: oral (tablet), inject, snort, smoke |

*Note.* DOA=duration of action; GHB=γ-hydroxybutyrate; LSD=lysergic acid diethylamide; MDMA=3,4-methylenedioxymethamphetamine; OOA=onset of action; ROA=route of administration.

[a]The dissolved form is the most commonly used form.

[b]Snorting is the most common ROA.

[c]Blotting paper is the most commonly used form.

[d]Tablet is the most commonly used form.

than OTC preparations, such as 200–1,500 mg. Physical signs of intoxication include mydriasis, nystagmus, tachycardia, elevated blood pressure, diaphoresis, slurred speech, ataxia, and loss of coordination. Toxicity may manifest as serotonin syndrome in the absence of other serotonergic drugs (Williams and Lundahl 2019). The presence of dextromethorphan may result in false-positive urine drug screens for PCP.

### Inhalants

Inhalant use is a more prevalent problem in youth because use generally decreases with advancing age. Very little inhalant use is seen beyond age 20. The use by youth has been attributed to the fact that volatile products are widely available, inexpensive, easily concealed, and legal for their intended purposes. Volatile solvents, fuels, and anesthetics are the most common inhalants used among youth; the remaining two subclasses of inhalants are nitrous oxide and volatile alkyl nitrates (Williams and Lundahl 2019). The onset of action occurs rapidly, inducing a high, lightheadedness, and disinhibition for several minutes. Continuous use leads to slurred speech, dizziness, disorientation, and ataxia, which can last for several hours. Clinical suspicion should be raised with the smell of inhalants on the breath, chemical stains or paint on skin or clothes, facial or airway frostbite from aerosol computer cans, and perinasal or perioral rash. Sudden death can result from repeated use because each use sensitizes the myocardium and can precipitate a fatal cardiac arrhythmia.

# Diagnosis

The diagnosis of SUDs in adolescents mirrors that of adults and is based on the criteria set forth by DSM-5 (American Psychiatric Association 2022; see Chapter 2, "General Approach to Patients With Multi-substance Use Disorders"). The presence of at least two criteria that reflect a pathological pattern of behavior in four main categories (diminished control, social impairment, hazardous use, pharmacological properties) within a 12-month period is required. The severity of the SUD is based on the number of criteria present (two or three for mild, four or five for moderate, and six or more for severe). There is concern that these criteria (and other SUD criteria) are too high for the adolescent population and, as a result, delay appropriate intervention, even though youth often begin to accumulate problems early. Substance-induced disorders are diagnoses that are separate from but related to SUDs and reflect substance intoxication, substance withdrawal, and substance-induced mental disorders. They are generally thought to be reversible conditions, but some reports indicate persistent long-term psychological consequences may sometimes occur in genetically vulnerable persons (McCabe et al. 2022).

# Screening

Clinical impressions of adolescents' substance use involvement are often underestimated. Structured screening tools significantly improve detection of substance-related problems in primary care and mental health settings and should be considered for use with all adolescent patients (Wilson et al. 2004). Screening tools are brief questionnaires or procedures that help identify persons who are at risk of developing or have already developed a certain disease. Screening is not diagnostic but is indicative of the need to initiate further assessment and potentially treat for conditions that may have been overlooked. For adolescents, a few screening measures for substance use have been well validated.

## CRAFFT

CRAFFT (Car, Relax, Alone, Forget, Friends, Trouble) is one of the most well studied tools and has been validated for youth (ages 12–21) from diverse socioeconomic and ethnic backgrounds (Knight et al. 2002). It helps identify high-risk behaviors such as operating a motor vehicle while under the influence of alcohol or drugs. The current version, CRAFFT 2.1+N, includes evidence-based revisions that increase its sensitivity and specificity. Vaping was added as an administration method for cannabis use and additional questions about tobacco and nicotine use. Higher scores indicate a higher likelihood that an adolescent will meet the DSM-5 criteria for an SUD of any level. On the basis of the score, a risk level category (i.e., low, medium, high) is available to help direct provider care, which is in line with the Screening, Brief Intervention, and Referral to Treatment (SBIRT) approach, which aims to deliver early intervention and treatment to persons with and at risk for SUDs.

## Alcohol Use Disorders Identification Test

The AUDIT was developed by the World Health Organization and includes 10 questions to assess alcohol-related problems. It has been consistently validated across sexes and in various ethnic groups and ages, including adolescents ages 12–17 years (Liskola et al. 2021). A shorter version with only three questions, the AUDIT-C, is also available. AUDIT has become the world's most widely used alcohol screening tool and is available in 40 languages. On the basis of the patient's score, the AUDIT also provides suggestions for intervention to help guide care in line with the SBIRT model.

## Screening to Brief Intervention and Brief Screener for Tobacco, Alcohol, and Other Drugs

The National Institute on Drug Abuse has two brief, online, evidence-based screening tools that assess the risk of SUDs in adolescents ages 12–17. The Screening to Brief Intervention (S2BI) and Brief Screener for Tobacco, Alcohol, and other Drugs (BSTAD) inquire about the frequency of use during the past year, and results are categorized into three levels of risk for SUD (i.e., no reported use, lower risk, higher risk). Results are followed with suggested actions in line with the SBIRT model. Both screening tools have the option of self-administration or clinician administration. S2BI has a gradient response (e.g., weekly, monthly). It has been empirically validated in pediatric primary care settings and is especially useful for identifying AUD and cannabis use disorder (CaUD), two common substance use problems among adolescents presenting for primary care (Levy et al. 2021). The BSTAD asks for days of use (i.e., 0–365) and is empirically validated for use in primary care settings (Kelly et al. 2014).

## Drug Abuse Screening Test

The Drug Abuse Screening Test (DAST-10) is a brief (10 questions), self-administered screening measure that assesses drug use in the past 12 months, excluding alcohol and tobacco use. For patients receiving a score greater than 3, further investigation is recommended. DAST-10 has been condensed from the original DAST, which has 28 questions (Skinner 1982). Both are best used in older youth and adults. DAST-A is best used in adolescents.

# Drug Testing

In adolescence, drug testing can be used to detect, deter, or delay drug use. However, its utility is limited by a variety of factors. A positive drug test does not confirm drug use, and a negative drug test does not exclude drug use. Drug tests detect the presence of drugs above a certain level and within a specific time window. Routine drug tests detect a limited number of substances and do not detect newer designer substances. Furthermore, drug tests do not reflect the severity of the SUD. Specimen types include urine, which is the most common type in the primary care setting; blood; breath; saliva; sweat;

and hair. Breath testing is used mainly by law enforcement and alcohol treatment programs. Hair testing is most useful for heavy, frequent, and past use and is not reliable for recent or occasional drug use. Home drug testing kits are readily available in retail drug stores. They may serve as a deterrent to drug use in youth. Conversely, they could result in a false sense of security because false negatives can occur. If the home drug test is available, a savvy youth will evade detection by altering samples or using substances not detectable by the specific drug test. Currently, the American Academy of Pediatrics does not endorse home testing because of the limited evidence that it reduces drug use among adolescents and concern that it may have a negative impact on the relationship between parents and their children (Levy et al. 2014). Regardless of these factors, drug tests should be considered for treatment monitoring in adolescents with SUDs.

# Treatment

After using appropriate screening measures and gathering a detailed clinical history, clinicians may identify an SUD that requires intervention. In addition, adolescents who are not diagnosed with an SUD or as being addicted to a substance may still benefit from some aspects of the intervention. Adult and youth substance problems manifest differently and require separate treatment approaches. Treatment programs created specifically for teenagers materialized in the 1980s and slowly continued to grow throughout the 1990s. Since then, advances have been made to improve treatment and outcomes. Treatment should be customized to the specific needs of the adolescent and should include an early assessment of strengths and weaknesses. The adolescent's biological, psychological, and social development must also be considered; these include school performance, family and peer relationships, sex and gender, cultural factors, and physical or mental issues. To achieve adequate improvement, treatment of co-occurring mental health conditions cannot be ignored. A treatment gap exists among adolescents struggling with substance use–related problems and those who receive treatment. Of those meeting criteria for an SUD, only 6% of adolescents and 8% of young adults receive treatment. This low number is thought to be due to various factors, including low motivation by youth or parents, a lack of specialized adolescent treatment programs, inconsistent quality of adolescent treatment services, and poor health care coverage (Winters et al. 2011). Components of a comprehensive substance use program include multiple services: mental health, medical (including treatment for infectious disease), educational, legal, vocational, and family. The setting of the treatment depends on the adolescent's severity of symptoms (e.g., intoxication, withdrawal), presence of comorbid medical or mental health conditions, readiness to change, risk of recurrence, and recovery environment.

## Medications

Pharmacotherapy research for substance use in adolescents is limited because research has focused largely on the adult population, and medications' safety and efficacy cannot be inferred from adult studies. As a result, except for buprenorphine, which is currently indicated for the treatment of OUD in adolescents ages 16 and older, no medications are approved by the FDA to treat SUD in persons younger than 18 years. Consequently, some health care providers may use medications for SUD treatment in adults off-label for youth, particularly older youth. Studies indicate that using pharmacological agents to reduce comorbid psychopathology can result in a milder reduction in SUD symptoms. The most robust evidence for this exists for treating SUD comorbid with affective disorders. Studies suggest that the use of pharmacological interventions may also increase the effectiveness of psychosocial strategies for SUD in adolescents (Waxmonsky and Wilens 2005).

### Alcohol Use Disorder

Pharmacotherapy in adults with AUD is focused on decreasing cravings and withdrawal symptoms, which is expected to decrease the likelihood of recurrence. Of the three FDA-approved medications (disulfiram, acamprosate, naltrexone) in adults for AUD, naltrexone has some literature that suggests it has good tolerability in adolescents and may be a potentially promising medication for adolescent AUD (Squeglia et al. 2019). Naltrexone can be administered orally daily or given intramuscularly monthly. It must be used with caution and careful monitoring, especially in individuals with severe hepatic or renal impairment, because hepatocellular injury is possible.

### Nicotine Use Disorder

Although cigarette use has declined among adolescents over the past several years, vaping has rapidly increased, having the largest 1-year increase of any substance use reported in the prior month in 2017 (Johnston et al. 2022). Nicotine replacement therapy (NRT), bupropion, and varenicline are three FDA-approved treatments for nicotine use disorder in adults. NRT is available via five different delivery methods: patch, gum, lozenge, inhaler, and nasal spray. Randomized trials involving adolescents have evaluated tobacco cessation pharmacotherapies, and the combination of bupropion with psychosocial interventions has had the most promising findings (Squeglia et al. 2019). Although used for its norepinephrine and dopamine reuptake inhibition, bupropion also acts as a nicotinic receptor antagonist, allowing it to block the effects of nicotine while mitigating withdrawal symptoms by increasing dopamine and norepinephrine in the brain. Bupropion is contraindicated in individuals with a history of eating disorders or seizure disorders, including seizures induced by alcohol withdrawal. No studies are available that have assessed using electronic nicotine delivery systems as a tool for smoking cessation, and it is thought that these systems have high misuse potential and may lead to the use of cigarettes.

## Cannabis Use Disorder

Cannabis use is the most common reason for substance use treatment referrals among adolescents. No pharmacotherapies are FDA-approved for CaUD in adults or adolescents, but some clinical trials assessing medication-assisted treatment for adolescent CaUD are available. *N*-acetylcysteine (NAC) combined with behavioral strategies has shown promising results compared with placebo (Squeglia et al. 2019). NAC can be obtained OTC and is most often prescribed as a mucolytic or for acetaminophen overdose. It has an established safety record in both adult and pediatric populations. Administration forms include oral, intravenous, and inhaled. NAC repairs glutamate homeostasis via upregulation of the glutamate transporter (GLT-1), which clears excess glutamate from the nucleus accumbens and reduces substance seeking and self-administration of substances. Topiramate is another agent studied in adolescent CaUD, but the results were not favorable compared with those for placebo because of its limited efficacy and substantial side effect profile.

## Opioid Use Disorder

Despite the low prevalence of opioid use among adolescents compared with adults, morbidity and mortality rates for adolescent OUD remain high and warrant effective treatment options. As stated in the "Medications" section, buprenorphine is the only FDA-approved medication-assisted treatment option for any SUD with an indication for OUD in adolescents age 16 years or older (Squeglia et al. 2019). Buprenorphine is a synthetic opioid developed in the late 1960s. It acts as a partial agonist at the μ receptor. Because of this unique pharmacological property, its analgesic properties plateau at higher doses and become antagonistic. It also has slow dissociation kinetics at the receptor, allowing for milder withdrawal symptoms than a full opioid agonist. The goal is to use buprenorphine as a substitute for more potent full μ opioid agonists (e.g., heroin, fentanyl, oxycodone), gradually tapering it over time to allow patients to withdraw with minimal discomfort. This substitution gives patients the opportunity to focus more on psychosocial interventions than on withdrawal symptoms, which are known to be highly uncomfortable.

## Psychosocial Interventions

Psychosocial interventions are the primary means of adolescent SUD treatment, given the limited data available for pharmacotherapies in this demographic. These interventions consist of various psychotherapeutic modalities and are necessary for successful treatment outcomes. Numerous evidence-based studies support their effectiveness (Fadus et al. 2019).

### Cognitive-Behavioral Therapy

The focal point of cognitive-behavioral therapy (CBT) is that thoughts about oneself, others, and the environment, if distorted, can negatively influence behavior. As it relates to substance use, CBT is used to help patients develop self-regulation and coping skills. CBT techniques help youth identify emotional or behavioral signs that may precede substance use, use diverse strategies to avoid situations that may precipitate the desire to use, and develop better communication and problem-solving skills (Winters et al. 2009).

### Contingency Management

Contingency management follows the operant conditioning model by providing positive reinforcement (e.g., tangible incentives such as rewards or privileges) for remaining sober and engaging in treatment (Boustani et al. 2019).

### Motivational Interviewing and Brief Intervention

Motivational interviewing and brief intervention use a person-centered, non-confrontational approach to help patients examine different aspects of their substance use patterns and create goals to attain a healthier lifestyle. The relationship between the therapist and adolescent is framed as a partnership, and the adolescent's autonomy regarding their substance use is respected. However, the therapist retains a directive role to encourage a change in behavior and resolve ambivalence using a noncoercive approach.

## Group Therapy

The peer support offered in group therapy can serve as an advantage and enhance motivation to remain sober. It is important to note that this method can have adverse outcomes if not implemented properly. Poor outcomes can be avoided by ensuring a heterogeneous group that includes prosocial youth, having well-trained therapists, maintaining appropriate supervision, and conducting manualized interventions that include ways to prevent or reduce harmful and verbally offensive references to group members.

## Family Therapy

Family therapy centers on the idea that an adolescent's family has a profound and enduring influence on their development. It includes the adolescent and at least one parent or guardian to assess and mediate family risk factors such as poor communication and problem-solving. Table 13–5 describes the various types of family therapy models.

# Microprocessor Disorders

Microprocessors include any electronic devices capable of carrying out the functions of a computer's central processing unit. Microprocessor addiction is described as recurrent use of microprocessors to the extent that it results in clinically significant impairment or distress, with disruption in various aspects of the individual's life. Microprocessor addiction has various synonyms, including problematic electronics use, problematic gaming, gaming disorder or addiction, and internet gaming disorder. It is also sometimes referred to as process addiction. Microprocessors, including smartphones and computers, are an important part of the modern adolescent's world, essential for their education, safety, social connection, and entertainment. A significant contributor to microprocessor addiction is electronic gaming, which is within the interactive entertainment industry and is estimated to have generated $128.3 billion in 2020, a figure that is twice the revenue generated by the movie industry and 5 times the revenue of the music industry (Alabama News Network 2021).

Estimates indicate that more than 95% of adolescents use the internet. Adolescent males engage more on gaming websites than do females (80.3% vs. 28.8%), who engage more on social media. About 8% of video game players ages 8 to 18 manifested pathological play patterns (Gentile 2009; Lee et al. 2017). Youth with pathological gaming were more likely to be male, have poorer grades in school, spend twice as much time playing, and have more

Table 13–5.　Types of family therapy

| Family therapy model | Description |
|---|---|
| Multidimensional family therapy | Focuses on four interdependent treatment domains: adolescent, parent, interactional, and extrafamilial. Considered a comprehensive, but flexible, system of treatment that adapts to individual circumstances. Duration: 4–5 months. |
| Multisystemic therapy | Addresses multiple factors of adolescent and family problems by targeting elements at the individual, family, peer, school, and community levels. Based on practical, goal-oriented techniques and problem-based treatment strategies. Duration: 16 weeks. |
| Functional family therapy | Aims to change dysfunctional family patterns that contribute to adolescent substance use. Structured therapy that is delivered in two phases: engaging and motivating families toward change and effecting behavioral changes. May use behavioral interventions such as contingency management. Duration: 24 weeks. |
| Brief strategic family therapy | Aims to reduce problematic adolescent behavior by improving relationships with the family, peers, and school. A manual-based intervention that is problem focused and directive and follows a structured format that is delivered in phases with specific goals. Duration: 12 weeks. |
| Adolescent community reinforcement approach | Based on the philosophy of using the community to reward sobriety and encourage prosocial behaviors, including family, social, educational, and vocational reinforcers. Case management services are usually included. Duration: 12 weeks. |
| Assertive continuing care | Home-based program that is usually offered after residential treatment. Uses an operant reinforcement and skills training module to assist the adolescent and their family with developing prosocial behaviors and navigating community services. Duration: 12–14 weeks. |

attentional problems compared with youth without gaming problems. They have also been discovered to have lower social competence and higher rates of ADHD, disruptive mood dysregulation disorder, depression, and social anxiety (Salerno et al. 2022). Furthermore, some studies have revealed that ADHD symptoms were associated with the severity of internet gaming disorder symptoms, with inattention showing the strongest association, followed by impulsivity (Park et al. 2017). The behavioral traits of hostility and narcissistic personality traits are also higher in such youth (Baer et al. 2012).

## Neurobiology

Like other addictions, microprocessor addictions are thought to stimulate synaptic dopaminergic transmission, resulting in activation of brain areas related to reward and enhancing attentional capacity. During gaming, repetitive activation of the brain's dopaminergic reward system and working memory system induces complex competitions and interactions between interhemispheric neurons. Additionally, the repetitive visuospatial working memory and executive function activation may promote increased neuronal connectivity. The anterior cingulate cortex, the central hub in top-down attentional processes that results in selective or focused attention, consistently shows functional activity during video game playing (Han et al. 2012). Habitual gamers have been found to have more efficient top-down resource allocation during demanding attentional tasks, allowing them to hyperfocus on gaming for longer periods. However, this is to the detriment of other stimuli in their immediate and remote environment. As such, they are often unaware of the need to eat, sleep, and self-care, invariably neglecting vital aspects of their life.

## Diagnosis and Treatment

Given that smart devices with internet connections are omnipresent in the modern individual's life, treating microprocessor addictions is a challenge. Scales commonly used to measure levels of symptoms include the 20-item Young's Internet Addiction Scale (YIAS) and the short and long forms of the Internet Gaming Disorder Scale (IGDS), with 9 and 27 items, respectively. Currently, no medication has received FDA approval for treating microprocessor disorders. However, treatment studies have yielded positive responses to bupropion, methylphenidate, atomoxetine, and escitalopram (Han et al. 2009, 2010; Park et al. 2016; Song et al. 2016). Treatment of gaming disorder is more efficacious when the underlying symptoms of ADHD are controlled (Chang et al. 2020). Psychological treatment studies include CBT; motivational interviewing; eclectic psychotherapy intervention, which includes a combination of CBT, family therapy, and motivational interviewing; and solutions-focused therapy (Kim et al. 2012).

# Conclusion

Adolescence is a unique period filled with physical, emotional, and social growth. The separation from parental figures and exploration of personal identity naturally involve experimentation. Although this process is expected and healthy, this stage increases the adolescent's vulnerability to potentially harmful activities. Screening, diagnosis, and treatment of underlying psychiatric conditions and SUDs strike a balance between patient autonomy and familial involvement. Although counterintuitive, a clinician working with this population may go further by approaching the adolescent with an open mind, mentoring rather than commanding.

# References

Alabama News Network: Global digital video game industry sees 40% jump in 2021. Alabama News Network, May 3, 2021. Available at: https://www.alabamanews.net/2021/05/03/global-digital-video-game-industry-sees-40-jump-in-2021. Accessed March 26, 2022.

American Psychiatric Association: Diagnostic and Statistical Manual of Mental Disorders, 5th Edition. Arlington, VA, American Psychiatric Association, 2022

Baer S, Saran K, Green DA, Hong I: Electronic media use and addiction among youth in psychiatric clinic versus school populations. Can J Psychiatry 57(12):728–735, 2012

Basedow LA, Kuitunen-Paul S, Wiedmann MF, et al: Verbal learning impairment in adolescents with methamphetamine use disorder: a cross-sectional study. BMC Psychiatry 21(1):166, 2021

Bhatia D, Mikulich-Gilbertson SK, Sakai JT: Prescription opioid misuse and risky adolescent behavior. Pediatrics 145(2):e20192470, 2020 31907292

Biederman J: Pharmacotherapy for attention-deficit/hyperactivity disorder (ADHD) decreases the risk for substance abuse: findings from a longitudinal follow-up of youths with and without ADHD. J Clin Psychiatry 64(Suppl 11):3–8, 2003 14529323

Blanco C, Flórez-Salamanca L, Secades-Villa R, et al: Predictors of initiation of nicotine, alcohol, cannabis, and cocaine use: results of the National Epidemiologic Survey on Alcohol and Related Conditions (NESARC). Am J Addict 27(6):477–484, 2018 30088294

Bourque J, Afzali MH, Conrod PJ: Association of cannabis use with adolescent psychotic symptoms. JAMA Psychiatry 75(8):864–866, 2018 29874357

Boustani MM, Henderson CE, Liddle HA: Family-based treatments for adolescent substance abuse: advances yield new developmental challenges, in The Oxford Handbook of Adolescent Substance Abuse. Edited by Zucker RA, Brown SA. New York, Oxford University Press, 2019, pp 675–716

Boykan R, Messina CR, Chateau G, et al: Self-reported use of tobacco, e-cigarettes, and marijuana versus urinary biomarkers. Pediatrics 143(5):e20183531, 2019 31010908

Caldwell LC, Schweinsburg AD, Nagel BJ, et al: Gender and adolescent alcohol use disorders on BOLD (blood oxygen level dependent) response to spatial working memory. Alcohol Alcohol 40(3):194–200, 2005 15668210

Chadwick B, Miller ML, Hurd YL: Cannabis use during adolescent development: susceptibility to psychiatric illness. Front Psychiatry 4(Oct):129, 2013 24133461

Chambers RA, Taylor JR, Potenza MN: Developmental neurocircuitry of motivation in adolescence: a critical period of addiction vulnerability. Am J Psychiatry 160(6):1041–1052, 2003 12777258

Chang C-H, Chang Y-C, Cheng H, et al: Treatment efficacy of internet gaming disorder with attention deficit hyperactivity disorder and emotional dysregulation. Int J Neuropsychopharmacol 23(6):349–355, 2020 32047929

Charach A, Yeung E, Climans T, et al: Childhood attention-deficit/hyperactivity disorder and future substance use disorders: comparative meta-analyses. J Am Acad Child Adolesc Psychiatry 50(1):9–21, 2011 21156266

Chen K, Kandel DB: The natural history of drug use from adolescence to the mid-thirties in a general population sample. Am J Public Health 85(1):41–47, 1995 7832260

Chung T, Martin CS, Cornelius JR, et al: Cannabis withdrawal predicts severity of cannabis involvement at 1-year follow-up among treated adolescents. Addiction 103(5):787–799, 2008 18412757

Crum RM, Green KM, Storr CL, et al: Depressed mood in childhood and subsequent alcohol use through adolescence and young adulthood. Arch Gen Psychiatry 65(6):702–712, 2008 18519828

Dalsgaard S, Mortensen PB, Frydenberg M, et al: ADHD, stimulant treatment in childhood and subsequent substance abuse in adulthood: a naturalistic long-term follow-up study. Addict Behav 39(1):325–328, 2014 24090624

Deas-Nesmith D, Brady KT, Campbell S: Comorbid substance use and anxiety disorders in adolescents. J Psychopathol Behav Assess 20(2):139–148, 1998

Disney ER, Elkins IJ, McGue M, et al: Effects of ADHD, conduct disorder, and gender on substance use and abuse in adolescence. Am J Psychiatry 156(10):1515–1521, 1999 10518160

Dumontheil I: Adolescent brain development. Curr Opin Behav Sci 10:39–44, 2016

Dwyer JB, McQuown SC, Leslie FM: The dynamic effects of nicotine on the developing brain. Pharmacol Ther 122(2):125–139, 2009 19268688

Fadus MC, Squeglia LM, Valadez EA, et al: Adolescent substance use disorder treatment: an update on evidence-based strategies. Curr Psychiatry Rep 21(10):96, 2019

Field M, Christiansen P, Cole J, et al: Delay discounting and the alcohol Stroop in heavy drinking adolescents. Addiction 102(4):579–586, 2007 17309540

Gentile D: Pathological video-game use among youth ages 8 to 18: a national study. Psychol Sci 20(5):594–602, 2009 19476590

Goldenson NI, Leventhal AM, Stone MD, et al: Associations of electronic cigarette nicotine concentration with subsequent cigarette smoking and vaping levels in adolescents. JAMA Pediatr 171(12):1192–1199, 2017 29059261

Goldstein BI, Bukstein OG: Comorbid substance use disorders among youth with bipolar disorder: opportunities for early identification and prevention. J Clin Psychiatry 71(3):348–358, 2010

Grace AA, Floresco SB, Goto Y, et al: Regulation of firing of dopaminergic neurons and control of goal-directed behaviors. Trends Neurosci 30(5):220–227, 2007 17400299

Griesler PC, Hu M-C, Wall MM, et al: Assessment of prescription opioid medical use and misuse among parents and their adolescent offspring in the US. JAMA Netw Open 4(1):e2031073, 2021 33410876

Griffith-Lendering MFH, Wigman JTW, Prince van Leeuwen A, et al: Cannabis use and vulnerability for psychosis in early adolescence: a TRAILS study. Addiction 108(4):733–740, 2013 23216690

Han DH, Lee YS, Na C, et al: The effect of methylphenidate on internet video game play in children with attention-deficit/hyperactivity disorder. Compr Psychiatry 50(3):251–256, 2009 19374970

Han DH, Hwang JW, Renshaw PF: Bupropion sustained release treatment decreases craving for video games and cue-induced brain activity in patients with internet video game addiction. Exp Clin Psychopharmacol 18(4):297–304, 2010 20695685

Han DH, Kim SM, Lee YS, et al: The effect of family therapy on the changes in the severity of on-line game play and brain activity in adolescents with on-line game addiction. Psychiatry Res 202(2):126–131, 2012 22698763

Hanson KL, Cummins K, Tapert SF, et al: Changes in neuropsychological functioning over 10 years following adolescent substance abuse treatment. Psychol Addict Behav 25(1):127–142, 2011 21443308

Johnston LD, Miech RA, O'Malley PM, et al: Monitoring the Future national survey results on drug use, 1975–2021: overview, key findings on adolescent drug use. Bethesda, MD, National Institute on Drug Abuse, January 2022. Available at:

https://monitoringthefuture.org/wp-content/uploads/2023/01/mtfoverview2022.pdf. Accessed February 25, 2023.

Kelly SM, Gryczynski J, Mitchell SG, et al: Validity of brief screening instrument for adolescent tobacco, alcohol, and drug use. Pediatrics 133(5):819–826, 2014 24753528

Kim SM, Han DH, Lee YS, et al: Combined cognitive behavioral therapy and bupropion for the treatment of problematic on-line game play in adolescents with major depressive disorder. Comput Human Behav 28:1954–1959, 2012

Knight JR, Sherritt L, Shrier LA, et al: Validity of the CRAFFT substance abuse screening test among adolescent clinic patients. Arch Pediatr Adolesc Med 156(6):607–614, 2002 12038895

Langlois S, Zern A, Kelley ME, et al: Adversity in childhood/adolescence and premorbid tobacco, alcohol, and cannabis use among first-episode psychosis patients. Early Interv Psychiatry 15(5):1335–1342, 2021 33289325

Lee HH, Sung JH, Lee JY, et al: Differences by sex in association of mental health with video gaming or other nonacademic computer use among US adolescents. Prev Chronic Dis 14:E117, 2017 29166250

Lee LK, Mannix R: Increasing fatality rates from preventable deaths in teenagers and young adults. JAMA 320(6):543–544, 2018 29852050

Levy S, Siqueira LM, Ammerman SD, et al: Testing for drugs of abuse in children and adolescents. Pediatrics 133(6):e1798–e1807, 2014 24864184

Levy S, Weitzman ER, Marin AC, et al: Sensitivity and specificity of S2BI for identifying alcohol and cannabis use disorders among adolescents presenting for primary care. Subst Abus 42(3):388–395, 2021 32814009

Liskola J, Haravuori H, Lindberg N, et al: The predictive capacity of AUDIT and AUDIT-C among adolescents in a one-year follow-up study. Drug Alcohol Depend 218(Jan):108424, 2021 33257195

Marshall EJ: Adolescent alcohol use: risks and consequences. Alcohol Alcohol 49(2):160–164, 2014 24402246

McCabe SE, Dickinson K, West BT, et al: Age of onset, duration, and type of medication therapy for attention-deficit/hyperactivity disorder and substance use during adolescence: a multi-cohort national study. J Am Acad Child Adolesc Psychiatry 55(6):479–486, 2016 27238066

McCabe SE, Schulenberg JE, Schepis TS, et al: Longitudinal analysis of substance use disorder symptom severity at age 18 years and substance use disorder in adulthood. JAMA Netw Open 5(4):e225324, 2022

McGrath JJ, Alati R, Clavarino A, et al: Age at first tobacco use and risk of subsequent psychosis-related outcomes: a birth cohort study. Aust N Z J Psychiatry 50(6):577–583, 2016 25991762

McNeill AD, West RJ, Jarvis M, et al: Cigarette withdrawal symptoms in adolescent smokers. Psychopharmacology (Berl) 90(4):533–536, 1986 3101108

Medina KL, Schweinsburg AD, Cohen-Zion M, et al: Effects of alcohol and combined marijuana and alcohol use during adolescence on hippocampal volume and asymmetry. Neurotoxicol Teratol 29(1):141–152, 2007 17169528

Meier MH, Caspi A, Danese A, et al: Associations between adolescent cannabis use and neuropsychological decline: a longitudinal co-twin control study. Addiction 113(2):257–265, 2018 28734078

Miech R, Leventhal A, Johnston L, et al: Trends in use and perceptions of nicotine vaping among US youth from 2017 to 2020. JAMA Pediatr 175(2):185–190, 2021 33320241

Molina BSG, Hinshaw SP, Eugene Arnold L, et al: Adolescent substance use in the multimodal treatment study of attention-deficit/hyperactivity disorder (ADHD) (MTA) as a function of childhood ADHD, random assignment to childhood treatments, and subsequent medication. J Am Acad Child Adolesc Psychiatry 52(3):250–263, 2013 23452682

Nguyen-Louie TT, Matt GE, Jacobus J, et al: Earlier alcohol use onset predicts poorer neuropsychological functioning in young adults. Alcohol Clin Exp Res 41(12):2082–2092, 2017 29083495

O'Donnell P: Adolescent maturation of cortical dopamine. Neurotox Res 18(3–4):306–312, 2010 20151241

O'Neil KA, Conner BT, Kendall PC: Internalizing disorders and substance use disorders in youth: comorbidity, risk, temporal order, and implications for intervention. Clin Psychol Rev 31(1):104–112, 2011

Park JH, Lee YS, Sohn JH, et al: Effectiveness of atomoxetine and methylphenidate for problematic online gaming in adolescents with attention deficit hyperactivity disorder. Hum Psychopharmacol 31(6):427–432, 2016 27859666

Park JH, Hong JS, Han DH, et al: Comparison of QEEG findings between adolescents with attention deficit hyperactivity disorder (ADHD) without comorbidity and ADHD comorbid with internet gaming disorder. J Korean Med Sci 32(3):514–521, 2017 28145657

Peters J, Bromberg U, Schneider S, et al: Lower ventral striatal activation during reward anticipation in adolescent smokers. Am J Psychiatry 168(5):540–549, 2011 21362742

Quigley J, Committee on Substance Use and Prevention: Alcohol use by youth. Pediatrics 144(1):e20191356, 2019 31235610

Rubino T, Parolaro D: Long lasting consequences of cannabis exposure in adolescence. Mol Cell Endocrinol 286(1–2)(Suppl 1):S108–S113, 2008 18358595

Ryan SA: Cocaine use in adolescents and young adults. Pediatr Clin North Am 66(6):1135–1147, 2019 31679603

Salerno L, Becheri L, Pallanti S: ADHD-gaming disorder comorbidity in children and adolescents: a narrative review. Children (Basel) 9(10):1528, 2022

Schepis TS, Adinoff B, Rao U: Neurobiological processes in adolescent addictive disorders. Am J Addict 17(1):6–23, 2008 18214718

Schumann G, Loth E, Banaschewski T, et al: The IMAGEN study: reinforcement-related behaviour in normal brain function and psychopathology. Mol Psychiatry 15(12):1128–1139, 2010 21102431

Skinner HA: The drug abuse screening test. Addict Behav 7(4):363–371, 1982 7183189

Song J, Park JH, Han DH, et al: Comparative study of the effects of bupropion and escitalopram on internet gaming disorder. Psychiatry Clin Neurosci 70(11):527–535, 2016 27487975

Spear LP: The adolescent brain and age-related behavioral manifestations. Neurosci Biobehav Rev 24(4):417–463, 2000 10817843

Squeglia LM, Fadus MC, McClure EA, et al: Pharmacological treatment of youth substance use disorders. J Child Adolesc Psychopharmacol 29(7):559–572, 2019 31009234

Substance Abuse and Mental Health Services Administration: Key Substance Use and Mental Health Indicators in the United States: Results From the 2020 National Survey on Drug Use and Health. Rockville, MD, Substance Abuse and Mental Health Services Administration, 2021. Available at: https://www.samhsa.gov/data/sites/default/files/reports/rpt35325/NSDUHFFRPDFWHTMLFiles2020/2020NSDUHFFR1PDFW102121.pdf. Accessed February 15, 2023.

Volkow N: Suicide deaths are a major component of the opioid crisis that must be addressed. Nora's Blog, September 19, 2019. Available at: https://nida.nih.gov/about-nida/noras-blog/2019/09/suicide-deaths-are-major-component-opioid-crisis-must-be-addressed. Accessed March 26, 2022.

Volkow ND, Wargo EM: Association of severity of adolescent substance use disorders and long-term outcomes. JAMA Netw Open 5(4):e225656, 2022 35363272

Volkow ND, Han B, Einstein EB, et al: Prevalence of substance use disorders by time since first substance use among young people in the US. JAMA Pediatr 175(6):640–643, 2021 33779715

Waxmonsky JG, Wilens TE: Pharmacotherapy of adolescent substance use disorders: a review of the literature. J Child Adolesc Psychopharmacol 15(5):810–825, 2005 16262597

Wetherill RR, Squeglia LM, Yang TT, et al: A longitudinal examination of adolescent response inhibition: neural differences before and after the initiation of heavy drinking. Psychopharmacology (Berl) 230(4):663–671, 2013 23832422

Williams JF, Lundahl LH: Focus on adolescent use of club drugs and "other" substances. Pediatr Clin North Am 66(6):1121–1134, 2019 31679602

Williams NJ, Scott L, Aarons GA: Prevalence of serious emotional disturbance among U.S. children: a meta-analysis. Psychiatr Serv 69(1):32–40, 2018 28859585

Wilson CR, Sherritt L, Gates E, et al: Are clinical impressions of adolescent substance use accurate? Pediatrics 114(5):e536–e540, 2004 15520086

Winstanley EL, Steinwachs DM, Stitzer ML, et al: Adolescent substance abuse and mental health: problem co-occurrence and access to services. J Child Adolesc Subst Abuse 21(4):310–322, 2012 24532964

Winters KC, Botzet AM, Fahnhorst T, et al: Adolescent substance abuse treatment: a review of evidence-based research, in Adolescent Substance Abuse: Evidence-Based Approaches to Prevention and Treatment (Issues in Children's and Families' Lives). Edited by Leukefeld CG, Gullotta TP. New York, Springer, 2009, pp 73–96

Winters KC, Botzet AM, Fahnhorst T: Advances in adolescent substance abuse treatment. Curr Psychiatry Rep 13(5):416–421, 2011 21701838

# 14

# Substance Use Disorders in the LGBTQ+ Population

## Daryl Shorter, M.D.

*Persons* identifying as lesbian, gay, bisexual, transgender, and queer/questioning (LGBTQ+) represent a particularly vulnerable community with an increased risk for developing substance use disorders (SUDs). Compared with cisgender and/or heterosexual persons, people who are LGBTQ+ have higher rates of smoking than the general population, are more likely to use alcohol recreationally and to use other substances, have higher rates of SUDs, and are less likely to abstain from substance use (Eliason et al. 2012; Substance Abuse and Mental Health Services Administration 2001). Rather than considering this increased risk to be secondary or related to factors inherent within LGBTQ+ identity, however, clinicians must first understand this heightened vulnerability in relation to the forces of discrimination that contribute to psychosocial stress among LGBTQ+ persons.

*Heteronormativity* refers to rules of "correct" behavior that are both explicitly and implicitly communicated and imply that social and cultural appropriateness is achieved primarily by identifying with and leading a heterosexual lifestyle. These messages are transmitted from an early age and are carried forward throughout the life cycle. Operating from within the framework of heteronormativity, it is assumed, for example, that men and women will *marry* and have children, among other expectations and values. Behavior also may be rooted in rigid and inflexible gender roles, sometimes referred to as *toxic masculinity* and *toxic femininity*. Furthermore, outright discrimination and hatred of LGBTQ+ persons can take the form of homophobia or transphobia and are associated with increased risk for bullying and violence, victimization, and worsened health and psychosocial outcomes (Meyer 2008). Taken together, these forces increase the overall stress (historically referred to as *minority stress*) under which LGBTQ+ individuals live and represent a significant factor in their predisposition to, and perpetuation of, substance use (Dyar et al. 2019). A number of factors are protective against LGBTQ+-related mental health challenges and SUDs, including family acceptance of the LGBTQ+ identity, social support from friends, the presence of gay-straight alliances in schools, and specific nondiscrimination policies protecting LGBTQ+ persons (Hall 2018; Hatzenbuehler 2011; Ryan et al. 2010).

# General Approach to Treatment

## Discuss LGBTQ+ Identity With Patients

When working with LGBTQ+ patients who use substances or have SUDs, it is critically important to understand the context under which the person is presenting for evaluation and treatment. This includes understanding their relationship to their own sexual orientation and/or gender identity. For example, clinicians should inquire whether the person is "out," meaning they have shared with others their LGBTQ+ status. In addition, clinicians should assess for any past rejection or lack of acceptance within the family or community. This information may help the clinician understand historical trauma as well as the patient's process of self-acceptance. Although some studies have found that gay and bisexual males who are out are less likely to engage in substance use because they have disclosed their identity to others and perhaps gained support or acceptance, other studies suggest that those who are out are more likely than closeted males to engage in substance use, which is commonly performed in club settings (Petersson et al. 2016). Therefore, it is important to avoid making assumptions regarding whether a person is more or less likely to engage in substance use just on the basis of their out status. These distinctions may also reflect other aspects of their identity (e.g., race or ethnicity) or social factors such as employment, socioeconomic status, or geographical location.

When discussing substance use with LGBTQ+ patients, a focus on both initiation and trajectory of use over time is warranted. Because LGBTQ+ safe spaces have historically been associated with nightlife, bars, or clubs, patients may have first encountered or used substances within those environments. More recently, with the advent of online dating, the generalized spread and expansion of hookup culture, and the reduction in the number of LGBTQ+-specific bars and clubs, many individuals connect via smartphone apps and online websites. These virtual spaces can also serve as access points to obtain substances, encounter other substance users, and engage in sexual activities enhanced by substance use (see "Assess History and Current Risk for Participation in Chemsex" section). Clinicians should talk with patients about their use of smartphone or dating apps because working with patients to develop a social life and connections within the community that do not involve bars and clubs or certain online spaces can be an important treatment element when working with LGBTQ+ patients with SUD.

Just as some people may be out, others do not easily or readily identify with an LGBTQ+ identity. When patients are reluctant to discuss LGBTQ+ identity or do not feel their sexual orientation or gender identity is related to their substance use, rather than argue with or confront them, clinicians should accept their perspective and allow the door to remain open to future conversations. Clinicians should reassure patients that the treatment relationship is a safe place for them, regardless of whether they feel comfortable discussing sex or sexuality-related topics.

Finally, for some members of the LGBTQ+ community, concealing sexual orientation or gender identity may not be easily accomplished, contributing even further to possible discrimination and marginalization and perhaps placing them at risk for victimization. Thoroughly discussing with patients their feelings about their LGBTQ+ status can enhance the therapeutic alliance, create opportunities for them to feel seen and better understood, and provide clues for potential areas of focus during treatment.

## Assess History and Current Risk for Participation in Chemsex

The use of psychoactive substances during sexual encounters, also referred to as *chemsex*, has been an area of particular focus among providers caring for members of the LGBTQ+ community. Chemsex has also been increasingly associated with increased risk of HIV seroconversion and of contracting other sexually transmitted infections (see Chapter 11, "HIV and Substance Use Disorders"). It is important to recognize, however, that substance use during sexual encounters is neither exclusive to LGBTQ+ persons nor a new phenomenon.

When we discuss chemsex in this chapter in relation to LGBTQ+ persons with SUD, we are referring to a specific type of sexualized drug use among LGBTQ+ individuals (predominantly, men who have sex with men [MSM] but also women who have sex with women and transgender individuals) that is intended not only to enhance the quality and duration of the sexual encounter but also to reduce feelings of guilt and shame associated with same-sex and/or transgender sexual practices. Although chemsex broadly refers to sex involving substances of any kind, the drugs most commonly associated with sex (and studied by researchers) include cannabis, methamphetamine, and amyl nitrate (commonly known as poppers). Other substances that may be involved in the realm of chemsex include cocaine, $\gamma$-hydroxybutyrate (GHB) or $\gamma$-butyrolactone (GBL), 3,4-methylenedioxymethamphetamine (MDMA), ketamine, and erectile dysfunction medications such as sildenafil. Ultimately, the relationship of LGBTQ+ persons with chemsex is quite complicated. Despite the known risks of HIV seroconversion and other sexually transmitted infections, rates of chemsex appear to be increasing (Rosner et al. 2021).

## Acknowledge Intersectional Identity

Clinicians must remember that LGBTQ+ identity can be further complicated by the presence of other intersecting marginalized or minoritized identities, such as those based on race/ethnicity, sex/gender, disability, geographical location, and socioeconomic status. Not all LGBTQ+ people experience the same types and levels of discrimination, and those with multiple identities may feel discriminated against more on the basis of group identifications than on LGBTQ+ identity. Ultimately, acknowledging the possibility of this complicated experience and allowing it to play a role in both diagnostic formulation and treatment planning can be a vital component in establishing rapport, demonstrating cultural competency and humility, and promoting treatment retention.

## Combine Pharmacotherapy With Motivational Enhancement and Skills-Building

When working with LGBTQ+ patients with SUDs, the clinician should approach treatment from a patient-centered perspective, helping them identify their goals and values and working with them to understand and articulate the goals of treatment. In some cases, abstinence may not be a goal, and patients may only hope to change their relationship with a particular substance or to reduce the potential for harm related to substance use. By combining motivational interviewing with skills building, clinicians can help patients begin to work toward their self-defined goals. When possible, supporting their work with pharmacotherapy can be helpful with treatment retention and harm reduction.

# Substance Use Disorder Pharmacotherapy

Much of the research on treating SUD in LGBTQ+ populations has focused on psychotherapeutic interventions. Novel modifications of more classical forms of psychotherapy consider inclusion of LGBTQ+ identity to be a critical component of the overall therapeutic process. Treatment goals are neither to change nor to alter sexual orientation or gender identity (as with conversion therapies) but rather to inform an approach that focuses on the patient's self-acceptance and identity integration. Additional work may be needed in relation to coming to terms with family or other community members, such as those with church or religious affiliations, who are not accepting of LGBTQ+ identity. Therapists may also work with patients to reduce feelings of shame related to LGBTQ+ identity and increase shame resilience.

When focused primarily on SUDs, in addition to including their patients' LGBTQ+ identity, therapists should employ motivational interviewing to clarify patients' values and goals related to substance use and to enhance their desire to change. Therapists should also assist patients with developing skills to tolerate, reduce, or resist drug craving and to bolster self-efficacy. Therapeutic interventions offer practical information related to harm reduction; promote safer sexual practices; encourage medication adherence for HIV preexposure prophylaxis, postexposure prophylaxis, or antiretroviral therapy; and promote other behaviors related to health care screening, nutrition, and exercise. Despite these innovations, however, the therapeutic approach toward LGBTQ+ persons with SUDs remains a much-needed area of research.

Unfortunately, addiction pharmacotherapy has been even less studied in clinical trials of LGBTQ+ persons in SUD treatment. Currently no clinical trials focusing on buprenorphine or methadone treatment of opioid use disorder (OUD) in this population have been published, despite a need for LGBTQ+-specific OUD treatment programs and substantial barriers to care among LGBTQ+ persons with OUD (Paschen-Wolff et al. 2022). Examination of off-label pharmacotherapy for treatment of cannabis use disorder

(CaUD), hallucinogen use disorder, and sedative, hypnotic, or anxiolytic use disorder is also absent from the literature. Perhaps even more alarming, strikingly few studies focus on lesbian females, and even in cases in which lesbian females are included in the study, the outcomes specific to this group are not reported (Kidd et al. 2022).

Clinical trials among LGBTQ+ persons with SUDs have focused primarily on alcohol, tobacco, and methamphetamine (Table 14–1). Alcohol studies range from those aimed at reducing alcohol consumption among persons with problematic or heavy episodic drinking to treating DSM-5-defined alcohol use disorder (AUD) (American Psychiatric Association 2022). Trials involving pharmacotherapy for smoking cessation among LGBTQ+ persons include nicotine replacement therapy (NRT) alone or in combination with bupropion; however, studies focus primarily on behavioral intervention, with pharmacotherapy used as a pillar of the overall treatment program. There are currently no randomized, placebo-controlled studies of medications such as bupropion or varenicline for treating nicotine use disorder among LGBTQ+ persons. Studies focusing on methamphetamine typically focus on gay and bisexual males or MSM, with non-Hispanic white males making up most of the respective samples. Other investigational agents that may hold promise in the treatment of SUD among LGBTQ+ persons include oxytocin for methamphetamine use disorder (MUD), which has been shown in clinical trials to increase treatment attendance and be safely tolerated (Stauffer et al. 2020).

# Guiding Principles

When working with LGBTQ+ patients with SUDs, clinicians should consider the role of pharmacotherapy in the development of a comprehensive treatment plan.

1. Because rates of smoking are higher among LGBTQ+ persons in comparison with their cisgender and/or heterosexual counterparts, specific interventions are needed that apply motivational enhancement in relation to tobacco and nicotine use within the context of their sexual- and gender-identity minoritized status. Medications with FDA approval for the treatment of nicotine use disorder, such as NRT, bupropion, and varenicline, should be offered along with smoking cessation counseling, group therapy, and tobacco quitlines and text lines. Response rates among gay and bisexual men may be higher at the initiation of treatment.

**Table 14–1.  Summary of clinical pharmacotherapy trials for treatment of substance use disorder among LGBTQ+ persons**

| Study | Participants | Trial duration | Intervention | Findings |
|---|---|---|---|---|
| **Alcohol** | | | | |
| Morgenstern et al. 2012 | 200 MSM with "problem drinking" seeking to reduce, not quit | 12 weeks | Four groups: <br>1) MBSCT + naltrexone <br>2) MBSCT + placebo <br>3) Medication counseling + naltrexone <br>4) Medication counseling + placebo (12 weeks) | Decreased drinks per week and decreased HDD in MBSCT groups compared with others <br><br> Decreased likelihood of nonhazardous drinking in naltrexone vs. placebo |
| Santos et al. 2016 | 30 MSM with methamphetamine use and heavy episodic alcohol (binge) consumption | 8 weeks | Two groups: naltrexone 50 mg vs. placebo (+ SUD counseling, behavioral assessment q 2 weeks) | No differences in methamphetamine use or drinking <br><br> Greater reduction in serodiscordant RAI and serodiscordant condomless RAI in naltrexone group <br><br> Greater decrease in methamphetamine use days and HDD in frequent methamphetamine users in naltrexone group |

**Table 14–1.** Summary of clinical pharmacotherapy trials for treatment of substance use disorder among LGBTQ+ persons (*continued*)

| Study | Participants | Trial duration | Intervention | Findings |
|---|---|---|---|---|
| **Alcohol** (*continued*) | | | | |
| Gonzales et al. 2020 | 155 persons (both MSM and transgender women) with AUD and HIV, newly initiating ART | 48 weeks | Naltrexone 50 mg/day initiated concomitantly with ART ($n=103$) vs. ART + placebo ($n=52$) for 24 weeks, followed by ART alone for 24 weeks | Drinking effects not reported  No difference in adverse events with naltrexone + ART in comparison with naltrexone + placebo |
| **Tobacco** | | | | |
| Covey et al. 2009 | 54 gay/bisexual and 243 heterosexual males | 8 weeks | Open-label: nicotine patch, bupropion, and counseling | Higher initial abstinence among gay/bisexual smokers in first 2 weeks; abstinence rates converged and were identical by end of treatment |
| **Methamphetamine** | | | | |
| Das et al. 2010 | 30 methamphetamine-dependent MSM | 12 weeks | Double-blind, randomized: bupropion XL 300 mg/day vs. placebo | Greater decrease in methamphetamine-positive urine samples in bupropion group but no significant difference  Decreased sexual risk behavior observed in both groups |

**Table 14–1.** Summary of clinical pharmacotherapy trials for treatment of substance use disorder among LGBTQ+ persons *(continued)*

| Study | Participants | Trial duration | Intervention | Findings |
|---|---|---|---|---|
| **Methamphetamine** *(continued)* | | | | |
| McElhiney et al. 2009 | 16 methamphetamine-dependent HIV+ gay men | 18 sessions over 16 weeks | Single-blind: modafinil (up to 200 mg/day) for 12 weeks, followed by placebo for 4 weeks + CBT | 10/16 (77%) completed<br>6/10 reduced methamphetamine use by >50%<br>2/10 discontinued modafinil due to side effects |
| Colfax et al. 2011 | 60 methamphetamine-dependent, sexually active MSM | 12 weeks | Double-blind, randomized: mirtazapine 30 mg/day vs. placebo | Greater reduction in methamphetamine-positive urine samples (73% vs. 44%) in mirtazapine group than in placebo group (67% vs. 63%)<br>Significantly greater reduction in sexual risk behaviors in mirtazapine group:<br>Fewer partners with whom methamphetamine was used<br>Fewer episodes of anal intercourse with serodiscordant partner<br>Fewer episodes of UAI with serodiscordant partner<br>Fewer episodes of IAI with serodiscordant partner |

**Table 14–1.** Summary of clinical pharmacotherapy trials for treatment of substance use disorder among LGBTQ+ persons (*continued*)

| Study | Participants | Trial duration | Intervention | Findings |
|---|---|---|---|---|
| **Methamphetamine** (*continued*) | | | | |
| Coffin et al. 2018 | 100 sexually active, methamphetamine-dependent MSM | 12 weeks | Double-blind, randomized: naltrexone XR 380 mg (*n*=50) vs. placebo (*n*=50) | No significant differences between groups in regard to methamphetamine-positive urine screens<br><br>Decreased sexual risk behaviors in both arms<br><br>High medication adherence, but no advantage compared with placebo |
| Coffin et al. 2020 | 120 community-recruited, sexually active cisgender men (*n*=115) and transgender women (*n*=5) who have sex with men, have MUD, and are actively using | 24 weeks + 12-week follow-up | Double-blind, randomized: mirtazapine 30 mg/day vs. placebo | Greater reduction in methamphetamine-positive urine samples in mirtazapine group at weeks 12, 24, and 36<br><br>At week 24, significantly greater reduction in sexual risk behaviors in mirtazapine group:<br><br>Fewer sexual partners<br><br>Fewer episodes of condomless anal intercourse with serodiscordant partner |

**Table 14–1.** Summary of clinical pharmacotherapy trials for treatment of substance use disorder among LGBTQ+ persons *(continued)*

| Study | Participants | Trial duration | Intervention | Findings |
|---|---|---|---|---|
| **Methamphetamine** *(continued)* | | | | |
| Coffin et al. 2020 *(continued)* | | | | Fewer episodes of condomless RAI<br><br>Fewer depression symptoms, insomnia severity reduced |

*Note.* ART = antiretroviral therapy; AUD = alcohol use disorder; CBT = cognitive-behavioral therapy; HDD = heavy-drinking days; IAI = insertive anal intercourse; MBSCT = modified behavioral self-control therapy, with counseling sessions held weekly; MSM = men who have sex with men; MUD = methamphetamine use disorder; RAI = receptor anal intercourse; SUD = substance use disorder; UAI = unprotected anal intercourse; XL = extended release; XR = extended release.

2. Naltrexone should be included in the medication regimen of LGBTQ+ persons with AUD. This medication can be safely administered to persons with HIV, including concomitant addition with newly initiated antiretroviral therapy. Patient-centered goals that naltrexone may support include both harm reduction (through moderation management) and abstinence initiation.

3. Off-label pharmacotherapy for psychostimulant use and MUD should be provided, particularly given the impact of these medications on reducing HIV risk behaviors in clinical trials. Mirtazapine, in particular, represents a promising option given its additional potential benefits in reducing depression and insomnia.

4. Much investigation of the pharmacological treatment of SUDs among LGBTQ+ persons is needed. There is a surprising lack of research into pharmacotherapy for lesbian and bisexual women and transgender persons. The additional impact of other identities must also be a focus of future investigational study.

# Conclusion

In summary, the treatment of SUDs in people identifying as LGBTQ+ requires a comprehensive understanding of the many factors at play. Heightened vulnerability in this community contributes significantly to substance use and SUD. Treatment approaches must therefore not only address these unique stressors but also factor in the nuances of LGBTQ+ identity, intersectional identities, and the history and trajectory of substance use. Future research efforts must address the striking dearth of knowledge on LGBTQ+ specific treatment. Concurrently, treatment providers must prioritize building safe and accepting environments to foster mutual respect and effective therapeutic alliances.

# References

American Psychiatric Association: Diagnostic and Statistical Manual of Mental Disorders, 5th Edition, Text Revision. Washington, DC, American Psychiatric Association, 2022

Coffin PO, Santos G-M, Hern J, et al: Extended-release naltrexone for methamphetamine dependence among men who have sex with men: a randomized placebo-controlled trial. Addiction 113(2):268–278, 2018 28734107

Coffin PO, Santos G-M, Hern J, et al: Effects of mirtazapine for methamphetamine use disorder among cisgender men and transgender women who have sex with men: a placebo-controlled randomized clinical trial. JAMA Psychiatry 77(3):246–255, 2020 31825466

Colfax GN, Santos GM, Das M, et al: Mirtazapine to reduce methamphetamine use: a randomized controlled trial. Arch Gen Psychiatry 68(11):1168–1175, 2011 22065532

Covey LS, Weissman J, LoDuca C, et al: A comparison of abstinence outcomes among gay/bisexual and heterosexual male smokers in an intensive, non-tailored smoking cessation study. Nicotine Tob Res 11(11):1374–1377, 2009 19778993

Das M, Santos D, Matheson T, et al: Feasibility and acceptability of a phase II randomized pharmacologic intervention for methamphetamine dependence in high-risk men who have sex with men. AIDS 24(7):991–1000, 2010 20397286

Dyar C, Newcomb ME, Mustanski B: Longitudinal associations between minority stressors and substance use among sexual and gender minority individuals. Drug Alcohol Depend 201(August):205–211, 2019 31252354

Eliason MJ, Dibble SL, Gordon R, et al: The last drag: an evaluation of an LGBT-specific smoking intervention. J Homosex 59(6):864–878, 2012 22853185

Gonzales P, Grieco A, White E, et al: Safety of oral naltrexone in HIV-positive men who have sex with men and transgender women with alcohol use disorder and initiating antiretroviral therapy. PLoS One 15(3):e0228433, 2020 32134956

Hall WJ: Psychosocial risk and protective factors for depression among lesbian, gay, bisexual, and queer youth: a systematic review. J Homosex 65(3):263–316, 2018 28394718

Hatzenbuehler ML: The social environment and suicide attempts in lesbian, gay, and bisexual youth. Pediatrics 127(5):896–903, 2011 21502225

Kidd JD, Paschen-Wolff MM, Mericle AA, et al: A scoping review of alcohol, tobacco, and other drug use treatment interventions for sexual and gender minority populations. J Subst Abuse Treat 133(February):108539, 2022 34175174

McElhiney MC, Rabkin JG, Rabkin R, et al: Provigil (modafinil) plus cognitive behavioral therapy for methamphetamine use in HIV+ gay men: a pilot study. Am J Drug Alcohol Abuse 35(1):34–37, 2009 19152204

Meyer D: Interpreting and experiencing anti-queer violence: race, class, and gender differences among LGBT hate crime victims. Race Gend Cl 15(3/4):262–282, 2008

Morgenstern J, Kuerbis AN, Chen AC, et al: A randomized clinical trial of naltrexone and behavioral therapy for problem drinking men who have sex with men. J Consult Clin Psychol 80(5):863–875, 2012 22612306

Paschen-Wolff MM, Velasquez R, Aydinoglo N, et al: Simulating the experience of searching for LGBTQ-specific opioid use disorder treatment in the United States. J Subst Abuse Treat 140(September):108828, 2022 35749919

Petersson FJM, Tikkanen R, Schmidt AJ: Party and play in the closet? Exploring club drug use among Swedish men who have sex with men. Subst Use Misuse 51(9):1093–1103, 2016 27158751

Rosner B, Neicun J, Yang JC, et al: Substance use among sexual minorities in the US—linked to inequalities and unmet need for mental health treatment? Results from the National Survey on Drug Use and Health (NSDUH). J Psychiatr Res 135(Mar):107–118, 2021 33472121

Ryan C, Russell ST, Huebner D, et al: Family acceptance in adolescence and the health of LGBT young adults. J Child Adolesc Psychiatr Nurs 23(4):205–213, 2010 21073595

Santos G-M, Coffin P, Santos D, et al: Feasibility, acceptability, and tolerability of targeted naltrexone for nondependent methamphetamine-using and binge-drinking men who have sex with men. J Acquir Immune Defic Syndr 72(1):21–30, 2016 26674372

Stauffer CS, Moschetto JM, McKernan S, et al: Oxytocin-enhanced group therapy for methamphetamine use disorder: randomized controlled trial. J Subst Abuse Treat 116(Sept):108059, 2020 32741502

Substance Abuse and Mental Health Services Administration: A Provider's Introduction to Substance Abuse Treatment for Lesbian, Gay, Bisexual, and Transgender Individuals (HHS Publ No SMA-12-4104). Rockville, MD, Substance Abuse and Mental Health Services Administration, 2001. Available at: https://store.samhsa.gov/sites/default/files/SAMHSA_Digital_Download/sma12-4104.pdf. Accessed February 27, 2023.

# 15

# Pain and Substance Use Disorders

Benjamin Li, M.D.
Britney Lambert, M.D.
Thanh Thuy Truong, M.D.

## Chronic Pain Evaluation and Management for Patients With Opioid Use Disorder

Many patients who have developed opioid use disorder (OUD) are likely to have chronic pain conditions. One recent estimate in 2022 indicated a 45.3% prevalence of chronic pain among patients with OUD who are receiving opioid substitution therapy, compared with a prevalence of about 30% in the general population (Delorme et al. 2023). Identifying, empathetically understanding, and treating underlying pain conditions are a crucial part of helping someone in recovery, even when pharmacotherapy for the treatment of OUD is already involved. Opioid tolerance, opioid-induced hyperalgesia (OIH), and pseudoaddiction are all processes that may lead to increased doses of opioids that increase harm.

## Tolerance and Opioid-Induced Hyperalgesia

Particularly for those who have OUD and are actively using full opioid agonists, clinicians must be vigilant for signs of OIH and tolerance and how these phenomena may perpetuate the use of the opioid agonist. These are both distinct and separate processes. *Tolerance* is the effect reduction with prolonged opioid use at the same dosage or increased opioid use required over time to maintain the same effect. *OIH* is a hypersensitivity to painful stimuli that occurs in a state of hyperexcitation (Mercadante et al. 2019). In other words, OIH is a decreased pain threshold after long-term opioid use. Signs of OIH include a waning treatment effect of opioids in the absence of disease progression, unexplained pain or diffuse allodynia unassociated with the original pain, and increased pain levels despite escalating dosages of opioids (Lee et al. 2011; Powell et al. 2021). Thus, one key difference between tolerance and OIH is that increasing the dosage can overcome tolerance, whereas it could continue to worsen OIH. Unacknowledged OIH has significant clinical implications: it often influences a patient's perception that despite taking a high dosage of opioids, the treatment is not effective enough for analgesia. As a result, the patient may request even higher dosages of medication to meet the perceived need for pain control that OIH initially worsened. If the prescriber is unaware of potential opioid-induced analgesia, they may fulfill the request, with an unacknowledged detriment to the patient. A cycle may then ensue that leads to consistent dosage elevations, placing the patient at risk while not helping them better tolerate pain. Treatment of OUD with FDA-approved medication such as methadone or buprenorphine may help to reverse OIH. *N*-methyl-D-aspartate (NMDA) receptor activation has been implicated in the development of OIH, and as a weak NMDA receptor antagonist, methadone has been shown to be effective in reducing high-dose-related OIH (Lee et al. 2011). The antihyperalgesic properties of buprenorphine can also reduce pain in patients who transition from long-term opioid treatment. Thus, methadone and buprenorphine, despite being opioids themselves, can reduce hyperalgesia induced by other chronic opioid therapy and improve quality of life.

# Pseudoaddiction

The concept of pseudoaddiction is a debated topic in pain management that may influence the treatment dynamic between the patient and clinician. The term *pseudoaddiction* was coined by Weissman in a 1989 case report, in which he described a patient as exhibiting opioid-seeking behaviors because of undertreated pain. The treatment team misconstrued these behaviors as behavioral symptoms of addiction (Weissman and Haddox 1989). Proponents of pseudoaddiction believe that undertreatment of pain is an iatrogenic cause of medication-seeking behaviors. However, when the pain requirements are adequately met, the patient's requests for medication adjustment diminish or even cease. Although it is essential to acknowledge and empathize with the patient's pain perception, overindulgent prescribing of opioids to a patient with inadequate analgesia may also lead to a host of undesired medical risks, including OIH. Pharmacological tolerance and OIH can develop as soon as 1 month after a patient starts taking opioids (Greene and Chambers 2015).

# Medication for Treatment of Opioid Use Disorder in Pain Management

Medication for treatment of opioid use disorder (MOUD) includes naltrexone, buprenorphine, and methadone, but these medications all have different neurobiological effects within the pain pathways. Compared with buprenorphine (a partial μ agonist) and naltrexone (a μ antagonist), methadone may theoretically have the most benefit for treating pain because it is a full μ opioid receptor agonist. As part of patient-centered treatment, a patient's underlying chronic pain conditions must be considered when choosing which modality of MOUD may be the most appropriate. Although the main objective of using the FDA-approved agents is to treat OUD (as opposed to strict pain management), uncontrolled pain in a patient leads to a high risk of opioid cravings or a return to opioid use. One study found that greater pain predicted greater subsequent use of opioids due to stronger opioid cravings. The risk for poor treatment outcomes associated with ongoing pain is largely due to cravings (Messina and Worley 2019). Another study found that in treatment-seeking patients with opioid use and a history of chronic pain, 43.2% cited pain as a driving force for recurrence (Ellis et al. 2021). Thus, in OUD treatment, even if strict pain management is not the primary target, treating pain will at least indirectly decrease cravings, which is 1 of the 11 DSM criteria for OUD (American Psychiatric Association 2022).

In general practice, patients with co-occurring OUD and severe chronic pain may prefer methadone and buprenorphine. A growing number of studies indicate some analgesic properties of naltrexone, even though it is a μ receptor antagonist. Referred to as low-dose naltrexone (LDN) at 1–5 mg, it blocks toll-like receptor 4 (*TLR4*), which leads to the inhibition of proinflammatory cytokines and pain-sensitizing nitric oxide production (Patten et al. 2018; Trofimovitch and Baumrucker 2019). However, LDN has been studied in only a few chronic conditions associated with pain. There is insufficient evidence to draw definitive conclusions about its efficacy for analgesia or anti-inflammation (Patten et al. 2018). Another limitation of LDN is that the dosage is significantly lower than those seen for treatment of OUD (typically at least 50 mg/day orally), and it is not available at standard pharmacies. Only a compounding pharmacy may be able to make such a low dosage.

The first review to evaluate all randomized controlled trial (RCT) data on methadone's analgesic properties found that methadone may be an analgesic for certain pain types, including postprocedural, cancer-related, and nociceptive pain. However, data on its effectiveness for neuropathic pain are limited (Hanna and Senderovich 2021). Comparisons have been made between analgesic outcomes in patients taking methadone versus those taking buprenorphine. Neumann et al. (2013) found that treatment retention and analgesia did not differ between methadone and buprenorphine groups after 6 months; however, this study was limited by a small sample, was not double-blind, and had heterogeneous etiology of chronic pain syndromes. The literature supports using buprenorphine for analgesia in patients receiving long-term opioid treatment. A systematic review from 2021 found that buprenorphine was associated with reduced chronic pain in patients receiving long-term opioid treatment who transitioned to buprenorphine; perhaps this outcome is related to the drug's antihyperalgesic properties (Powell et al. 2021). In fact, its antihyperalgesic effects have a significantly longer duration than its analgesic effects, which is the reverse of what is seen for full μ receptor agonists (Koppert et al. 2005). One theory is that buprenorphine, as a κ receptor antagonist, can counteract the hyperalgesia from chronic opioids caused by upregulated dynorphin signaling (associated with the κ receptor) and indirect NMDA receptor activation (Infantino et al. 2021).

# Evaluation and Management of Pain for Patients Taking Buprenorphine

Despite many patients with OUD taking buprenorphine products for treatment, many continue endorsing significant pain that leads to life dysfunction and reduced quality of life. Some may experience near to complete remission of pain while taking buprenorphine. However, for those who are experiencing either continued or exacerbated pain during treatment, several factors should be considered.

During treatment, an inadequate dosage of opioid agonist to meet the patient's opioid tolerance may lead to withdrawal symptoms, including pain. Use of withdrawal scales such as the Clinical Opiate Withdrawal Scale (COWS) can help identify the withdrawal syndrome, particularly when a patient is not yet at a stabilizing dosage of buprenorphine or is not taking buprenorphine correctly. In our experience, some patients adjust the manner in which they administer the medication sublingually (as a result of taste aversion, nausea, or dry mouth), which could affect its bioavailability. Chewing or swallowing the film or tablet can reduce the absorption of sublingual buprenorphine and therefore reduce its effectiveness for analgesia and control of cravings and withdrawal symptoms. Reviewing the patient's urinary buprenorphine and norbuprenorphine levels may provide clues about the consistency of compliance. Further details about buprenorphine laboratory testing are discussed in Chapter 4, "Laboratory Testing." Finally, one can consider whether the local pharmacy might have changed the generic buprenorphine medication. In our experience, some patients who switched between different brands of sublingual buprenorphine products reported a change in pain control with different products. This has also been seen in some case reports, in which a slight dosage increase helped reduce withdrawal symptoms that occurred during the transition from brand-name to generic buprenorphine (Cedeño et al. 2022). Those who have higher addiction severity seem to prefer the brand-name to the generic formulation (Binder et al. 2016).

If the patient is already taking the maximum dosage of buprenorphine or there are specific clinical reasons for not increasing the overall buprenorphine dosage, one option is to keep the same total daily dosage but divide it into more frequent smaller doses. Buprenorphine has more analgesic properties than its metabolite norbuprenorphine; a study in rats found the analgesic effect of norbuprenorphine is one-fiftieth that of buprenorphine. Norbuprenorphine may also have low intrinsic analgesic effects and low permeability into the brain (Ohtani 2007; Ohtani et al. 1995). Thus, more frequent dosing theoretically allows more exposure to the parent compound buprenorphine. Nevertheless, debate is ongoing about the benefit of divided doses of buprenorphine compared with single daily doses in OUD outcomes. One study found that those who took single doses had better outcomes (in terms of the percentage of negative urine drug screens and average number of recurrences) than patients taking multiple daily doses; however, the study had significant limitations, such as the patients taking multiple daily doses requiring higher total buprenorphine dosages and having significantly more methamphetamine use (Allen et al. 2022).

An increase in the daily dosage of buprenorphine is another option for acute pain, possibly on a short-term basis depending on risks versus benefits.

The literature, however, is conflicting about whether an analgesia ceiling effect exists for buprenorphine. Some articles cite a ceiling effect to analgesic properties (Walsh et al. 1994), whereas others report no ceiling effect (Dahan et al. 2006). Whether any additional analgesia at higher dosages is secondary to a direct physiological response versus a psychological or placebo-based response is unclear. If their pain is unmanageable and opioid cravings remain intense and chronic despite maximum dosages of buprenorphine (24–32 mg/day), some patients may be better suited for a methadone clinic. The full opioid agonist properties of methadone may then improve the patient's quality of life by reducing their pain and therefore their cravings and opioid use related to the pain. We suggest initially experimenting with buprenorphine dosages exceeding 16 mg/day before considering a switch to methadone.

## Adjunct Medications

Combining adjunct pharmacological treatments with buprenorphine may also be helpful and is discussed later (see "Alternatives to Opioids for Chronic Pain Management"). A multidisciplinary approach, including direct discussion with the patient's primary care physician, can raise awareness of the unmet pain control for the patient. In fact, among patients who receive chronic pain management, 75.2% receive care in the form of biomedical interventions (Ellis et al. 2021). However, providers outside of addiction treatment programs may be hesitant to add or prescribe any additional analgesic medication (even nonnarcotic) options under the assumption that buprenorphine alone should be adequate to manage the pain. The literature is abundant with nonnarcotic treatment adjuncts such as nerve blocks, steroids, nonsteroidal anti-inflammatory drugs (NSAIDs), cyclooxygenase (COX) inhibitors, and muscle relaxants. However, special caution must be taken when prescribing medication such as gabapentin and pregabalin. Although they may potentiate the analgesic effects of buprenorphine, they pose an overdose risk when combined. In addition, the OUD population is particularly vulnerable to misusing gabapentinoids (Smith et al. 2016).

Other options to consider include methocarbamol and cyclobenzaprine. However, like gabapentinoids, muscle relaxants are susceptible to misuse. Carisoprodol, for example, metabolizes to meprobamate, a drug with known addictive potential. These drugs also pose a risk of overdose when combined with opioids and a risk of unintentional harm from reduced alertness (e.g., medicated while driving). The amount of nonnarcotic adjuncts used must be monitored and asked about routinely because patients may not proactively share how they take them. To avoid taking opioids, many patients may resort to large, potentially harmful doses of NSAIDs for pain management. Education is crucial in these situations to inform patients of the potential for gastric ulcers (which would inadvertently create another source of pain) and paradoxical headaches from NSAID overuse. In such situations, the risks may outweigh the benefits of chronic NSAID therapy. Some patients resort to using substances they perceive to be less dangerous than opioids, such as cannabis. However, cannabis has diminishing returns for pain control in many patients because they may develop cannabis hyperemesis syndrome with associated abdominal pain (Galli et al. 2011). If more conservative medications are ineffective in treating acute pain, then alternative opioids can be supplemented in addition to the patient's buprenorphine dosing. In cases in which full μ opioid receptor agonists are needed, they may compete against buprenorphine for unoccupied receptors because buprenorphine occupies most of, but not all, μ opioid receptors (Gudin and Fudin 2020).

## Role of Pain Perception

There is high association between anxiety and depression and how they affect pain perception. Clinicians must explore with patients how heightened anxiety and depression affect their pain perception and whether more aggressive psychiatric treatment is warranted. Treatment of anxiety and depression reduces the risk of chronic pain development and vice versa (Michaelides and Zis 2019). Fortunately, psychotropic options are available that can treat both anxiety and depression and certain pain syndromes simultaneously (e.g., duloxetine). In combination with other psychotropic treatments, psychotherapy can help rectify maladaptive cognitive beliefs about pain. For example, a common misconception is that sciatic pain requires more bed rest, but evidence recommends staying active over bed rest (Valat et al. 2010). This an example of the fear-avoidance model of pain, in which catastrophized views of pain and hypervigilance to physical stressors lead to the avoidance of exercise and activity that catalyzes deconditioning and worsening of the physical state (Linton and Shaw 2011). Expectations of pain control could also be addressed. Reframing a patient's expectations of a chronic pain condition could include how to live life *with* pain and maintain the best quality of life and productivity as opposed to expecting 100% pain remission. Cognitive-behavioral therapy and acceptance and commitment therapy are options that can be included to address these maladaptive beliefs. Essentially, clinicians guide patients in separating their *suffering* from their *pain*.

Exploration of a patient's social and occupational environments helps identify any risks for future injury as part of prevention efforts. Often, an occupation may put someone at risk because lifting heavy objects or poor posture is required. Lack of self-care leading to suboptimal dietary patterns may lead to a higher risk of dental issues that cause severe pain. Obesity and weight gain may theoretically place more pressure on the joints from walking, leading to pain and reduced functionality from lack of exercise. A study by Chen et al. (2022) found a causal relationship between BMI and hip, back, and knee pain. Furthermore, avoiding occupational and physical therapy following an injury may lead to overcompensating by using another muscle group, causing pain in an additional or contralateral body site. Identifying these maladaptive patterns may prevent the counterproductive erosion of any gains from pain management.

Finally, overendorsement of pain for secondary gain should be considered in some cases. Although it should not immediately be assumed in any patient with pain receiving MOUD, diversion is a risk with buprenorphine. Unfortunately, accurately assessing and detecting malingering of pain can be challenging (Fishbain et al. 2002; Greve et al. 2009). However, diversion should be on the differential when clinical cues, such as a pattern of discordant buprenorphine levels, exist in conjunction with inadequate film counts and reports of severe pain symptoms that appear to be consistently incongruent with mental status examination. Overendorsement of pain may also have a role in primary gain; for example, a patient may need clinical attention from pain treatment as a form of validation. These interventions are summarized in Table 15–1.

# Managing Acute Pain for Procedures in Patients Taking Medication for Opioid Use Disorder

## Buprenorphine

Views on the preoperative and perioperative management of buprenorphine have evolved over the years. Initially, one preference was to hold buprenorphine products before surgery and then start full opioid agonists for maximal analgesic response perioperatively. However, the caveat was that doing so required a traditional induction for the patient back onto buprenorphine after the postoperative acute opioid course was completed. This process exposed patients to a heightened risk of opioid withdrawal and recurrence. A variety of microinduction protocols were developed to facilitate the transition be-

**Table 15–1.** Approaches to evaluating pain in context of buprenorphine therapy for opioid use disorder

| Clinical history item | Intervention examples | Desired outcome |
| --- | --- | --- |
| Withdrawal symptoms | Check for withdrawal symptoms; may use clinical scales such as COWS | Withdrawal-related pain diminishes or ceases |
| | Titrate dosage of buprenorphine as indicated to minimize withdrawal symptoms | |
| Dose scheduling | Consider split dosing of buprenorphine product | Improved analgesia due to more exposure to parent compound buprenorphine |
| General compliance | Monitor buprenorphine and norbuprenorphine levels | Improved compliance, including not overtaking medication or running out early, which may lead to more consistent analgesia |
| | Ask patient if they are running out of buprenorphine early | |
| Buprenorphine formulation | Check the National Drug Code for taken buprenorphine | Continue the identified National Drug Code that best works for patient |
| New medical history | Refer to primary care physician if appropriate for new-onset injuries | Can use adjunct therapies for pain |
| Other analgesic use, including OTC medication | Assess for overuse of NSAIDs, for example | Reduce or eliminate counterproductive excessive analgesic use causing rebound pain |
| Prescribed drug interactions with buprenorphine | Adjust use of CYP3A4 inducers or buprenorphine dosage | Reduce acceleration of buprenorphine metabolism |

**Table 15–1.  Approaches to evaluating pain in context of buprenorphine therapy for opioid use disorder (*continued*)**

| Clinical history item | Intervention examples | Desired outcome |
|---|---|---|
| Other illicit substance use | Request urine drug screen to detect other substance use | Reduce or discontinue other substance use that is responsible for pain or having drug interaction with buprenorphine |
| | Assess change in cannabis use because cannabis is a potent CYP3A4 inhibitor (Vierke et al. 2021) | |
| Depression and anxiety assessment | Initiate or adjust antidepressants and/or anxiolytics | Reduced depression leads to reduced cravings |
| Cognitive distortions related to pain | Use cognitive-behavioral therapy or acceptance and commitment therapy, brief interventions | Patient learns to better cope with pain even when it is chronic |
| Environmental risks | Work on prevention measures | Reduced risk of pain exacerbation |
| Primary gain | Obtain good clinical history, remain empathetic | Patient has improved insight into the role of pain in their life |

*Note.*   COWS=Clinical Opiate Withdrawal Scale; CYP3A4=cytochrome P450 3A4; NSAIDs=nonsteroidal anti-inflammatory drugs; OTC=over-the-counter.

tween taking full opioid agonists and buprenorphine without redoing a traditional buprenorphine induction. A systematic review by Spreen et al. (2022) found that 95.6% of patients in the traditional initiation group and 96% of those following a microinduction protocol successfully resumed sublingual buprenorphine.

Previous recommendations were to withhold buprenorphine preoperatively so that enough μ receptors were available for binding with full opioid agonists for analgesia; however, this trend has changed to the current recommendation of continuing buprenorphine during the perioperative period. On the basis of clinical studies, even at higher dosages of buprenorphine (24–32 mg/day total), μ receptors are still available with which additional full opioid agonists can bind (Kohan et al. 2021). Continuing buprenorphine treatment perioperatively has three benefits: increasing evidence of the ability to achieve sufficient analgesia in buprenorphine-maintained patients, reducing risk of recurrence preoperatively, and reducing risk of overdose from full opioid agonists when buprenorphine is discontinued (Buresh et al. 2020). In addition, maintaining a patient on buprenorphine postoperatively spares the necessity of traditional reinduction from full opioid agonists back onto buprenorphine, a process that increases the risk of recurrence. Although some believe that the dosage of buprenorphine should be reduced below 16 mg/day preoperatively (for those taking a maintenance dosage of 16 mg/day or more) (Hickey et al. 2022), other experts recommend maintaining buprenorphine dosage prior to surgery (Quaye and Zhang 2019).

Management of perioperative mild breakthrough pain includes nonopioid analgesics and splitting the once-daily buprenorphine dose to three doses per day (Buresh et al. 2020). Moderate or severe pain may benefit from increasing buprenorphine dosage to 24–32 mg/day or continuing buprenorphine while adding full opioid agonists such as oxycodone, hydromorphone, or fentanyl in addition to regional blocks and nonopioid analgesia. Nonopioid medications can include, but are not limited to, NSAIDs, acetaminophen, duloxetine, lidocaine, steroids, gabapentinoids, ketamine, clonidine, dexmedetomidine (Buresh et al. 2020; Harrison et al. 2018).

## Methadone

Because methadone is a full opioid agonist, it already provides analgesia for acute injury. A patient should be continued on at least the same methadone maintenance dosage as preinjury. A temporary dosage increase could be considered while monitoring respiratory function or drug interactions with QT-prolonging agents. If a patient spends a prolonged time in the hospital with a higher methadone dosage, this dosage change should be communicated with the outpatient opioid treatment program that will administer the methadone doses after discharge.

## Naltrexone

Naltrexone may pose various challenges depending on whether the patient is prescribed the oral or intramuscular formulation. Oral naltrexone can be discontinued 2–3 days before anticipated or elective surgery, but the extended-release formulation, naltrexone XR, must be stopped 30 days preoperatively. For unexpected or unplanned procedures, the next oral dose should be held. Note that the effectiveness of any opioid analgesic options could be diminished initially until an adequate amount of naltrexone is displaced from the μ receptors. If naltrexone is to be restarted again after completion of opioid agonist therapy, the patient should wait at least 7–10 days to ensure that naltrexone will not precipitate withdrawal.

For those taking naltrexone XR, blockade of opioid receptors will likely continue, especially if the patient is well into maintenance therapy with steady state plasma levels. Achieving adequate analgesia can be particularly challenging in this circumstance because there is less literature for guidance on this topic. In some animal studies, levels 6–20 times typical opioid dosages are needed to achieve analgesia. Because complete lack of analgesia to opioids may occur in the first 2 weeks of treatment, other opioid-sparing techniques (e.g., regional and neuraxial anesthetics) should be employed (Harrison et al. 2018).

# Cannabis and Pain

## Efficacy of Cannabis in Pain Management

Despite many patients anecdotally citing pain relief through cannabis product use, none of the FDA-approved cannabis-related products are indicated for use in chronic pain. In 2018, the CDC determined that opioids were involved in more than 69.5% of all drug overdose deaths; thus, alternative options have been sought for chronic pain management, including the two components of interest in the cannabis plant, Δ-9-tetrahydrocannabinol (Δ-9 THC) and cannabidiol (CBD). Nabiximols, which contain a ratio of THC to CBD, have shown promise for chronic pain treatment, but the efficacy of isolated CBD is unknown. In addition, limited regulation in the United States may lead to inaccurate quantities of ingredients in CBD products (Urits et al. 2020).

As of November 2022, the FDA has approved one cannabis-derived and three cannabis-related drug products. Epidiolex contains a purified form of CBD for treating seizures associated with Lennox-Gastaut syndrome, tuberous sclerosis complex, or Dravet syndrome in patients age 1 year or older. The FDA has also approved Marinol and Syndros, both of which contain dronabinol (synthetic THC), for nausea associated with cancer chemotherapy and treatment of anorexia associated with weight loss in patients with AIDS. Cesamet, which contains nabilone, is indicated for nausea associated with cancer chemotherapy. Despite many patients anecdotally citing pain relief through cannabis product use, none of the FDA-approved cannabis-related products are indicated for use in chronic pain. A review reported that inhaled cannabis might be clinically valuable for the treatment of chronic neuropathic pain, whereas oral cannabinoids seem to be less effective and less tolerable than inhaled cannabis to reduce pain intensity (Romero-Sandoval et al. 2017). However, many studies on this topic are heterogeneous, with small sample sizes, a short study duration, or a high risk of bias.

A 2018 Cochrane systematic review rigorously filtered through studies (including unpublished ones) examining the efficacy and safety of cannabis-based medicines compared with placebo or conventional drugs for treatment of chronic neuropathic pain conditions in adults. When only RCTs of at least 2 weeks' duration were included, only 16 studies qualified for inclusion in the quantitative analysis. The findings revealed low-quality evidence for substantial ($\geq$50%) pain relief; global improvement; and reduction of mean pain intensity, sleep problems, and psychological distress. On the other hand, there was moderate-quality evidence that more people dropped out because of adverse events with cannabis-based medicines, which included somnolence, confusion, and psychosis. The authors concluded that potential harms may outweigh potential benefits of cannabis-based medications in chronic neuropathic pain (Mücke et al. 2018). Given the lack of high-quality evidence for the use of cannabis-related products in chronic neuropathy, we do not recommend cannabis for neuropathic pain management.

## Buprenorphine and Cannabis

Despite the lack of FDA-approved indication for cannabis-related products for pain syndromes, many patients receiving buprenorphine for OUD may self-medicate their chronic pain, anxiety, depression, low appetite, or insomnia with cannabis. Although data on the prevalence of cannabis use among adults receiving MOUD are lacking, the 30-day prevalence of current cannabis use in a Massachusetts adult sample receiving MOUD was 41% in 2020 (Streck et al. 2022). The use of cannabis while taking MOUD may have significant clinical implications; one study found that patients using cannabis had elevated buprenorphine levels and decreased metabolite-to-parent drug ratios compared with the control group. This elevation may occur because cannabis use reduces buprenorphine metabolism through cytochrome P450 (CYP) 3A4 inhibition. A case report included in this study described a patient who experienced withdrawal symptoms and cravings, with a concomitantly reduced buprenorphine level, following abstinence from cannabis use (Vierke et al. 2021). Thus, although cannabis use should be monitored while patients are receiving MOUD, ongoing use does not necessarily mean that patients should be discontinued from MOUD treatment. From a harm reduction approach, maintaining the patient on the MOUD may be more productive to help bolster treatment retention and decrease risk of overdose death from opioids. Retention in treatment could be used to gradually replace cannabis with other treatments that have higher-quality evidence for pain control. However, when cannabis use decreases while patients are taking MOUD, they may need increased pain management due to any (if at all) reduced analgesic effect from cannabis cessation and reduced buprenorphine levels from the previous cannabis-buprenorphine interactions.

# Alcohol and Pain

Few studies have examined the overlap of alcohol use disorder (AUD) and pain despite significant concern about the intersection as a public health burden. A literature review indicated that patients with AUD have a higher risk of developing pain disorders than those without AUD (Hung et al. 2021). A 2015 Polish study of patients with AUD showed 34% of patients reported moderate to severe physical pain in the past 4 weeks (Jakubczyk et al. 2015). In the United States, up to 25% of individuals presenting for pain have been found to have a history of heavy drinking. To complicate matters further, it is estimated that 25%–66% of individuals with AUD also have alcohol-related neuropathic pain (Kim et al. 2013; Lawton and Simpson 2009).

Clinicians who are treating patients with AUD and comorbid pain should first address acute alcohol withdrawal. Following an assessment and appropriate management of the acute withdrawal, maintenance treatment should be considered for AUD where appropriate. Currently, three medications are

FDA-approved for the treatment of AUD in the United States: disulfiram, naltrexone (oral and long acting), and acamprosate. Unfortunately, none of these is indicated for pain management. Clinicians should begin with one of the FDA-approved medications for AUD and combine that with acetaminophen or NSAIDs for pain management. For specific pain conditions, interest is increasing in the use of off-label medications such as gabapentin, topiramate, and baclofen as comorbid treatment options. More information about medications used to treat AUD can be found in Chapter 5, "Alcohol and Co-occurring Substance Use."

## Gabapentin

Currently, gabapentin holds FDA approval for pain treatment of only postherpetic neuralgia. Interest in broader indications for pain treatment has revealed evidence in favor of gabapentin for treatment of acute postoperative pain and chronic neuropathic pain (Peckham et al. 2018). American Psychiatric Association treatment guidelines also suggest gabapentin for patients with moderate to severe AUD who want to reduce their alcohol consumption or achieve abstinence (Reus et al. 2018). Gabapentin has been shown to increase abstinence and reduce heavy drinking when taken at dosages between 900 mg and 1,800 mg (Burnette et al. 2022). Thus, clinicians can consider gabapentin for patients with moderate to severe AUD who experience specific pain syndromes related to postherpetic neuralgia, acute postoperative pain, and chronic neuropathic pain. Because of concern for gabapentin misuse and diversion in patients with comorbid OUD, careful examination of specific patient circumstances should occur prior to initiation (Smith et al. 2016).

## Topiramate

Topiramate has been studied as a repurposed agent in the pharmacological treatment of AUD. As with gabapentin, the American Psychiatric Association suggests the use of topiramate in patients with moderate to severe AUD who have the goal of reducing alcohol consumption or achieving abstinence (Reus et al. 2018). A meta-analysis of seven RCTs showed statistically significant effects on abstinence and heavy drinking with topiramate (Blodgett et al. 2014). Doses ranged from 200 mg/day to 300 mg/day (Burnette et al. 2022). Topiramate also holds FDA approval for prophylactic treatment of migraine headaches. Consequently, it can be considered for patients with migraines and co-occurring moderate to severe AUD. Close monitoring of side effects during dosage titration should occur because previous trials showed concern for mental slowing and reductions in verbal fluency and working memory in patients with AUD (Knapp et al. 2015).

## Baclofen

Baclofen has approval for AUD in France but not in the United States. Its efficacy continues to be debated in the field. Multiple challenges exist in the current literature studies, including wide variations in dosing, heterogeneity in pharmacokinetics, sex variations, and treatment duration (de Beaurepaire et al. 2019). The American Psychiatric Association's current position remains that recent RCTs have not shown benefit in using baclofen for AUD (Reus et al. 2018). However, there is growing evidence of baclofen's utility in promoting abstinence and potential usefulness in patients with alcohol-related liver disease (Morley et al. 2018; Rolland et al. 2014). Regarding pain management, baclofen holds FDA approval for spasticity in multiple sclerosis and some value for patients with spinal cord injuries. Off-label, it has favorable evidence for back pain (Migliorini et al. 2021). Clinicians should share decision-making with their patients with co-occurring AUD when choosing baclofen for the treatment of spasticity in multiple sclerosis, spinal cord injuries, and lower back pain. Baclofen's efficacy remains contentious, and the safety considerations surrounding the potential for dangerous withdrawal and tolerance are necessary to balance in a risk-benefit discussion.

# Alternatives to Opioids for Chronic Pain Management

Multimodal approaches to pain management include medications, physical therapy, and psychotherapy. Medication selection is dependent on the type of pain:

- Nociceptive pain arises from threatened or actual damage to nonneural tissue (e.g., joints, bones) and is often experienced as aching at the site of injury. Treatment includes NSAIDs and acetaminophen.
- Neuropathic pain is caused by an injury to nerve tissue and is experienced as burning, lancinating, or electrical sensations. Causes include diabetes, hypothyroidism, and nerve compressions. Central sensitization is when nociceptive neurons in the CNS respond more strongly to their normal peripheral input.

- Nociplastic pain is pain arising from abnormal nociception despite no evidence of injury. Initial treatment involves antidepressants, such as serotonin-norepinephrine reuptake inhibitors and tricyclics; antiepileptics; and localized topical therapy (Table 15–2) (Center for Substance Abuse Treatment 2012).

# Summary of Nonpharmacological Interventions

The level of impairment associated with chronic pain depends on a combination of physiological and psychological factors. Many patients develop negative beliefs that precipitate and perpetuate their mood changes around pain. Treatment goals include reducing not only pain but also the suffering and functional impairment from the pain. Cognitive-behavioral therapy, mindfulness, meditation, and biofeedback can improve coping and functionality. A physical activity plan may be tailored to the individual's current ability and be designed to have achievable challenges. Yoga, stretching, aquatic therapy, Pilates, and tai chi are activities with easily accessible programs that vary in intensity. Patients who have difficulty leaving their homes may access programs online. Patients may also integrate other therapies into their rehabilitation, such as acupuncture, massage therapy, and spinal manipulation (musculoskeletal pain).

# Conclusion

Pain and substance use have a bidirectional relationship. Increased physical and psychological pain sensitivity may drive opioid-seeking behaviors, particularly in patients taking chronic opioid medications. Managing chronic pain requires a multimodal approach that empowers patients to function despite pain and, ultimately, to separate pain from suffering.

**Table 15–2.** Nonnarcotic medications for chronic pain

| Medication | Type of pain | Comments |
|---|---|---|
| Nonsteroidal anti-inflammatory drugs | Nociceptive | Use with caution in patients with renal insufficiency. |
| Acetaminophen | Nociceptive | Long-term use may be associated with liver toxicity. Limit dosage to 3,000 mg/day (2,000 mg/day for older patients or patients with liver disease). |
| Antidepressants | Neuropathic, nociplastic, central sensitization | |
| Duloxetine 60–120 mg/day | | Avoid in patients with hepatic or severe renal insufficiency. |
| Levomilnacipran 20–80 mg/day | | Avoid in patients with end-stage kidney disease; use with caution in patients with angle-closure glaucoma and liver disease. Dosages of 120 mg/day have been used. |
| Venlafaxine ER 75–225 mg/day | | Induced hypertension may occur. Caution and monitoring should be used in patients with cardiac disease. Discontinuation symptoms are common. |
| Nortriptyline 25–75 mg/day | | Less sedation than other tricyclic antidepressants. |
| Amitriptyline 25–125 mg/day | | Increased sedation may be helpful for patients with insomnia. Monitor for anticholinergic effects (constipation, blurry vision, cognitive effects). |
| Antiepileptic medications | Neuropathic, nociplastic, central sensitization | Combination with opioids, benzodiazepines, and other sedatives may increase risk of respiratory depression. Use lower doses in older adults and in patients with renal insufficiency. |
| Gabapentin IR 300–1,200 mg tid | | |
| Gabapentin ER 600–1,200 mg bid | | |
| Pregabalin 150–300 mg bid | | |

**Table 15–2. Nonnarcotic medications for chronic pain** (*continued*)

| Medication | Type of pain | Comments |
|---|---|---|
| Localized topical therapy | Neuropathic, nociplastic, central sensitization | |
| Lidocaine patch | | Apply for 12 hours or less per day. |
| Capsaicin cream or gel, 0.75% applied to affected area qid | | May cause burns or irritation and CNS depression. Caution patients about performing tasks that require alertness and attention. Onset of action is delayed 2–4 weeks. |
| Capsaicin patch, applied to most painful areas for 30 minutes q 3 months | | May cause burns or irritation and CNS depression. Caution patients about performing tasks that require alertness and attention. Up to four patches may be applied. Onset of action is delayed 1 week. |

*Note.* ER=extended release; IR=immediate release.

# References

Allen SM, Nichols TA, Fawcett J, Lin S: Outcomes associated with once-daily versus multiple-daily dosing of buprenorphine/naloxone for opioid use disorder. Am J Addict 31(3):173–179, 2022 35226393

American Psychiatric Association: Diagnostic and Statistical Manual of Mental Disorders, 5th Edition, Text Revision. Washington, DC, American Psychiatric Association, 2022

de Beaurepaire R, Sinclair JMA, Heydtmann M, et al: The use of baclofen as a treatment for alcohol use disorder: a clinical practice perspective. Front Psychiatry 9(Jan):708, 2019 30662411

Binder P, Messaadi N, Perault-Pochat M-C, et al: Preference for brand-name buprenorphine is related to severity of addiction among outpatients in opioid maintenance treatment. J Addict Dis 35(2):101–108, 2016 26745033

Blodgett JC, Del Re AC, Maisel NC, et al: A meta-analysis of topiramate's effects for individuals with alcohol use disorders. Alcohol Clin Exp Res 38(6):1481–1488, 2014 24796492

Buresh M, Ratner J, Zgierska A, et al: Treating perioperative and acute pain in patients on buprenorphine: narrative literature review and practice recommendations. J Gen Intern Med 35(12):3635–3643, 2020 32827109

Burnette EM, Nieto SJ, Grodin EN, et al: Novel agents for the pharmacological treatment of alcohol use disorder. Drugs 82(3):251–274, 2022 35133639

Cedeño E, Cruz A, Cortés J, et al: Experiences and preferences of opioid-use-disorder patients who switched from brand to generic buprenorphine/naloxone films: a case series. Patient Prefer Adherence 16(January):69–78, 2022 35046643

Center for Substance Abuse Treatment: Managing Chronic Pain in Adults With or in Recovery From Substance Use Disorders. Rockville, MD, Substance Abuse and Mental Health Services Administration, 2012. Available at: https://www.ncbi.nlm.nih.gov/books/NBK92048. Accessed November 14, 2022.

Chen X, Tang H, Lin J, et al: Causal relationships of obesity on musculoskeletal chronic pain: a two-sample Mendelian randomization study. Front Endocrinol (Lausanne) 13(Aug):971997, 2022 36082069

Dahan A, Yassen A, Romberg R, et al: Buprenorphine induces ceiling in respiratory depression but not in analgesia. Br J Anaesth 96(5):627–632, 2006 16547090

Delorme J, Kerckhove N, Authier N, et al: Systematic review and meta-analysis of the prevalence of chronic pain among patients with opioid use disorder and receiving opioid substitution therapy. J Pain 24(2):192–203, 2023 36220483

Ellis MS, Kasper Z, Cicero T: Assessment of chronic pain management in the treatment of opioid use disorder: gaps in care and implications for treatment outcomes. J Pain 22(4):432–439, 2021 33197581

Fishbain DA, Cutler RB, Rosomoff HL, et al: Does the conscious exaggeration scale detect deception within patients with chronic pain alleged to have secondary gain? Pain Med 3(1):39–46, 2002 15102217

Galli JA, Sawaya RA, Friedenberg FK: Cannabinoid hyperemesis syndrome. Curr Drug Abuse Rev 4(4):241–249, 2011 22150623

Greene MS, Chambers RA: Pseudoaddiction: fact or fiction? An investigation of the medical literature. Curr Addict Rep 2(4):310–317, 2015 26550549

Greve KW, Etherton JL, Ord J, et al: Detecting malingered pain-related disability: classification accuracy of the test of memory malingering. Clin Neuropsychol 23(7):1250–1271, 2009 19728222

Gudin J, Fudin J: A narrative pharmacological review of buprenorphine: a unique opioid for the treatment of chronic pain. Pain Ther 9(1):41–54, 2020 31994020

Hanna V, Senderovich H: Methadone in pain management: a systematic review. J Pain 22(3):233–245, 2021 32599153

Harrison TK, Kornfeld H, Aggarwal AK, et al: Perioperative considerations for the patient with opioid use disorder on buprenorphine, methadone, or naltrexone maintenance therapy. Anesthesiol Clin 36(3):345–359, 2018 30092933

Hickey T, Abelleira A, Acampora G, et al: Perioperative buprenorphine management: a multidisciplinary approach. Med Clin North Am 106(1):169–185, 2022 34823729

Hung H-Y, Chien W-C, Chung C-H, et al: Patients with alcohol use disorder increase pain and analgesics use: a nationwide population-based cohort study. Drug Alcohol Depend 229(Pt A):109102, 2021 34634646

Infantino R, Mattia C, Locarini P, et al: Buprenorphine: far beyond the "ceiling." Biomolecules 11(6):816, 2021 34072706

Jakubczyk A, Ilgen MA, Bohnert AS, et al: Physical pain in alcohol-dependent patients entering treatment in Poland—prevalence and correlates. J Stud Alcohol Drugs 76(4):607–614, 2015 26098037

Kim CH, Vincent A, Clauw DJ, et al: Association between alcohol consumption and symptom severity and quality of life in patients with fibromyalgia. Arthritis Res Ther 15(2):R42, 2013 23497427

Knapp CM, Ciraulo DA, Sarid-Segal O, et al: Zonisamide, topiramate, and levetiracetam: efficacy and neuropsychological effects in alcohol use disorders. J Clin Psychopharmacol 35(1):34–42, 2015 25427171

Kohan L, Potru S, Barreveld AM, et al: Buprenorphine management in the perioperative period: educational review and recommendations from a multisociety expert panel. Reg Anesth Pain Med 46(10):840–859, 2021 34385292

Koppert W, Ihmsen H, Körber N, et al: Different profiles of buprenorphine-induced analgesia and antihyperalgesia in a human pain model. Pain 118(1–2):15–22, 2005 16154698

Lawton J, Simpson J: Predictors of alcohol use among people experiencing chronic pain. Psychol Health Med 14(4):487–501, 2009 19697258

Lee M, Silverman SM, Hansen H, et al: A comprehensive review of opioid-induced hyperalgesia. Pain Physician 14(2):145–161, 2011 21412369

Linton SJ, Shaw WS: Impact of psychological factors in the experience of pain. Phys Ther 91(5):700–711, 2011 21451097

Mercadante S, Arcuri E, Santoni A: Opioid-induced tolerance and hyperalgesia. CNS Drugs 33(10):943–955, 2019 31578704

Messina BG, Worley MJ: Effects of craving on opioid use are attenuated after pain coping counseling in adults with chronic pain and prescription opioid addiction. J Consult Clin Psychol 87(10):918–926, 2019 31556668

Michaelides A, Zis P: Depression, anxiety and acute pain: links and management challenges. Postgrad Med 131(7):438–444, 2019 31482756

Migliorini F, Maffulli N, Eschweiler J, et al: The pharmacological management of chronic lower back pain. Expert Opin Pharmacother 22(1):109–119, 2021 32885995

Morley KC, Baillie A, Fraser I, et al: Baclofen in the treatment of alcohol dependence with or without liver disease: multisite, randomised, double-blind, placebo-controlled trial. Br J Psychiatry 212(6):362–369, 2018 29716670

Mücke M, Phillips T, Radbruch L, et al: Cannabis-based medicines for chronic neuropathic pain in adults. Cochrane Database Syst Rev 3(3):CD012182, 2018 29513392

Neumann AM, Blondell RD, Jaanimägi U, et al: A preliminary study comparing methadone and buprenorphine in patients with chronic pain and coexistent opioid addiction. J Addict Dis 32(1):68–78, 2013 23480249

Ohtani M: Basic pharmacology of buprenorphine. Eur J Pain Suppl 1(S1):69–73, 2007

Ohtani M, Kotaki H, Sawada Y, et al: Comparative analysis of buprenorphine- and norbuprenorphine-induced analgesic effects based on pharmacokinetic-pharmacodynamic modeling. J Pharmacol Exp Ther 272(2):505–510, 1995 7853163

Patten DK, Schultz BG, Berlau DJ: The safety and efficacy of low-dose naltrexone in the management of chronic pain and inflammation in multiple sclerosis, fibromyalgia, Crohn's disease, and other chronic pain disorders. Pharmacotherapy 38(3):382–389, 2018 29377216

Peckham AM, Evoy KE, Ochs L, et al: Gabapentin for off-label use: evidence-based or cause for concern? Subst Abuse 12(Sept):1178221818801311, 2018 30262984

Powell VD, Rosenberg JM, Yaganti A, et al: Evaluation of buprenorphine rotation in patients receiving long-term opioids for chronic pain: a systematic review. JAMA Netw Open 4(9):e2124152, 2021 34495339

Quaye AN, Zhang Y: Perioperative management of buprenorphine: solving the conundrum. Pain Med 20(7):1395–1408, 2019

Reus VI, Fochtmann LJ, Bukstein O, et al: The American Psychiatric Association practice guideline for the pharmacological treatment of patients with alcohol use disorder. Am J Psychiatry 175(1):86–90, 2018 29301420

Rolland B, Paille F, Fleury B, et al: Off-label baclofen prescribing practices among French alcohol specialists: results of a national online survey. PLoS One 9(6):e98062, 2014 24887094

Romero-Sandoval EA, Kolano AL, Alvarado-Vázquez PA: Cannabis and cannabinoids for chronic pain. Curr Rheumatol Rep 19(11):67, 2017 28983880

Smith RV, Havens JR, Walsh SL: Gabapentin misuse, abuse and diversion: a systematic review. Addiction 111(7):1160–1174, 2016 27265421

Spreen LA, Dittmar EN, Quirk KC, et al: Buprenorphine initiation strategies for opioid use disorder and pain management: a systematic review. Pharmacotherapy 42(5):411–427, 2022 35302671

Streck JM, Regan S, Bearnot B, et al: Prevalence of cannabis use and cannabis route of administration among Massachusetts adults in buprenorphine treatment for opioid use disorder. Subst Use Misuse 57(7):1104–1110, 2022 35410577

Trofimovitch D, Baumrucker SJ: Pharmacology update: low-dose naltrexone as a possible nonopioid modality for some chronic, nonmalignant pain syndromes. Am J Hosp Palliat Care 36(10):907–912, 2019 30917675

Urits I, Gress K, Charipova K, et al: Use of cannabidiol (CBD) for the treatment of chronic pain. Best Pract Res Clin Anaesthesiol 34(3):463–477, 2020 33004159

Valat J-P, Genevay S, Marty M, et al: Sciatica. Best Pract Res Clin Rheumatol 24(2):241–252, 2010 20227645

Vierke C, Marxen B, Boettcher M, et al: Buprenorphine-cannabis interaction in patients undergoing opioid maintenance therapy. Eur Arch Psychiatry Clin Neurosci 271(5):847–856, 2021 31907614

Walsh SL, Preston KL, Stitzer ML, et al: Clinical pharmacology of buprenorphine: ceiling effects at high doses. Clin Pharmacol Ther 55(5):569–580, 1994 8181201

Weissman DE, Haddox DJ: Opioid pseudoaddiction: an iatrogenic syndrome. Pain 36(3):363–366, 1989 2710565

# Index

Page numbers printed in **boldface** type refer to figures and tables.